Global Perspectives
on Health Promotion Effectiveness

Global Perspectives
on Health Promotion
Effectiveness

Edited by

David V. McQueen
Centers for Disease Control and Prevention (CDC)
Atlanta, Georgia, United States

and

Catherine M. Jones
International Union for Health Promotion and Education
Saint-Denis, France

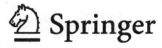 Springer

Editors:
David V. McQueen
National Center for Chronic Disease
Prevention and Health Promotion
US Centers for Disease Control and
Prevention (CDC)
Atlanta, GA, USA

Catherine M. Jones
IUHPE
42, Blvd. de la Libération
Saint-Denis Cedex 93203
France
www.iuhpe.org

ISBN-13: 978-1-4419-2428-5   eISBN-13: 978-0-387-70974-1

Printed on acid-free paper.

9 8 7 6 5 4 3 2 1

springer.com

About the Editors

David V. McQueen is Senior Biomedical Research Scientist and Associate Director for Global Health Promotion at the National Center for Chronic Disease Prevention and Health Promotion (NCCDPHP), at the US Centers for Disease Control and Prevention (CDC) in Atlanta, Georgia. Before joining the Office of the Director, he was Director of the Division of Adult and Community Health at NCCDPHP. From 1983 to 1992, he was Professor and Director of the Research Unit in Health and Behavioral Change at the University of Edinburgh, Scotland and, prior to that, Associate Professor of Behavioral Sciences at the Johns Hopkins University School of Hygiene and Public Health in Baltimore, USA. He has also served as Director of WHO Collaborating Centers as well as a technical consultant with the World Bank.

Over the past 30 years, he has maintained an active interest in health promotion. In the 1980s, he chaired the WHO (EURO) committee that developed the document on the "Concepts and Principles of Health Promotion"; organized and participated in many conferences and meetings concerned with the fostering of health promotion in Europe; actively participated in the development of the Ottawa Charter; and established a collaborating center with EURO concerned with the evaluation of health promotion, healthy cities, and other health promoting activities. During the 1990s his concerns focused on (1) the challenges raised by the efforts to promote an evidence-based health promotion; (2) the efforts to build health behavior monitoring systems to establish a public health infrastructure for health promotion globally; and (3) the development of a broad theoretical base for health promotion.

Since 2001, he has served on the IUHPE Board of Trustees as an elected global member with two consecutive terms as Vice-President for Scientific and Technical Development. It is in this capacity, in addition to his recognized expertise and passion for the subject area, that he has provided leadership and guidance for the Global Programme on Health Promotion Effectiveness.

Catherine M. Jones, a graduate of the American University of Paris with a Bachelor of Arts in International Affairs and a minor in Philosophy, has been a staff member at the IUHPE Headquarters for over 7 years and a resident of Paris since 1995. She has served the IUHPE in a number of roles where her duties included membership development, communications, and project management. She also acted as the Managing Editor of the IUHPE's quarterly multi-lingual journal, *Promotion & Education*, from the end of the year 2000 to the middle of 2006. In her present capacity as the Programme Director, she is responsible for the design, development, implementation, supervision, and evaluation of the IUHPE's main programmatic areas, including a diverse range of global and regional projects, many of which are carried out in close collaboration with key IUHPE member organizations across the world.

Since early 2003, she has been accountable for the coordination of the Global Programme on Health Promotion Effectiveness (GPHPE). She carries out this role, capitalizing on her experience with the network and having a global perspective of the IUHPE's activities in all regions, independently from the GPHPE, in order to be able to create direct links forging partnerships when opportunities emerge, and having a comprehensive knowledge of the GPHPE, of the relationships with its partners, and of the key people involved.

Acknowledgements

The editors would like to extend thanks and appreciation to the following people who generously volunteered their time and expertise as either readers in the review process, copy editors, consultants in the publication's development process, or regional participants in targeted consultations for updating material. Volume I of Global Perspectives on Health Promotion Effectiveness would not have been possible without their professional assistance and contributions.

Thomas Abel
Marco Akerman
Laurie M. Anderson
Janine Cadinu
Stefano Campostrini
Simon Carroll
Clara-Rachel Casséus-Eybalin
Janet Collins
Linnea Evans
Vincent T. Francisco
Chuck Gollmar
Lawrence W. Green
Spencer Hagard
Mary Hall
Marcia Hills
Maurice B. Mittelmark
Fu Hua
Jack Jones

Robert Karch
Marie-Claude Lamarre
Diane Levin-Zamir
Leandris C. Liburd
Debra Lightsey
Peter Makara
Nella Mikkonen
Masaki Moriyama
Eun Woo Nam
Andrea Neiman
Paivi Nykyri
Fran Perkins
Martha W. Perry
Louise Potvin
Mika Pyykkö
Louise Rowling
Michael Sparks
Erio Ziglio

Foreword

The issue of effectiveness in health promotion became a concern in Europe in the late 1980's, spread to other developed countries in the 90's and has become global in the early years of the 21st Century. Key milestones marking the development and escalation of this concern were the first European conference on health promotion quality and effectiveness in 1989, the establishment of the WHO-EURO Working Group on Health Promotion Evaluation in 1995, the first International Symposium on Health Promotion Effectiveness in 1996, the initiation of the IUHPE project on the evidence of health promotion effectiveness in 1998 and the IUHPE Global Program on Health Promotion Effectiveness in 2001.

This interest in the effectiveness of health promotion interventions is not just a casual one but rather, is critical to the future of health promotion and is likely to continue and grow in the decades ahead. This is due to the fact that governments throughout the world are increasingly demanding evidence that their investments are worthwhile and that they pay both financial and social dividends. In addition, people working in the field of health promotion are increasingly interested in knowing if their efforts are effective and efficient and how they might be made better. These demands are not going to disappear in the foreseeable future and therefore organizations and individuals working in health promotion are going to need to address them with increasing effort, rigor, resources and imagination.

The IUHPE Global Program on Health Promotion Effectiveness has a critical role to play in improving and sustaining our efforts to provide credible evidence on the effectiveness of health promotion interventions. One of the reasons why this is the case is that health promotion is a unique enterprise which requires unique and appropriate evaluation approaches. It has become abundantly clear over the past couple of decades, that the RCT has only limited relevance in the evaluation of health promotion interventions and that we need to give credibility to a whole range of other approaches including quasi-experimental designs, observational studies and even story-telling. This means that these approaches will need to be carried out as rigorously as possible and that our capacity needs to be enhanced in order to do so. It also means that we need to find better ways to synthesize the knowledge that we obtain though the use of multiple approaches. In all of these efforts, the IUHPE is in a position to facilitate the exchanges of information and international collaboration that is needed to further develop and sustain this work around the world.

This volume is tangible evidence of the IUHPE's ability to do so. It reflects work of people from a wide range of countries, both developed and less developed, as well as from a variety of disciplines necessary for appropriate evaluations of health promotion interventions. I would personally like to thank the IUHPE for all the work that it has done to develop the foundations for sound evaluations of health promotion work and to provide the critical information required by those who are on the ground to do their work in the most effective and efficient way possible. I look forward to discussing these issues further at the 19th IUHPE World Conference on Health Promotion and Health Education in Vancouver in June 2007 and hope to see you there helping the IUHPE in furthering these important efforts to make health promotion more effective.

Irving Rootman
Vancouver, British Columbia, Canada
December 2006

Preface

During the past decade, the demand for evidence-based practice in medicine has influenced health policy, practice and research in profound ways. Health promotion has also been affected, through calls for evidence-based practice and increased attention to quality and effectiveness in all we do. Much of the funding that supports health promotion research comes from bio-medical funding programmes, and there has been an understandable, but inappropriate tendency to apply bio-medical standards in the evaluation of health promotion research. Therefore, a core project for health promotion is to decide what research standards are appropriate, to conduct quality research in accordance with those standards, and to disseminate evidence of what works to practitioners and policymakers.

The International Union for Health Promotion and Education's contribution to this work has been to stimulate dialogue about what types of knowledge are most meaningful in evaluating the effectiveness of planned health promotion actions. Because health promotion engages in action spanning individual-level to policy-level interventions, the standards of any single discipline are too narrow to provide a single framework for judging the quality of health promotion research and evidence. This book makes an important contribution to the dialogue, but it is not intended as a summary or an authoritative position on the question of what constitutes effective health promotion.

To the contrary, the IUHPE is committed to continue the work of the Global Programme for Health Promotion Effectiveness, as a permanent and core activity of the organisation. Readers may anticipate with confidence future publications in a series, of which this volume is the first. Readers' reactions to this volume will have important consequences for the way the IUHPE carries the work forward. We envisage that IUHPE conferences in the regions and the triennial world conferences will be discussion arenas where a wide range of ideas will be exchanged, about the future directions of the Global Programme for Health Promotion Effectiveness. In addition to our conferences, the IUHPE print and online journals and our web site enable health promoters from around the world to engage in discussion about the critical questions that lie at the heart of this volume: what health promotion actions are effective and why? How can the quality and effectiveness of health promotion be improved? How can we communicate convincingly with decision-makers, so that they support effective health promotion? How can the interplay of practice, policy and research be managed, to produce better health outcomes for all?

Maurice B. Mittelmark
IUHPE President
Bergen, Norway
December 2006

Contents

Section 2. Reports from the Field

Section 3. Global Areas of Interest that Challenge the Assessment of Health Promotion Effectiveness

Section 4. Global Debates about Effectiveness of Health Promotion

List of Contributors

Mary Amuyunzu-Nyamongo
African Institute of Health and Development (AIHD), Nairobi, Kenya

Margaret M. Barry
Department of Health Promotion, National University of Ireland, Galway, Ireland

Adrian Bauman
Centre for Physical Activity, School of Public Health, University of Sydney, Australia

Ursel Broesskamp-Stone
Health Promotion Switzerland, Bern, Switzerland

Fiona Bull
BHF National Centre for Physical Activity and Health, School of Sport & Exercise Sciences, Loughborough University, United Kingdom

Anne W. Bunde-Birouste
School of Public Health and Community Medicine, University of New South Wales, Sydney, Australia

Cynthia Callard
Physicians for a Smoke-Free Canada, Ottawa, Ontario, Canada

Stefano Campostrini
Department of Statistics, University of Venice, Italy

J. Hope Corbin
Research Centre for Health Promotion, University of Bergen, Norway

Evelyne de Leeuw
School of Health and Social Development, Faculty of Health, Medicine, Nursing and Behavioural Sciences, Deakin University, Burwood, Australia

Treena Delormier
Department of Social and Preventive Medicine, University of Montreal, Canada

Ligia de Salazar
University of Valle and Director, Center for the Development and Evaluation of Public Health Policy and Technology (CEDETES), Cali, Colombia

Mark Dooris
Healthy Settings Development Unit, Lancashire School of Health and Postgraduate Medicine, United Kingdom

Randy Elder
National Center for Injury Prevention and Control, Division of Unintentional Injury, US Centers for Disease Control and Prevention (CDC), Atlanta, Georgia, United States

Steve Fawcett
WHO Collaborating Centre for Community Health and Development, University of Kansas, United States

Ghislaine Goudreau
Sudbury and District Health Unit, Ontario, Canada

Marcia Hills
Canadian Consortium for Health Promotion Research and School of Nursing, Centre for Community Health Promotion Research, University of Victoria, Canada

Mary Hall
National Center for Chronic Disease Prevention and Health Promotion, US Centers for Disease Control and Prevention (CDC), Atlanta, Georgia, United States

Peter Howat
Centre for Behavioural Research in Cancer Control, Division of Health Sciences, and National Drug Research Institute, Curtin University, Perth, Western Australia

Eva Jané-Llopis
WHO Regional Office for Europe, Copenhagen, Denmark

Lloyd Kolbe
Indiana University, Bloomington, United States

Ronald Labonte
Institute of Population Health, University of Ottawa, Canada

Marie-Claude Lamarre
International Union for Health Promotion and Education (IUHPE), Saint-Denis, France

Albert Lee
Centre for Health Education and Health Promotion, and Department of Community and Family Medicine, The Chinese University of Hong Kong, China

Tim Lobstein
Child Obesity Programme, International Obesity TaskForce, London, United Kingdom SPRU - Science and Technology Policy Research, University of Sussex, United Kingdom

Pascale Mantoura
Léa-Roback Research Centre on Social Health Inequalities, University of Montreal, Montreal, Canada

Bruce Maycock
Western Australian Centre for Health Promotion Research, School of Public Health and National Drug Research Institute, Curtin University, Perth, Western Australia

Douglas S. McCall
Canadian Association for School Health, British Columbia, Canada

Marilyn Metzler
Community Health and Program Services Branch, National Center for Chronic Disease Prevention and Health Promotion, US Centers for Disease Control and Prevention (CDC), Atlanta, Georgia, United States

Maurice B. Mittelmark
Research Centre for Health Promotion, University of Bergen, Norway,

Alok Mukhopadhyay
Voluntary Health Association of India (VHAI), New Delhi, India

Andrea Neiman
National Center for Chronic Disease Prevention and Health Promotion, US Centers for Disease Control and Prevention (CDC), Atlanta, Georgia, United States

Vikram Patel
London School of Hygiene and Tropical Medicine, United Kingdom

Martha W. Perry
International Union for Health Promotion and Education (IUHPE), Saint-Denis, France

Louise Potvin
Community Approaches to Health Inequalities, Department of Social and Preventive Medicine, University of Montreal, and Léa-Roback Research Centre on Social Health Inequalities, Montreal, Canada

Blake Poland
Department of Public Health Sciences, Faculty of Medicine, University of Toronto, Canada

John Raeburn
University of Auckland, New Zealand

Valéry Ridde
International Health Unit, University of Montreal, Canada

Jan Ritchie
School of Public Health and Community Medicine, University of New South Wales, Sydney, Australia

Bungon Rithiphakdee
South-East Asia Tobacco Control Alliance (SEATCA), Bangkok, Thailand

Irving Rootman
University of Victoria, Canada

Yussuf Saloojee
National Council against Smoking, Johannesburg, South Africa

Olga Sarmiento
School of Medicine, Department of Social Medicine, University of the Andes, Bogota, Colombia

Trevor Shilton
National Heart Foundation of Australia, Western Australia

David Sleet
National Center for Injury Prevention and Control, Division of Unintentional Injury, US Centers for Disease Control and Prevention (CDC), Atlanta, Georgia, United States

Viv Speller
Health Development Consulting Ltd., Hampshire, United Kingdom

Lawrence St. Leger
School of Health and Social Development, Faculty of Health and Behavioural Sciences, Deakin University, Melbourne, Australia

Karen Slama
Tobacco Prevention Division, International Union against Tuberculosis and Lung Disease, Paris, France

Boyd Swinburn
School of Exercise and Nutrition Sciences, Deakin University, Melbourne, Australia

Marianne van der Wel
Research Centre for Health Promotion, University of Bergen, Norway

Joan Wharf-Higgins
School of Physical Education, University of Victoria, Canada

Marilyn Wise
Australian Centre for Health Promotion, School of Public Health, University of Sydney, Australia

Ian M. Young
NHS- Health Scotland, Edinburgh, Scotland

Section 1
The Global Programme on Health Promotion Effectiveness

1
Global Perspectives on Health Promotion Effectiveness
An Introduction

Davᴀᴠɪᴅ V. McQuᴇᴇɴ* ᴀɴᴅ Cᴀᴛʜᴇʀɪɴᴇ M. Jᴏɴᴇs

General Remarks on the Monograph

It has been both a great opportunity and a challenge to put together this first volume of the global monograph on health promotion effectiveness for the Global Programme on Health Promotion Effectiveness (GPHPE) of the International Union for Health Promotion and Education (IUHPE). The pleasure has been to work with so many skilled and knowledgeable people who are zealously concerned with health promotion effectiveness. The result, hopefully, is a document that reflects the skill, knowledge and dedication of these authors.

As with all such undertakings, we faced a number of decisions about what to include, what to postpone, what to define, and in general how to structure this product of the GPHPE. First and foremost one should note that this document is just one of numerous existing and future products of the GPHPE. It is not intended to be a "final report" or even an "interim report" of the GPHPE; rather it should be seen as one of numerous products of the GPHPE. To date the GPHPE has produced many different papers, documents, presentations, symposia and conferences and all of these combined are "products" of an ambitious programme. This monograph represents a taking stock perspective in the middle of a long term programme to address issues around evidence, effectiveness and evaluation. This document is, in itself, a by-product of many papers, documents, discussions, presentations, symposia and conferences held in the last decade.

One oft asked question is about the target audience for this monograph. This question is more easily asked than answered. The question itself echoes an effectiveness type question if one transforms it to a viewpoint of who one wants to influence. Having concentrated on thinking about what is evidence and what is effectiveness for several years, the question becomes much more challenging and at the same time less obvious to answer. It is a question of marketing, that embodies the challenges of how to address a field that is concerned with how to promote health. The simple answer is that this is a book addressed to health promotion

---

* The views and opinions in this chapter are those of the authors and do not necessarily reflect the views of the Centers for Disease Control and Prevention of the Department of Health and Human Services.

students, researchers, practitioners and other professionals concerned with promoting health. The editors tried to design it as a critical and self-reflexive piece about one of the most important issues in health promotion, namely demonstrating the effectiveness of the work being done. It is not intended for policy makers or decision takers in the first instance, although it will hopefully be read by some of these key people as well. The intended readership is a wide and diverse one.

A suggestion that was frequently submitted to the editors was to be very exclusive and precise about what kind of evidence or what kind of effectiveness we are seeking. It was even suggested that this introductory chapter should be very specific about this. However, it is now clear that any attempt to be so specific would undermine the wide diversity of opinion and discourse that is contained in the individual chapters and in the book as a whole. It is the fervent hope of many that evidence can be finally, accurately and absolutely defined for the field of health promotion. Unfortunately, this remains merely an area of hope at this time. Those anticipating a final definition will have to remain perseverant and wait for Volume II or perhaps III or IV. Those who are familiar with a majority of health promotion literature will recognize that most of the published literature only covers and presents the "success" stories, not the failures; it is our desire that future volumes will give due attention to both, as it is our opinion that we have as much, if not more, to learn from our disappointments than from our achievements.

Topics Arising in the Preparation of the Monograph

In the discussions that have taken place in the time since the GPHPE began, many critical topics have arisen. A significant number of these topics are discussed in the chapters that follow. However there are three topics that continue to be salient to the GPHPE that warrant notice here: size of interventions, level of economic development in places where interventions occur, and the understanding of the relationship between effectiveness and evidence. Hereafter, we briefly touch on each of these critical topics.

Essentially, an intervention is an organized effort to change the course of development of some object over a period of time. That is, the intervention hopes to either decrease, increase or stabilize some process that is occurring either naturally or as a result of any external concerted efforts. A simple example from health promotion illustrates this. A smoking cessation intervention in a small population of smokers can be seen as an effort to intervene in their routine of smoking so many cigarettes a day. The intervention is designed to bring them to stop this habit and/or to greatly reduce the number of cigarettes smoked over some defined period of time. The evidence that the intervention is successful is often defined by the number of people who successfully, for some period of time, stop smoking after the intervention as measured at some later, but specific, point in time. The effectiveness of the intervention is often defined by how the intervention as a whole was carried out by those conducting the intervention (more will be said about this relationship below). In any case, this intervention example can be seen as rather simple and straightforward. Although there are various problems of validity, reliability and measurement that arise, these remain rather trivial. On the other hand, there are many interventions in health promotion that seek to change large and complex dynamic systems. Another example illustrates this. The healthy cities initiatives comprise a health promotion action area that seeks to change the dynamics of very complex systems related to urbanization, economics, globalization, governance, to name just a few of the components relevant to interventions related to the healthy cities movement. Suddenly, in this example, the assessment of evidence of effectiveness becomes extremely complicated, as our ability to demonstrate evidence then relates to the size of the parameters surrounding the intervention.

A common claim that is incessantly reiterated in health promotion is the lack of resources. There is a broadly held belief that economically poor countries have far fewer resources with which to engage in interventions to promote health. Moreover, this issue of resources seems to be a feature that distinguishes the practice of health promotion in the economically developed world from that of the economically poor world. However, this may not accurately represent the situation. The argument can surely be made that resources are more than purely financial, and that communities throughout the world have many different kinds of resources with which to support and carry out interventions that are health promoting. In fact, an entire area of research and practice has arisen on how to recognize, foster and benefit from assets for health promotion. Nonetheless, in terms of the visibility of health promoting interventions, financial resources seem to be the cornerstone for subsistence and dissemination. It has come our attention quite often that there are important and critical interventions occurring in the less economically developed world that are indeed very effective, but we cannot see them because the financial issues associated with evaluation, publication, diffusion, et cetera are not available. The assumption that there are noteworthy and vital excellent effective interventions occurring in the developing world has come to be an accepted belief among many in the field of health promotion. However, the GPHPE has not been sufficiently effective at uncovering them to a wide enough extent in order to discover whether this belief rests on solid or weak ground.

Perhaps the most critical point arising in the preparation of this monograph has been trying to locate the nexus between evidence and effectiveness. How do these concepts relate to each other? To fully address this topic here would be duplicative of thorough discussions found elsewhere in the monograph, but it is imperative to note the critical relationship between these two ideas. In trying to understand the change processes that occur as a result of an intervention, one must ask what are the dimensions that belong to evidence and those that belong to effectiveness. In the simplest form, with respect to an intervention, evidence relates to the certainty about what works and effectiveness relates to the agreement about how to do what works. That is to say, you can have perfect evidence that if you do intervention "x" that outcome "y" will follow; however the execution of intervention "x" may not be carried out appropriately, thus "y" does not happen. Some refer to this as the problem of translation of evidence into practice, yet however one conceptualizes this problem (the process of carrying out an intervention) cannot be isolated from success that should occur based on all the best evidence. With evidence, we are faced with dealing with the certainty of what works, and our evidence can be very strong or very weak. At the same time we are faced with coming to agreement about how to conduct the intervention and that agreement can also be very high or low. In an ideal situation, we would have wide certainty (or proof) about what works and high agreement on how to conduct the intervention; in that ideal situation, we could then easily develop standards or guidance documents on how the evidence should be implemented into practice. The reality for health promotion, unfortunately, is that we are often working in areas with some uncertainty about what works and considerable disagreement about how to carry out an intervention. The challenge for the understanding of effectiveness in relation to evidence for health promotion is to focus on the proportion of work to pursue that lies on this continuum of certainty to uncertainty.

Topics Arising in the Chapters

In the reading, editing and reviewing of the chapters in this monograph many additional and critical topics have arisen. We propose here three topics that need to be highlighted because they occur in one form or another in practically every chapter, namely: methodology, measurement and the Ottawa Charter. Here, we only briefly comment on these and encourage the reader to keep them in mind while reading the monograph.

With regard to methodology, it becomes clear that there is no single methodological approach that dominates the search for effectiveness in health promotion. The widespread variation is remarkable. During the initial stages of preparing this monograph, there was an expectation that some clear methodological directions for assessing evidence and establishing effectiveness would emerge. Quite the opposite has occurred. Many methodologies range from judgment to qualitative approaches to highly quantitative approaches. One might have expected a preponderance of quasi-experimental designs for example, but such is not the case. The best conclusion we can make is that the given methodological approach is mainly driven by the topic area and backgrounds of those searching for evidence of effectiveness.

Measurement, although an entire chapter is devoted to the subject, is another topic that is implicit in many of the chapters, but seldom addressed with adequate specificity. Many chapters deal with areas or variables that should be measured or measurable, but rarely concentrate on the problem in any technical way. In many chapters there is an implied plea for recognition of a need for indicators, but few specifics of how these might be obtained. Chapters in the final section of this monograph provide stimulus to open up new debate and encourage the development of innovative research agendas that could attempt to bridge this gap.

Finally, there is notably less citation of or recognition of the Ottawa Charter than was projected. When the Charter is discussed, it is often in only the most general terms, more or less a mention of it because it is expected. It is difficult to find much discussion of how the Charter relates directly to the questions of evidence and effectiveness. Perhaps this is because the Charter itself neither specifically calls for evidence nor addresses issues of effectiveness. After all, the Charter calls for what should be done and not how to evaluate or decide how effective what has been done in its name. It is only in retrospect that we can now see the challenge of research on effectiveness as related to the Charter.

Limitations of Volume I: Sins of Omission, Commission

In the work to produce a major monograph to reflect the efforts of the GPHPE, some things became clear. First, after considerable discussion and consideration it was recognized that we could not possibly cover all the breadth and scope of the topics relevant to the GPHPE in a single document. Thus was born the idea of having a series of monographs of which this is the first. To begin with, it is evident that, faced with real and stringent publisher deadlines, it is not possible to complete all the topics that one hopes for in the initial volume. These lacking chapters are "sins of omission" arising from many considerations, not just deadlines, but also the availability of obtaining the appropriate people to write on the topics. In addition, we did not have the resources to go further than what we have been able to produce at this time. At the same time, there are also certain "sins of commission", that is the inclusion of some topics that may not be as critical to the evidence and effectiveness debate at this point in time, but, because they were topic areas and chapters already well underway, meeting our deadlines, were ready to go into this first volume.

We well recognize the lack of chapters that address more fully the evidence and effectiveness debate in the less economically developed world, in particular given the fact that the inclusion of chapters of this nature was one of our main objectives for the monograph at its inception. Related to this is also lack of coverage of some major regions of the world. This is a pity, but in our opinion, probably reflects at least two factors. First, the primary editors and developers of the GPHPE were from the West and from economically highly advanced regions. It is interesting to note that in spite of efforts to engage as many readers from the less economically developed world as possible in the blind review process for the chapters at various stages of development, this was also found difficult, primarily for the aforementioned reason as well, with the exception of course of those who were trained in the West. Second, despite the best intentions and efforts of the GPHPE, less progress was made in those less represented regions. There is no simple solution to this; perhaps time, resources and greater representation and leadership from other regions will provide the answer. Of course, a debatable point is that perhaps the fixation with evidence and effectiveness is a peculiarly Western phenomenon that has much les relevance for the rest of the world, and that such efforts are a luxury that can be ill-afforded elsewhere.

The barriers that exist here are not solely ones of economics and financial resources or the technical divide, but other tiers of impediments exist such as those of culture and language. The challenges of working across cultures and languages on the issues of evidence and effectiveness are great. As we mentioned above, this can bring a great deal of diversity and a far-reaching breadth of perspectives; nevertheless, it can also hinder communication, information and data collection and obviously publication and dissemination. More "translation" in the pure sense of the word is not the only solution, as the profound conceptual issues are actually lying much deeper under the surface in terms of cultural perceptions of evidence and effectiveness, and then of course the specificity of the vocabulary available in that language to communicate them. This is an on-going challenge for the GPHPE, and to which the IUHPE is committed to working with its global network of partners and members to foster dialogue to help us better understand each others contexts beyond the physical environment.

A serious omission in this first volume is a careful and considered examination of evidence and effectiveness with regard to health promotion interventions at the community level. Obviously many of the following chapters address aspects that have to do with the community, but there is no single chapter focused on the community as a setting for health promotion practice. Particularly lacking is a careful analysis of the effectiveness of participatory community approaches. Of course, there are many other sources and organizations evaluating evidence in this area and they are referred to in many of the following chapters; nonetheless, this is a central topic that needs careful analysis in the GPHPE and is an obvious, distinct subject area for future volumes.

One area that was considered, but was not included is that of the translation and communication of evidence and effectiveness. Partially, this is because this it is an emerging area of importance that is developing rapidly in the West. It is a familiar problem to many working in the biomedical field: "Why is there such delay in adopting methods and approaches that are found to be effective"? Now, institutions in public health and health promotion, in a number of countries, are giving considerable attention and resources to this issue. The problem itself thus becomes one of finding the evidence of how to effectively translate knowledge in action. Thus it is kind of a secondary "evidence debate" about what is the best evidence of how to put forward evidence to those who need to have and use it for policy development and organizational change. The self examination necessary to address this secondary debate has not yet emerged, but clearly this is an important future topic for the GPHPE.

Future Topics for Consideration to be Addressed in Volume II

It is quite clear that in the development of this monograph many topics for potential inclusion were discussed by the editors, regional project leaders and coordinators and members of the GPHPE global steering group. In addition, in a number of ancillary meetings many additional topics were encouraged. Because of the scope of health promotion, there are a plethora of possible topics for inclusion, and we look forward to encouraging their development and seeing many of these topics in future volumes.

It has already been mentioned that this volume did not concentrate on the developing world as much as was originally hoped. Volume II will surely remedy this. However it will be largely up to those in the less economically developed world to carry this solution forward. The leadership for this effort must be found in that part of the world if it is to have the credibility that one hopes for. Volume II must also make a concerted effort to explore in depth the evidence of effectiveness around community based interventions.

New topics which we hope will emerge, based on considerable discussion include but are not limited to: health promotion effectiveness in the early stages of life, health promotion in the welfare state and the effectiveness of social services, health promotion and Aboriginal health, effective use of health promotion to combat chronic disease, the role of the arts in health promotion, health promotion effectiveness and ethics, the effectiveness of health promotion in addressing HIV and AIDS, consideration of the harmful and unintended effects in health promotion, the evidence of the effectiveness of the Healthy Cities movement, the impact of globalization (including demographic changes and sustainable development) at the community level and interventions to address that impact, communication and dissemination of health promotion interventions using new technologies, the evidence that decision-makers use evidence to make decisions, and a thorough analysis of the interventions arising from the recommendations of international organizations, notably the Ottawa and Bangkok Charters.

Undoubtedly there are many additional topics that the readers of this monograph will propose in the near future and these all need careful consideration. In addition, many will acknowledge the need to further examine many of the topics covered in Volume I. Indeed, it is quite clear that topics like urbanization, governance, inequity, empowerment, et cetera will continue to be critical to health promotion and continue to present challenges of effectiveness. Nevertheless, it is a challenge to the field of health promotion to bring forth fresh faces and a cadre of new committed researchers to address many of these issues. It is hoped that Volume II will be witness to many new authors, from a wide range of cultural and linguistic backgrounds, and some surprising and pioneering insights into evidence and effectiveness.

Conclusions

It is difficult to offer just a few conclusions to a first Volume publication of such a broad-based effort as the GPHPE; nonetheless, we will restrict ourselves to three overriding conclusions to this monograph and the GPHPE in general. First, it is apparent that the main people who are interested in assessing health promotion are those working in health promotion. What are the implications of this? Second, it is clear that evidence as a concept sits uncomfortably within the spectrum of health promotion practice. Finally, it is obvious that health promotion needs many more interventions based on the best practice and theory if it is to address all the difficult questions on evidence and effectiveness.

In the vast literature on evaluation there are many perspectives on who should carry out evaluation. One common premise is that evaluation should be carried out by people who have no connection with, or are relatively independent from, what is being evaluated. This idea of impartiality is the hallmark for much research evaluation. Evaluation is seen as most valid when it is carried out either by peers or knowledgeable "outsiders." Yet in the field of health promotion, such independent evaluation is rarely practiced. With regard to evidence and effectiveness this is also the case. Undoubtedly, this is once again a question of resources. Many health promotion projects and interventions often have very few funds to set aside for evaluation and even fewer for "external" evaluation. There are unfortunately few solutions available to this state of affairs. One hopeful direction, on a broader evaluation spectrum, is the further development and use of large scale monitoring/surveillance systems to routinely collect data on key variables of interest to those in health promotion. Such data could be very useful in the analysis of the impact of large-scale policy decisions related to health promotion. In the meantime careful self evaluation and scrutiny of health promotion interventions will provide the best hope for the evidence of effectiveness.

Many criticisms have been made of the concept of evidence as appropriate to the field of health promotion. Some argue that the requirements for evidence are too deeply based in the so-called hard sciences and are not necessarily applicable to the main interventions found in health promotion practice. Others have argued that many of the areas for health promotion practice, namely areas such as communities, cities, governance, globalization, and social health inequities, for example, are simply too complex for the testing of the effectiveness of interventions. The outcomes are either too multivariate or too distill to be successfully recognized on the short term timetable demanded by many seeking evidence of effectiveness. There is, of course, no simple answer to these legitimate concerns. However, it is unmistakable that evaluation must be carried out and this means that different ideas about how to assess evidence of effectiveness must be developed and embraced by those who demand it.

Finally, it is overwhelmingly obvious that the field of health promotion, with its vast subject area and multiple areas of concern, is still in early stages in terms of the number of interventions undertaken. A common theme, reiterated throughout this monograph, and supported by the experience of international evidence review groups, is that we simply do not have enough interventions to evaluate. This is the reason why the outcome "insufficient evidence" reoccurs so often. It is not necessarily for lack of good studies, but, rather, the lack of a sufficient number of studies. It is commonplace in many sciences for there to be dozens, if not hundreds, of similar studies replicating the success of a particular intervention or experiment. The paucity of interventions in the field of health promotion, coupled with their complex often multivariate nature, makes comparison exceedingly difficult. The only solution to this dilemma is the continued and persistent development and implementation of interventions that are designed to be appropriately evaluated in terms of evidence and effectiveness. We expect and trust that as the health promotion field evolves and matures this will be the plausible and natural resolution.

2
The Global Programme on Health Promotion Effectiveness (GPHPE)
A Global Process for Assessing Health Promotion Effectiveness with Regional Diversity

CATHERINE M. JONES, MARY AMUYUNZU-NYAMONGO,
URSEL BROESSKAMP-STONE, LIGIA DE SALAZAR, STEVE FAWCETT,
MARCIA HILLS, ALBERT LEE, ALOK MUKHOPADHAY, JAN RITCHIE,
VIV SPELLER AND DAVID V. MCQUEEN*

The GPHPE: A Framework for Effectiveness and Diversity

The Global Programme on Health Promotion Effectiveness is coordinated by the International Union for Health Promotion and Education (IUHPE) in collaboration with the World Health Organization and numerous other partners and supporters[†]. It is a unique worldwide programme which aims to raise standards of health-promoting policy-making and practice worldwide by reviewing evidence of effectiveness in terms of health, social, economic and political impact; translating evidence to policy makers, teachers, practitioners, researchers; and stimulating debate on the nature of evidence of effectiveness.

The GPHPE is an overarching programme that encompasses a number of regional projects and related activities being conducted across the globe. The significance of the GPHPE's global vision is not only in the programme's intent to examine and explore the differences among regions with respect to their approaches to assessing the effectiveness of health promotion in terms of health and social impact, but the distinct specificity is intrinsically related to the

---

[*] The views and opinions in this chapter are those of the authors and do not necessarily reflect the views of the Centers for Disease Control and Prevention of the Department of Health and Human Services.
[†] African Medical Research Foundation; Health Promotion Switzerland; IUHPE/ EuroHealthNet Joint Special Interest Group on Health Promotion Evidence, Effectiveness and Transferability; National Institute for Health and Clinical Excellence, England; The Netherlands Institute for Health Promotion and Disease Prevention; Pan-American Health Organization; Public Health Agency of Canada; US Centers for Disease Control and Prevention (an agency of the Department of Health and Human Services); Victorian Health Promotion Foundation; Voluntary Health Association of India, World Health Organization (Geneva), WHO/AFRO, among others.

programme's capacity to acknowledge the common factors, distinguish the differences in context and support the strengthening of linkages and interactive
exchange of this growing body of knowledge. Fundamentally, the GPHPE is concerned with how to stimulate the evaluation of effectiveness, champion the development of appropriate tools and methods to do so, and espouse the implementation
of this body of knowledge to its best use in practice and for advocacy.

The GPHPE is an on-going process, a long-term programme of work, which is
supported by a range of regional activities and projects. The global component of
the programme was designed to serve as a steering mechanism, a structure that
could be flexible enough to include and recognise a diverse range of perspectives
and approaches. The development of regional projects which have been carried
out under this global banner do not reflect a standard model, but rather represent
a collection of research projects, training programmes, publication and dissemination activities and advocacy initiatives. In this sense, one could see the GPHPE
as a field of wildflowers, none of which resemble each other, but when put
together, it is the diversity that enhances the depth of the beauty and creates an
overall image of unity. The ambiance of the GPHPE is one of mutual learning
wherein all partners and members have the opportunity to draw from the knowledge and lessons learned in other parts of the world.

At the core of this process, which allows for the incorporation of such a wide
array of work is the broad scope of definitions of evidence which the GPHPE has
adopted. A large portion of health promotion activities and interventions are
excluded from being evaluated for their effectiveness, discriminated against given
that they lie either linguistically or analytically outside the traditional boundaries of
Western-dominated science and research. The GPHPE attempts to create conditions
which bring the evidence from the non-English languages to the forefront, as well
as a more inclusive approach to the variety of interventions which might not be conventional choices for consideration in evaluation. Essentially, the GPHPE aims to
look at that which lies below the surface and remains invisible to the eyes of a
researcher, practitioner or decision-maker who adheres to the use of Western-biased
criteria for evaluation and review protocols and processes (McQueen, 2003).

The rationale used to encourage the development of regional projects on health
promotion effectiveness was that they would be geographically organised, they
would characterize the diversity of the regions and embody any specificity of issues
and approaches indigenous to the respective regions, and that they would move at
their own pace. The reality that each region operates in a unique linguistic, professional and cultural context is illustrated in the fact that they are all at different stages
of their projects. Some of the dimensions which contribute to this spectrum of development are resource differences (both human and financial), theoretical differences,
and ownership differences (various structures for partnership and entrepreneurship).

The GPHPE range of regional effectiveness projects are led and coordinated by
IUHPE collaborators working on the ground in their respective regions, and the
regional ownership of the established priorities and activities is what creates the
basis for a distinctive process to implement the research, evaluation results and
the accompanying activities. This kind of flexibility in the process is both an

advantage and a challenge. It is only through such a supple process that the programme can allow for the emergence of the local knowledge and practice on the effectiveness of health promotion in a given social, political, and cultural climate. However, the diversity of that which emanates from this process is often very complicated and complex to digest and relay in a more universal manner, making it difficult for the GPHPE to extract general lessons and make evidenced-based recommendations for policy-makers.

Supported by the Global Steering Group, the GPHPE coordinating team and leadership depend on all of the regional leaders and coordinators, as well as the members of an intricate web of institutional partners, interested groups, collaborators and independent scientific consultants across the globe to carry out the work at the level which corresponds to their interests and capacity. This set of connections also lays the groundwork for networking and exchange across regions, increasing opportunities to develop capacity. Without this foundation of people and organisations who epitomize the local, national and international expertise, the GPHPE process would be dubious and rendered weak. It is therefore not only the process which influences the practice, but undeniably vice-versa.

Assessing the Work of the Regions – Scanning the Globe via a Questionnaire

The aim of this chapter is to present the reader with an overview of the regions and the work which has been undertaken by the regional teams. Rather than present a set of separate regional reports, it was considered more useful to compile a comprehensive chapter that will provide regional feedback and highlight issues emanating from the various GPHPE regional projects. This section is intended as a conglomerate of all of the projects and has involved multiple authors. Each regional project team was contacted to provide answers to questions on what specific points and issues make their given region particular, on the state of the art in evaluation in their region, on the unique aspects for their region and what effectiveness means in their professional and cultural context. The authors considered this approach the best way to demonstrate the depth of the rich diversity (and similarities) and conditions under which these regional projects operate.

The project leaders and coordinators were sent a questionnaire containing six questions. The remainder of this chapter will provide a synthesis of their replies in order to show the range of experiences which have been accumulated over the course of the GPHPE since its inception in 2001.

Unique Regional Attributes Related to Assessing Evidence and Effectiveness of Health Promotion Interventions

The uniqueness of each region's exploits is primarily related to the interplay between any strategic priorities defined by the region as well as the resources available to address them. Resource availability has been dealt with in very creative ways by many of the regions who have initiated partnerships in order to carry out their work. For example in the South West Pacific region, the project has embarked on a very innovative project with a team from the School of Public Health and Community Medicine at the University of New South Wales (UNSW), to explore the links between health and peace-building and to develop a tool to help field workers work more effectively. The project is now in its third year and has been very productive. The tool, currently termed the Health and Peace-Building Filter, has been rigorously trialled and tested during its development to ensure it is as valid and reliable as possible in supporting field workers in the very difficult environment that exists in countries undergoing current or recent conflict. Funding for the Project has come through the Australian Agency for International Development (AusAID) and UNSW. Furthermore, a group in Western Australia has worked with the CDC to explore the local situation regarding alcohol related harm and road accidents. Both of these projects are described in more detail in separate chapters in this book, in Chapters 15 and 11, respectively. Finally, as a pre-requisite for developing effective interventions in mental health promotion in the region, a project was carried out with the purpose of developing a data base concerning the mental health promotion of young people. Entitled the "Child mental health promotion and prevention capacity mapping project", it uses a template from *HP-Source*[*] to achieve consistency in documenting activities in some selected countries in the region.

The question of resources can often be broken into two types of categories, too many or too few. For example, with the relative abundance of resources for research in North America, the North American region has a comparably large literature on the effectiveness of health promotion approaches. Initially, there were few dedicated resources for the North American Regional Effectiveness Project; this made it challenging to develop a brand new and complete knowledge synthesis. The team's strategy was hence twofold: 1) To obtain agreement on the overall direction through a shared mission and co-developed framework for creating conditions that promote health and address social determinants, and 2) To take advantage of ongoing efforts in knowledge synthesis by team members. The first strategy was fine-tuned to include a specific emphasis on multi-sectoral collaborations that seek to improve equity or reduce health disparities by addressing the social determinants or conditions for health. One development that significantly assisted the North American project was the initiation of a Canadian effectiveness project funded by the Public Health Agency of Canada. This has resulted in a framework for assessing the effectiveness of community interventions to promote health and the development of an alternative methodology for synthesizing evidence from complex community interventions (Hills, O'Neill, Carroll & MacDonald, 2004; Hills, 2004; Hills, 2005). As a result of the success of this

---

[*] http://www.hp-source.net/

federally funded program, two new research grants were obtained to further refine the methodology and to conduct a synthesis to assess the effectiveness of community interventions to ameliorate health inequities (details of the research grants are provided under the North American project achievements in Table 2.1).

This example is countered by that of the South East Asian region, which is one of the most underdeveloped regions of the world. It is home to 20% of the world's population with 40% of those living in absolute poverty. The challenge in making provisions for improved health care services is further compounded by its socio-cultural diversity and degree of governance. In most developing countries including India, millions of people die from diseases linked to unsafe water, sanitation and hygiene. The bulk of the burden of diseases lies upon the poor, women, scheduled castes and tribes. Voluntary agencies have played a significant role in developing flexible, community specific alternative models, as well as providing low cost and effective health services. They have succeeded in developing village based health cadres, appropriate educational materials and technologies filling gaps in the government health services; nevertheless their work is hampered due to a lack of a supportive climate and finances. The "for-profit" private sector's immense levels of resources make it an irresistible partner for public health initiatives. The public/private/non-profit partnership is becoming an essential reality as both the public and private sectors recognize their individual abilities to address emerging public health issues. Lastly, the grass roots democratic institutions like the Panchayati raj institutions (PRIs) in India and other countries have given power back to the local people to be change agents themselves. These institutions are more attuned to local realities, thus helping people better grapple with the host of problems linked to socio-economic condition, behaviour, social transition and change. Chapter 16 explores issues around the role that governance plays in the effectiveness of health promotion.

Regions' priorities are also shaped by the conditions in which they operate, and the professional and political structures which determine those conditions. The Northern Part of the Western Pacific and the Latin American regions are examples which attest to this. The uniqueness of Northern Part of the Western Pacific Regional project in assessing evidence and effectiveness of health promotion interventions is largely dependent upon how health promotion programmes are implemented. Broadly speaking, they can be divided into two main types in terms of putting policies and practice into evidence, the first being the Healthy Settings approach and the second that of health promotion interventions as a result of government policies. There is strong emphasis on investment in sustainable policies, actions and infrastructure to address the determinants of health; capacity building for policy development and leadership; regulation and legislation; and partnership and alliance building with public, private, non-governmental and international organizations and civil society to create sustainable actions. Frameworks have been established and resulting evidence demonstrating positive change in those areas should contribute to health promotion effectiveness. Chapter 19 introduces the challenges and future directions for building evidence for the effectiveness of whole system health promotion.

TABLE 2.1. Presentation of the GPHPE's regional effectiveness projects' major accomplishments

Region (listed alphabetically)	Accomplishments
Africa	1) Drafting a concept paper on health promotion and education effectiveness in the African Region, which called for a need to develop capacity in the region in terms of monitoring and evaluation, process documentation and advocacy.
	2) Conducting a comprehensive literature review on health promotion effectiveness in the Region, with a publication and dissemination of the full report.
	3) Commissioning a publication to review and synthesize evidence-based health promotion effectiveness, in a number of identified areas;
	4) Development of a comprehensive funding proposal for the African Regional Project, and fundraising for the African effectiveness activities.
	5) Planning research and training activities and other meetings (still in developmental stage):
	✓ Training in monitoring and evaluation: This is important in view of gathering evidence on effectiveness because we need to answer several questions: What evidence are we searching for? How shall we know the evidence we are looking for? How shall we package and share the evidence?
	✓ Holding a meeting to engage policy makers (including political leaders and managers from the health, education and other sectors).
	✓ Implement special research projects (e.g. health promotion schools, tobacco control, mitigation of HIV/AIDS, urbanization, youth and adolescent health, aging, malaria, epidemics, etc.).
Europe	IUHPE special reports:
	IUHPE (1999) *The evidence of health promotion effectiveness: Shaping public health in a new Europe.* Part 1: Core document. IUHPE (1999) *The evidence of health promotion effectiveness: Shaping public health in a new Europe.* Part 2: Evidence book. (This set of publications uniquely reviewed effectiveness in terms of not only 'health' outcomes but also social, economic, political outcomes, and was presented as both a comprehensive resource (review book) and a separate booklet for policy makers. These have also been translated into 7 languages.)
	Efficacité de la promotion de la santé: Actes du colloque organisé par l'INPES avec la collaboration de l'UIPES. Hors série 1 *Promotion & Education*, 2004.
	Speller, Viv. (2006) Synthesis of the knowledge at the international level in the field of evidence of effectiveness of health promotion and best practice. Report compiled by the IUHPE for Health Promotion Switzerland. (c) 2005 Health Promotion Switzerland. All rights reserved, reproduction with permission from Health Promotion Switzerland.

Products and deliverables from Getting Evidence into Practice project (GEP):

Bollars C, Kok H, Van den Broucke S & Molleman G (2005) *European Quality Instrument for Health Promotion (EQUIHP) and User Manual.*

Raty Sanna & Aro Arja R (2005) *European review protocol for health promotion.*

The challenge of getting evidence into practice: current debates and future strategies. Supplement 1 *Promotion & Education,* 2005.

Latin America	1. Design and implementation of the Latin American Program of Training on Effectiveness Evaluation in Health Promotion (two cohorts finished, two more currently in progress and inclusion of the topic in university academic programs).
	2. Literature review on the state of art of the evidences on health promotion effectiveness in Latin America.
	3. Regional Project of Evidence of Health Promotion Effectiveness' web portal (www.proyectoefectividad-iupes.com).
	4. Building a virtual network of institutions and persons interested in evaluation effectiveness in health promotion in Latin America.
	5. Design of methodologies of effectiveness evaluation appropriate for the Latin American context.
	The following are in progress:
	• Planning of a Latin American course integrating evaluation methodologies in health promotion.
	• Publication of a study on Latin American capacity for effectiveness evaluation in health promotion.
North America	1. Knowledge synthesis of the evidence base for 12 "best processes" or mechanisms by which communities create conditions for promoting community health and addressing social determinants [Published on the Community Tool Box http://ctb.ku.edu/ under the homepage feature, "Explore Best Processes and Practices"]
	2. Capacity-building resources for promoting community health and development community-based participatory research [Published on the Community Tool Box http://ctb.ku.edu/; including through its toolkits (e.g., for building collaborative partnerships, strategic planning, developing logic models, evaluation) and links to its 6,000 pages of practical how-to information]
	3. Recent papers on knowledge synthesis and capacity development including:
	a) Fawcett, S.B., Francisco, V., and Schultz, J. (2004). Improving and understanding the work of community health and development. (Pp. 209–242). In J. Burgos and E Ribes (Eds.). (2004). Theory, basic and applied research, and technological applications in behavior science. Guadalajara, Mexico: Universidad de Guadalajara.
	b) Boothroyd, R., Fawcett, S.B., and Foster-Fishman, P. (2004). Community development: Enhancing the knowledge base through participatory action research. (Pp. 37–52). In LA Jason et al. (2004). Participatory community research: Theories and methods in action. Washington, DC: American Psychological Association.

(Continued)

TABLE 2.1. (Continued)

Region (listed alphabetically)	Accomplishments
	c) Hills, M., & Carroll, S. (2004). Health promotion evaluation, realist synthesis and participation, Avaliacao em promocao de saude, sintese realista e participacao, Ciência & Saúde Coletiva, 9(3), 536–539, September 2004.
	d) Hills, M., Carroll, S., & O'Neill, M. (2004). Vers un modéle d'évaluation de l'efficacité des interventions communautaires en promotion de la santé: compte-rendu de quelques développements Nord-américains récents. *Promotion & Education*. Hors série – 1, Supplement – Edición especial, 17–21.
	4. Eighteen presentations at international and national conference and five reports to funding organizations (Hills, M. & Carroll, S.)
	5. Received five research grants to conduct synthesis reviews and refine methodology (Hills, M. & Carroll, S.): Hills, M., (PI) McQueen, D., Metzler, M., Rootman, I., & MacDonald, M. (2006). Building the Evidence Base for Reducing Health Disparities: An Alternative Methodology for Knowledge Synthesis. CIHR ($90,000).
	Hills, M., (PI) McQueen, D., Anderson, L., Metzler, M., Raphael, D., Jackson, S., & Pawson, R. (2006) Assessing the Effectiveness of Intersectoral Community Efforts to promote Health and Reduce Disparities. CIHR ($90,000).
	Phases 1,2 & 3 of the Public Health Agency of Canada's Effectiveness of Community Interventions Project (Hills, 2004; Hills, 2005a; Hills, 2005b).
Northern part of the Western Pacific	- *The Evidence of Health Promotion Effectiveness: Shaping Public Health in a New Europe* (IUHPE, 2000) translated and published in Japanese, Korean and Chinese languages.
	- Northern Part of the Western Pacific Regional Conference, June 24, 2006 with input from Europe as well as different countries in the region.
	- 2nd Asian Pacific Conference on Health Promotion, The Chinese University of Hong Kong, Nov 5–6, 2006, IUHPE Pearl River Liaison Office as co-organiser.
	Publications on evidence of Health Promoting Schools
	Lee A., Cheng F., Fung Y., St Leger L. Can Health Promoting Schools contribute to the better health and well being of young people: Hong Kong experience? *Journal of Epidemiology and Community* 2006; 60:530–536.
	Lee A., St Leger L., Moon AS. Evaluating Health Promotion in Schools meeting the needs for education and health professionals: A case study of developing appropriate indictors and data collection methods in Hong Kong. *Promotion & Education* XII (3–4): 123–130. (*Special issue reporting successful school health promotion programmes globally.*)

Publication on Lifestyle

Kawata C., Higuchi M., Yamamoto H., Sakamoto M., Kaneko N., Kusano E., De Silva S.D., Piyaseeli U.K.D., De Silva S., Handa Y. A study of the relationship between diabetes mellitus and lifestyle in Sri Lanka. *Grants in Aid for Scientific Research* 2002–2004 (Japan) 2005; 1–98.

Presentations

Lee A. *International Examples of School Health Programmes and Monitoring*. Comprehensive School Health: Understanding and Monitoring a Critical Mass of Programs to Benefit Children. Organised by Joint Consortium for School Health, Canadian Population Health Initiative and Canadian Council on Learning December 8–9, 2005, Ottawa, Canada.

Lee A. *Good practice of Healthy Schools leading to quality Healthy Cities*. Shanghai International Forum on Healthy Cities. Organised by Shanghai Municipal Committee of Health Promotion, WHO Kobe Centre and Shanghai Municipal Health Bureau, 20–22 November, 2005, Shanghai, China.

South East Asia	1. "KHOJ" publication, following which the Government of Arunachal Pradesh asked the Voluntary Health Association of India to take over the Primary Health Centres.
	2. Incorporation of recommendations into the National Rural Health Mission.
	3. Many State Governments have also come up with innovative schemes for community health to be funded by them.
	4. Indian experiences and others from South East Asia were also captured in the WHO film '*Paths are Made by Walking*'.
South West Pacific	1. Australian Health Promotion Association Conference April 2006: "A journey to peace building", Anne Bunde-Birouste, invited speaker, plenary presentation.
	2. IUHPE Board of Trustees presentation: The Role and Place of Health in Preventing Violence, Post-Conflict Recovery, and Peace Building, Anne Bunde-Birouste.
	3. Chapter for GPHPE global monograph: "Strengthening peace-building through health promotion: development of a framework" – a description of the AusAID-UNSW project, Anne Bunde-Birouste and Jan Ritchie.
	4. Completion of a report on the "Effectiveness of health promotion in preventing alcohol-related harm" (2006) which served as the basis for a chapter in the GPHPE global monograph.
	5. "Child mental health promotion and prevention capacity mapping project", using a template from *HP-Source*, coordinated by A/Prof Louise Rowling – ongoing.

Africa is a region where health promotion is becoming recognized as a critical approach in addressing the myriad of problems faced on the continent. Although health interventions and activities have been undertaken in the region over time, they have mainly been done within the Ministries of health but not recognized or documented as such. In addition, documentation and dissemination of information continues to be a big challenge in the region, hence the collection of evidence of effectiveness has a big role to play in influencing both policy and practice.

In the Latin American and the Caribbean region, a "unique" condition in relation to the evaluation of evidence of effectiveness in health promotion interventions is the search for evaluation approaches and models which, without losing the scientific character, manage to fit specific conditions of viability and feasibility in the region to assess health promotion effectiveness. Two strategies that have contributed to visualize the effectiveness project in the agenda of several Latin American countries have been: the strengthening of the regional capacity to develop effectiveness evaluations in health promotion and development of communications tools that have contributed to identify, recognize and disseminate the different evaluation initiatives and application of results to improve practice and reorient programs. The actions for the fulfillment of these objectives have been conditions necessary to make advance in systematic, productive and permanent evaluation initiatives in the different sub-regions of Latin America. Chapter 20 discusses the feasibility for health promotion under these various decision-making contexts.

The geographic organisation of the regional projects allows for a certain amount of synergy in approaches, but also brings a great deal of complexity into the process, given the state of the field in the individual countries and the historical development of health promotion and evaluation in those countries. For example, in order to respond to this question regarding uniqueness, the European Regional project had to take into account the status of both "evidence" about effective health promotion in Europe, and the wider set of conditions necessary to support "effectiveness" of health promotion. At least in part this separation is due to the discourse around evidence and effectiveness in Europe, where the terms are used differently in different health related disciplines, and may be used synonymously or interchangeably. The European team considers that, in order for a pan-European health promotion effectiveness movement to achieve success, a number of critical success factors would need to be fulfilled. These factors are closely linked with one another, to the extent that their full presence creates a virtuous cycle, whereas the absence of even one or two strongly mitigates against success. Six critical success factors were suggested: policy cogency of evidence-based, effective health promotion; completeness and competence of health promotion systems; researchers' interest in the field of evidence of health promotion effectiveness; health promotion funding, including *what* is funded; advocacy of effective health promotion; and the role of international organisations.

Factors which Contributed to the Feasibility, Utility and Productivity of the Regions' Work

Many of the regions acknowledged that existing networks were one of the strongest contributing factors to their work in terms of rendering their task possible. These networks included the global professional network of the IUHPE, other international networks and collaborations, and their own national and regional networks which could support and contribute to the development of multi-partner initiatives under the banner of the GPHPE. The GPHPE has served as a virtual forum that can unite these diverse networks and gives them a sense of purpose in collaborating on a specific programme, the results and reflections of which are equally available and valuable to all involved. Many regions cited the connectivity to other experts from around the world as being vital to their regional work to allow for cross-fertilization of ideas and sharing of results as well as providing opportunities for carrying out targeted consultations. This global network also makes it possible to share and contribute to the existing (yet expanding) knowledge base and expertise from around the world. Collaboration on the regional projects has also strengthened the relationships between these networks, often resulting in other spin-off collaborative projects or the establishment of more formalised and institutionalised agreements.

This is the case in the European Region where there now exist excellent connections and working relationships between key "players" that continue to be supported through IUHPE, encompassing and bringing together organizations, researchers, experts and practitioners. In the last few years, these networks have been expanded and supported through EuroHealthNet (representing contributing national agencies). There has been increasing exchange and cooperation developed between IUHPE and EuroHealthNet demonstrated particularly through their first joint EU co-funded project on Getting Evidence into Practice (GEP). This has led to the signature of a collaboration agreement to establish a Joint Special Interest Group on Health Promotion Evidence, Effectiveness and Transferability.

In addition to forging new partnerships, the GPHPE and the regional initiatives have tremendously benefited from the high levels of commitment and engagement of their members and partners. This includes the support of key institutional members to host meetings and symposia, to provide institutional support to advance the objectives and implement regional work plans and to create opportunities for synergy between the regions. These "in-kind" contributions, including availability and willingness of collaborators to participate voluntarily, are at the very core of the foundation for carrying out these activities and no regional project would be possible without them.

Finally, a variety of mechanisms were identified as being extremely supportive, most notably the opportunities linked to regional and world conferences. These events have been critical to the facilitation of exchange. While communication via the web, email or through publications is cited as fundamental, occasional face-to-face contact is also essential in order to provide a time to share, network, and plan in a way that helps maintain momentum.

Elements which Rendered the Task Difficult

A number of challenges have been evoked by the regional teams as having posed difficulties in the pursuit and implementation of their activities. These range from financial constraints, to dissemination channels not being completely fluid, to lofty goals being established when basic infrastructure was lacking to provide capacity for their realization. In some regions, where the IUHPE has a larger presence and representation with greater legitimacy, it was less of a challenge to marshal support, whereas in those where the IUHPE had a more conservative profile and less prominence, it was much more difficult.

The challenge of being under-resourced was a frustrating one for many, not only in its obstruction of carrying out an ideal work-plan, but also in that without sufficient funding, accountability to the project team's partners and objectives was difficult. Given that an overwhelming majority of the regional activity depends upon voluntary work, this also hinders the optimum development and implementation of the work. Although the generous support and donation of time and other resources has been an impetus, the opposite side of that fact results in a cycle of activity which can greatly vary in intensity. There was a good deal of consensus that the major challenge for regions was to weigh the objectives and scope of the GPHPE which are wide, in comparison to the minimal resources available to execute their projects. Even in some regions, such as Africa, where the propose areas of focus were perceived feasible, it has been difficult to raise adequate funds for most of the activities.

Communication challenges were also encountered but were of differing sorts. The sheer size of many regions, both in terms of geographic, population, cultural and linguistic coverage presented difficulties to regional teams in achieving their goals. In the North American region, although there are only three countries involved in the current project (Canada, the United States and the English speaking Caribbean) their cultures are extremely different from each other, making it difficult to have a united voice. This presents an enormous struggle for many of the regions and is also largely linked to resource-poor operations to meet these needs. This was also noted in the African region, where the different languages used on the continent (English, French, Portuguese) makes it a unique place for documenting evidence and also posed significant challenges for communication between the country focal points and the regional coordinating team. Often this led to a small number of countries that dominated the activities in some regions, in spite of efforts to reduce inequity in this respect. Furthermore, technical isolation and lack of access to IT also impeded developments. As projects of this nature, which aim to foster collaboration amongst people internationally, depend on distance communication, one must first ensure a baseline capacity to participate as well as to sensitize and train those who do not have the culture to work in this manner to use these technological methods of interacting and building collectivity.

There was also indication of challenges which could be classified as ideological, methodological or theoretical. For example, in Latin America, the unequal theoretical and technological developments about health promotion evaluation among the countries, as well as varying degrees of infrastructure and human resources to participate actively and willingly in project's activities, led to a pre-condition that participation be determined to a great extent by the activities that the project could help to finance in the countries and sub-regions. In the case of South-East Asia, the foundations of health promotion themselves were a challenge in that doing health promotion in deprived communities requires a re-thinking of the approach and an alteration of the aims to be that of ensuring the most basic needs. The North American region specifically acknowledged that there was a lack of expectation for a product that would support translation of knowledge to practice.

The European situation presents an interesting set of challenges which relate to a wave of policy shifts nationally as well as an on-going struggle between health promotion and public health about what constitutes evidence. More generally in the European context, there has been a repeated wave of reforms of public health and health promotion in countries. These reforms have threatened the development and implementation of effective health promotion repeatedly, and directly impacted upon individuals leading the European Regional Effectiveness Project. This lack of organizational stability has meant the lack of supportive infrastructures and resources for the GPHPE to draw upon. Although the region is rich in expertise, and indeed, activity in the realm of evidence-based health or health care, the amount and extent of activity and related "power bases" for public health and health promotion evidence in various countries and professional circles brings with it its own complications and difficulties. The complexity of connections necessary particularly in Europe with its high level of differentiation (e.g. IUHPE, EuroHealthNet, EUHPA, EPHA, WHO related networks, HP Settings networks, etc.) and the lack of resources to enable key individual experts and professionals to keep in touch with each other and with developments in knowledge, constrains the potential impact of GPHPE in Europe. This has led to a lack of profile for GPHPE in Europe – it may seem to be one voice amongst many; and possibly to a lack of a particular European flavor to the region's contributions to the overall project. There has also been a lack of focus on the use of evidence rather than just the generation of it, while there has been an expansion of the focus of research and evidence-generation side to include evidence coming out of daily practice and policy work. This work has also been conducted in the context of significant policy shifts in evidence-based public health and health promotion in Europe, where there is (at least in many European Union countries) a pronounced rhetoric about the use of evidence in developing policy and implementing effective practice. However strong the rhetoric, nevertheless there are often blind spots in terms of using evidence in policy if it does not seem to fit the political priorities.

How the Regions could have Accomplished More

The obvious response is resources! However, the more detailed response from many regions implied that an increase in resources would be necessary to increase participation and upscale efforts, and therefore they would be specifically targeted to communications. This included resources for more face-to-face meetings for reflection and dialogue, the recruitment of research assistants, and communications support (including the capacity for video conferencing and more translation services). Other gaps included the need for the provision of more opportunities to publish and disseminate experiences, regionally and globally. Dissemination support would ideally also include more training and capacity to plan, document, and evaluate experiences and interventions which would capitalize on the wealth of activity being undertaken in the regions.

In the European case, wherein the GPHPE regional project is just one of many endeavors in this arena, resources are needed in order to influence and organize in Europe where the need lies to position the GPHPE as a "leader", or at least as a strong partner, within a wider gamut of actors in the face of very strong and dominant "health care evidence" organizations at the national and European levels. Both of the Latin American and the European regions cited a need for clarity in order to leverage more political and institutional commitment for better use of the evidence in decision-making processes. In Africa, there was a call for the creation of a more strategic leadership structure to support the work of the African coordinating team. This could include, for example, the establishment of sub-regional hubs to better and more efficiently address the inherent differences between the linguistic and geographic sub-sectors of the continent.

The IUHPE has recognized the challenges to enhancing the effectiveness and quality of health promotion which have presented themselves over the course of the programme and the last chapter of this book presents some thoughts on the future of health promotion from the perspective of the IUHPE. The chapter is premised upon the recognition that health promotion has yet to contribute to equity in health to its full potential. The chapter aims to explore "what needs to happen if health promotion is to contribute to its full potential to improve health?" Although the IUHPE believes it is healthy to be self-critical in these reflections in order to stimulate growth and improvement, it continues to be committed to bridging the gap where health promotion professionals encounter obstacles as mentioned above. The IUHPE is open to respond and introduce suggestions for how we can advance together as a field to better meet these needs.

Major Regional Accomplishments

Each of the regions was requested to cite five major accomplishments. These could range from publications, to presentations, to seminars or other meetings. Table 2.1 presents those selected by the regions as examples.

In addition to the specific regional mentions, the GPHPE would like to give particular attention to the series of IUHPE regional conferences on the effectiveness and quality of health promotion. Whilst this series began as a European regional one in 1989, it has grown to become an internationally renowned event which brings together researchers, practitioners and policy and decision-makers from all over the world who are interested in the evidence of the quality and effectiveness of health promotion. Box 2.1 presents a list of the series chronologically beginning with the most recent one.

Box 2.1. IUHPE European conference series on the effectiveness and quality
of health promotion

6th IUHPE European Conference on the Effectiveness and Quality of Health
Promotion. *Best practice for better health.* June 1–4, 2005. Stockholm,
Sweden. (http://www.bestpractice2005.se/)
5th IUHPE European Conference on the Effectiveness and Quality of Health
Promotion. New Dimensions in Promoting Health: Linking health promoting
programmes with public policies. June 11–13, 2002. London, UK.
4th IUHPE European Conference on the Effectiveness and Quality of Health
Promotion. *Best practices.* May 16–19, 1999. Helsinki, Finland and Tallinn,
Estonia.
3rd IUHPE European Conference on Health Promotion Effectiveness. *Quality
Assessment in Health Promotion and Health Education.* 1996. Turin, Italy.
2nd IUHPE European Conference on Health Promotion Effectiveness. May
14–16, 1992. Athens, Greece.
The objectives of the Conference were:

a) to connect people working in the field and initiate multinational collaboration and networks;
b) to promote health promotion and health education evaluation techniques in
   all European countries;
c) to establish the idea of measurement of effectiveness, as a *sine qua non* of
   both health promotion and health education;
d) to introduce and elaborate on indicators of success and measures of
   performance;
e) to bridge the gap between academic and field workers.

1st IUHPE European Conference on Health Promotion Effectiveness.
December 12–15, 1989. Rotterdam, The Netherlands.
The objectives of the Conferences were threefold:

a) to provide insight into factors which determine the success of health education;
b) to make these insights accessible to policy makers, researchers and health
   education practitioners;
c) to inspire:
   policy makers – to make these insights in future policies for their own
   country;
   researchers – to do more research that is relevant for the health education
   practice;
   practitioners – to use the insights into their daily work.

A Cross-Cutting Vision of the Regional Work

Regional teams all found it difficult to reply to a question on how they might compare and contrast their own work with that of other regions. This is primarily due to the fact that there was a nearly unanimous feeling that they did not have enough information about what the other regions besides their own were doing. This is an interesting point, given that the benefits and strengths of the programme which were previously identified included global networking, exchange, and sharing of ideas and information. However, where the GPHPE has not been able to best serve the overall communication needs for the programme itself, is in the day-to-day easy access to regional products, publications, and reports. Circulation of this information is intermittent, and usually in direct response to requests. Partly this is due to the volunteer nature of the work done in most of the regions; however, it has also been a lack of capacity of the global coordinating body to implement a system that could respond to this need, that of a virtual storage and workspace where the GPHPE members can stock all types of relevant information from their regional projects and easily access and download that which others have posted.

Thanks to efforts of Alexandra Ricca who worked as a full-time intern at the IUHPE Headquarters in the fall of 2006, the GPHPE on-line workstation has become an operational tool and resource. The online GPHPE WorkStation space and services were generously provided by the University of Kansas, due to the voluntary contributions of Steve Fawcett and Rachel Oliverus. It is now positioned and underway to serve as a useful platform for the GPHPE regional projects and wide range of partners and participants to share information and keep up to date with the other regional developments (Fawcett, Schultz et al., 2003). This resource is intended to connect all of the GPHPE's partners and members, and its strength as a tool will be highly dependent on the feedback we receive from members and partners and their suggestions of items to upload. The call for having such an on-line workstation came from the need to share knowledge, information, and expertise across the regions and to encourage inter-regional exchange. It is the desire of the GPHPE to continue to build upon the existing on-line workstation in order to provide a strong possibility for the provision and exchange of both technical and operational support, both to the regions and across the regions. Regional Project Leaders' and Coordinators' investments to ensure that their respective regional project's level has the most up to date and pertinent information will help to guarantee that all of the members in the GPHPE are able to have access to the most recent activities and achievements and provide a basis from which the projects can cross-fertilize one another. The GPHPE team will aim to make this resource as informative, interesting and interactive as possible.

In addition to comparisons between regions, there is the more important dimension of synergy. There have been a couple of isolated examples of some inter-regional synergy, such as a specific joint-meeting held in 2004, in Puerto Rico, with the GPHPE team, and colleagues from the Latin American and North

American Regional Project teams, where the teams discussed their own work-plans in details as well as spending time to decipher specific areas which presented obvious opportunities for collaboration. This meeting did result in a set of inter-regional action points and activities which highlighted the particular importance of capacity development for community research and action. The strong call for capacity building, with an emphasis on equity, which emerged from this meeting was accompanied by the recognition that associated resources that would make it easier for evidenced-based practices to be adopted and used effectively by global partners. Another example is the case of the Canadian team from the North American project, who has recently submitted a research proposal to work more closely with the African effectiveness project.

It is recommended that as the GPHPE moves into the future, the Global Steering Committee should reflect on how to provide a set of guidelines and formal encouragement concerning how the regions can bring in new partners, especially young researchers and maybe even community members to bridge the researcher/researched divide, to foster creativity and to mentor the next generation of health promotion researchers. The GPHPE members recognise that the workstation will help immensely in this regard. The GPHPE's Global Steering Group approved a study to take place on synergy and the effectiveness of collaboration using the GPHPE as an example (Corbin, 2006). A condensed version of this research is contained in Chapter 4 of this publication.

Strengths and Weaknesses to Having Adopted a Regional Approach

The final section attempts to draw some general conclusions about the benefits and disadvantages of working in a regional approach from the perspective of the global coordinating team's viewpoint. Although the lack of resources was cited as an obstacle for many, the fact of the matter is that resources in general imply control. Resources given for a specific task automatically bring obligation to complete that task and therefore often lock people into one way of thinking from the beginning – thus the way usually being imposed or at least strongly suggested by the source of funding. Therefore, working through a regional approach in a very collegiate manner does offer a certain level of autonomy, flexibility and liberty to pursue the regional activities as deemed most appropriate by the regions themselves.

The global team has noticed over the course of the development of the regional projects that often the regional leaders, coordinators or steering group members have a great deal of difficulty getting out of their "national box", that is that they tend to be highly influenced by their own countries' framework of thinking. This relates to the roles of reflexivity and introspection which are absolutely crucial in such an undertaking, and only then can one reach beyond to understand one's own country's language, culture and contextual influences on scientific thinking. National perspectives can and do drive the way evidence is seen, health promotion is developed, and the professional workforce is trained. The regional teams are in a tough position in this respect, as while each individual brings with them their own national professional culture, they are also responsible for formulating a regional perspective and speaking with a regional voice, which is not necessarily a straightforward task.

Conclusion

As the search for evidence is primarily based upon the desire to reduce uncertainty, can one say that the regional projects within the GPHPE has achieved more certainty? The GPHPE has been able to substantiate the fact that all of the regions do face a certain number of common issues, such as questions around methodologies, measurement, equity, and transferability and applicability of both processes and programmes. These are all common entities and overarching headings to which all refer, ponder and reflect upon, irrespective of their context, culture, language, or nationality. It is for this reason that the final section of this book is dedicated to the exploration and discussion around topics which the GPHPE considers global debates about the effectiveness of health promotion. Section 4 is a discussion section, where key issues and questions are approached in a developmental, yet critical, manner. Authors of chapters included in this section were faced with the question as to whether or not one could even assess effectiveness in their respective area. The content areas of the chapters in this section are recognised as core values of the field of health promotion, but the question remains as to whether or not evidence, effectiveness, outcomes, or impact have any role in nurturing, guiding or developing these areas. And if so, why and where?

One thing is for certain, the widespread commitment of the Regional Project teams and their dedication to pursuing these reflections in their own regions, countries, cities and universities has brought a remarkable amount of diversity and energy into the GPHPE. Without them the GPHPE would resemble more of an isolated body of global experts; but with the regions, the GPHPE has its hands on the pulse of health promotion and the evaluation of effectiveness across the globe at a number of organisational levels. It is this collective heart beat that keeps the GPHPE alive.

References

Corbin, JH (2006). Interactive Processes in Global Partnership: A case study of the Global Programme on Health Promotion Effectiveness. *IUHPE Research Report Series* I (1). Accessible on www.iuhpe.org.

Fawcett, SB, Schultz, JA et al. (2003). Using Internet-based tools to build capacity for community-based participatory research and other efforts to promote community health and development. In: M Minkler and N Wallerstein (eds) *Community-based Participatory Research for Health.* (pp. 155–178). San Francisco: Jossey-Bass.

Hills, M, O'Neill, M, Carroll, S & MacDonald, M (2004). Effectiveness of Community Initiatives to Promote Health: An Assessment Tool Report. Submitted to Health Canada on behalf of the Canadian Consortium for Health Promotion Research/Le consortium canadien de recherché en promotion de la santé.

Hills, M (2004). Health Canada Effectiveness Report – Phase I, Public Health Agency of Canada.

Hills, M (2005a). Health Canada Effectiveness Report – Phase II, Public Health Agency of Canada.

Hills, M (2005b). Assessing the Effectiveness of Community Initiative to Promote Health: Best Practices. Public Health Agency of Canada.

McQueen, DV (2003). Judging the success of the Global Programme on Health Promotion Effectiveness. *Promotion & Education* X (3): 118.

3
The IUHPE Blueprint for Direct and Sustained Dialogue in Partnership Initiatives

CATHERINE M. JONES AND MAURICE B. MITTELMARK

The International Union of Health Promotion and Education (IUHPE) depends heavily on dialogue to build bridges of mutual understanding and direction with its partners. The "IUHPE Blueprint" for dialogue is based upon the premise that we must provide well-structured opportunities for experts and decision-makers to come together to better comprehend and integrate each others' needs and priorities. The aim of this chapter is to provide an overview of dialogue methodology and to illustrate its usefulness in IUHPE knowledge-based advocacy, in particular in the realm of health promotion effectiveness. Particular attention is given to the IUHPE's use of dialogue methodology in the original European Effectiveness Project from which the Global Programme on Health Promotion Effectiveness (GPHPE) emanated (IUHPE, 2007).

Defining Dialogue: Fundamental Distinctions

Dialogue is a distinct communication technique, a specialized form of conversation that forges a path to collective intelligence. As defined by the Co-Intelligence Institute (2007), dialogue *is shared exploration towards greater understanding, connection or possibility.* Dialogue should not, and must not, be confused with debate, discussion or training; many forms of communication do not qualify as dialogue. Unfortunately, dialogue is most frequently misused and confused with debate, when in fact these two communication forms are indeed diametrically opposed (Table 3.1).

Victory is the driver of debate, the inherent purpose of debate being to convince the other side, to win them over to agree with one's argument and claims. Dialogue, on the other hand, seeks camaraderie through finding common ground. Through a merging of ideas, dialogue aims to create an atmosphere of understanding. Dialogue can be visualized as a solvent, a powerful agent capable of dissolving barriers and unwrapping new avenues for cross-fertilization of concepts and ideas through mutual, open exploration. In the words of Edgar Shein (1998), *"Dialogue makes it possible not only to create a climate for more interpersonal learning, but also may be the only way to resolve*

TABLE 3.1. Dialogue versus debate

Dialogue	Debate
Collaborative	Oppositional
Common ground	Winning
Enlarges perspectives	Affirms perspectives
Searches for agreement	Searches for differences
Causes introspection	Causes critique
Looks for strengths	Looks for weaknesses
Re-evaluates assumptions	Defends assumptions
Listening for meaning	Listening for countering
Remains open-ended	Implies a conclusion

Source: Adapted from the Co-Intelligence Institute

interpersonal conflict when such conflict derives from differing tacit assumptions and different semantic definitions."

Thus, dialogue has tremendous value for the field of health promotion, as a field of research and practice in which productive partnerships and collaborations are fundamental. The usefulness of dialogue techniques has been demonstrated in diverse fields, including education, negotiation and mediation, psychology, environmental and development studies, inter-faith and inter-cultural work, community development, social work, policy development and futures technology (Sliska, Karelova & Mitrofanova, 2003; Brown & Bennett, 1995; Schatz, Furman, & Jenkins, 2003; VanWynsberghe, Moore, Tansey, &Carmichael 2003; de Haas, Algera, van Tuijl & Meulman, 2000; Ratner, 2004; Steinberg & Bar-On, 2002; Innes & Booher, 2000). In health promotion, the dialogue method is particularly suited to the many situations where collaboration involves practitioners, organizations and community members. It generates common understanding that bridges the special points of view that all actors bring to a collaborative endeavour, enhancing the "balance between the knowledge and power of institutions and professionals, and the knowledge and power of communities" (Labonte, Feather & Hills, 1999).

Dialogue can take many forms, but here we take up just one of those forms, *collaborative policy dialogue*. Innes and Booher (2000) have outlined a theory, informed by their vision of the world as a complex system, to help understand how and why collaborative policy dialogues work in practice and how they differ from traditional policy making. In our increasingly globalizing world, power is ever more fragmented, and there is an increasingly rapid flow of information across the globe, made possible in a matter of seconds, which dominates our communication processes. Although we are evermore intertwined with our fellow citizens in this global community, we cannot count on shared objectives and values as a basis to conduct business. Therefore, we must start from scratch in order to better understand each other and what is going on in our societies. Collaborative thinking and dialogue methods are capable of producing qualitatively different solutions and alternatives to those produced by traditional methods of policy making.

The IUHPE Blueprint: Dialogue among Researchers, Practitioners and Policy and Decision-Makers

Although not referred to as such in the early days, the IUHPE has been implementing various forms of dialogue methodology since the renowned European Effectiveness Project,[*] which produced a set of documents that have become an essential staple on many health promoters' bookshelves. This project was built upon an innovative process created to use evidence to initiate dialogue as a stimulus to lead to further understanding, rather than the search for evidence as an end product in and of itself. The GPHPE received important impetus from IUHPE work in Europe in the mid- to late 1990's, in the project and resulting publications entitled *The Evidence of Health Promotion Effectiveness: Shaping Public Health in a New Europe*, managed on behalf of a broad-based partnership by the IUHPE (IUHPE, 1999). The project had two aims: summarize twenty years of evidence on health promotion's effectiveness, and communicate the information directly to policy-makers in Europe. The starting point of the project was the acknowledgement of the following points:

- Health promotion has developed a growing range of low-cost, highly effective technologies for improving public health, but has had limited success in influencing key decision-makers to modify health policies and funding accordingly;
- Health promotion researchers and practitioners have been using professional language and arguments to try to influence political processes; this is the wrong language, leading to unpersuasive arguments;
- The root of the problem is therefore communications failure, not lack of sufficient evidence.

Addressing this problem, the IUHPE developed a communications strategy with these elements:

- Provide opportunities for experts and decision makers to come together to bridge gaps of understanding of each group's needs and priorities through collaborative dialogue. Early in the project, health promotion experts and European experts on policy-making and policy processes were brought together to decide the dimensions and the strategy of the project. Not surprisingly, there was discord. The subject-area experts used academic jargon and arguments to make their points, and often concluded that "more research was needed!" The politically savvy participants highlighted the self-defeating nature of this approach. They urged that the project summarize not just health impacts, but also social, economic, and political impacts of effective health promotion – and remain focused on what works. The vital component to this was the engagement of a communication expert who was hired to assist in facilitating the dialogue and transforming the outcome into a particularly readable and convincing document. In fact, this mix

---

[*] The "Impact and Effectiveness of Health Promotion Project" was funded by the European Commission [Project Number SOC 97 202247 05F03 (97CVVF3-443)].

of political, health promotion and communications expertise to me was key in the success of the project.[*]

- Value the priorities of decision-makers as legitimate concerns throughout this process conducted by the experts, leading them to recognize that their input may need re-directing to be understood. Initial drafts of evidence prepared by the subject-area experts were dismantled by the policy experts in face-to-face debates, and the experts gave way, re-drafting the evidence summaries in ways that communicated with the intended audience.
- Reject rigid guidelines about what counts as evidence and what does not. It was agreed from the outset that medical models of evidence generation – clinical trials to test new therapies for example – are rarely if ever suitable to generate evidence in community settings such as schools and workplaces, or to test policy interventions. What was needed was triangulation, agreement from evidence collected by various methods leading to prudent decisions about what works under real life conditions.
- Produce usable summaries for decision-makers and in-depth analyses to back them up. This led to the development of two books of evidence. A core document of only 28 pages crystallized the evidence and made concrete recommendations for action by decision-makers. A detailed report of 164 pages backed the core document, providing information about what works in workplace and school health promotion, what infrastructure is needed to mount effective health promotion at national and regional levels, health promotion for the aging population, oral health promotion, and mental health promotion.
- Engage decision-makers in face-to-face dialogue about health promotion policy, using the published evidence reviews as the stimulus – not the end product. An exhibition booth was set up at the European Parliament in Strasbourg from January 17–20, 2000. The booth consisted of two parts, highlighting both the IUHPE and the European Commission's activities in the area of health promotion; however, the overall emphasis was placed on the effectiveness documents described above. On January 18, a cocktail reception was held at the booth with the goal of introducing members of Parliament (MEPs) to the potential that health promotion can bring to addressing health and well-being. The reception gathered 20 members of the project team and approximately 60 MEPs. The reception provided MEPs with the chance to discuss European health issues and concerns with health promotion professionals. The reception was followed by a dinner at the Parliament for the MEPs and health promotion specialists. Dining tables were arranged to mix MEPs and members of the Effectiveness Project, providing for lively exchange. Commissioner David Byrne opened the evening with introductory remarks. The IUHPE Vice-President for Scientific and

---

[*] As the Project's Editor and communication expert, David Boddy, a leading European health lobbyist, served as an instrumental part of the bridge-building process between the political and health promotion communities.

Technical Development, Maurice Mittelmark at the time, introduced the pertinence of health promotion, concluded his remarks as follows:

I'll end by posing a question that we do not yet have a clear answer to, but desperately need: why is this proven health promotion technology under-utilised in Europe? Is it because the word 'health' in health promotion automatically takes us down the wrong path, by making us think immediately of other health technology, such as hospitals, doctors and curative medicine? Is it because the word 'promotion' has connotations that distract one's attention from the solid basis on which the technology is built? Is it because people think of health 'police' when they hear health promotion, misunderstanding our technology and approach? Is it because evidence on health promotion effectiveness is not presently in the right way, to the right people, at the right time? Is it all of these, or none of these? We hope that your discussions before and during dinner have included a focus on this issue, and we look forward to a lively dialogue this evening.

This was followed by several hours of discussion. Both the exhibit and the dinner-dialogue were sponsored by MEP John Bowis, who also participated in the entire length of the project. Following the dinner, one participant stated:

. . .at my table, where we had two MEPs from Italy, we talked a lot about health issues. They had some knowledge, of course, but they seemed to appreciate the evening. . . . Probably an evening of this kind is more useful than a traditional meeting to which MEPs would hardly come if they were invited. The reception before the dinner also attracted MEPs who normally might not attend a meeting about health. So, "non-traditional" ways should be tried and used a lot more.

Thus, the IUHPE communications approach followed a plan leading to direct and sustained dialogue with key decision-makers, using the evidence of health promotion effectiveness as the foundation for discussion. The participants judged the strategy as a success, so much so that the same strategy has been used by the IUHPE since to structure communications about mapping national capacity for health promotion in Europe, and about public-private partnerships for better health care in Europe and in India. For example, the IUHPE's HP-Source.net[*] is a discovery tool where health promotion capacity is mapped through an ongoing voluntary dialogue amongst researchers, policy makers and practitioners who share the goal of maximizing the efficiency and effectiveness of health promotion policies, infrastructures and practice. In another example, in the IUHPE-managed Indo/European Union dialogue[†] on public/private partnerships for sustainable health care systems, dialogue stimulated a two-way learning process that led to substantial consensus despite vast differences in European and Indian contexts.

Most recently, the IUHPE has employed a refined method of dialogue to engage the international Project Advisory Group of a project (in collaboration with the Canadian Consortium on Health Promotion Research) to renew commitment to the

---

[*] http://www.hp-source.net/
[†] This project was funded by the European Commission (IND SPF/191002/965/96-447).

Ottawa Charter, through the development of recommendations on the policy and system conditions necessary for sustainable and effective health promotion.[*]

The Effectiveness of Dialogue

A United Nations (UN) survey of good practice in public-private sector dialogue for a UN Conference on trade and development provides evidence about the validity of dialogue as a research tool, and provides a set of principles and effective mechanisms for promoting dialogue (United Nations, 2001). The results show that dialogue methodology can influence policy makers' and researcher's mindsets, helping them move from an orientation focused on data extraction to a participative orientation. Products from this UN work include indicators for maturity of dialogue, a paradigm for the management of dialogue, and a taxonomy for assisting dialogue. However, instead of presenting these in detail, it is more constructive in light of this chapter's aim to consider why dialogue is effective rather than merely focus on the principles of effective dialogue.

Schatz and colleagues (2003) at the Department of Social Work at Colorado State have published an interesting analysis of the effectiveness of dialogue in social work interventions and involving multi-cultural learning. They conclude that dialogue is effective because it satifies people's need for human connection and belonging; it leaves no room for a passive participant; it is a synergistic experience; it promotes the values and uniqueness of each member; it develops trust and intimacy; it promotes both individual and group reflections on values and vulnerabilities; and it cultivates interpersonal relationships.

While there is not adequate space available here to provide details, a number of organizations have developed practical tools and guidelines which are valuable resources for the practice of dialogue.[†]

Concluding Remarks

The IUHPE is committed to further developing dialogue as a central methodology in its knowledge-based advocacy for health, through an in-depth and on-going review of the relevant literature, and then through applied research on the use of dialogue methods in future IUHPE projects. This brief treatment of dialogue

---

[*] This project has received funding from the Public Health Agency of Canada.
[†] Some of the most practical ones include the National Coalition for Dialogue and Deliberation (http://thataway.org/), PublicPrivateDialogue.org (http://www.publicprivatedialogue.org/), The Co-Intelligence Institute (http://www.co-intelligence.org/P-dialogue.html), Viewpoint Learning Inc. (http://www.viewpointlearning.com/), The World Café (http://theworldcafe.com/), and the United Nations University Framework for Action for a Dialogue of Civilizations (http://www.unu.edu/dialogue/FrameworkForAction.pdf).

methodology is presented with the intention to stimulate discussions in the health promotion community about how increased use of dialogue can help improve the effectiveness of advocacy and policy development activities. The IUHPE's positive experiences with dialogue methodology give weight to the idea that health promotion training programmes should consider adding it to the list of core competencies of graduates. The ethical use of dialogue methodology requires careful attention and skill, especially to curb any tendency to slip "back" into ways of thinking and working that resemble debate more than dialogue. We are optimistic that the proper use of dialogue in the health promotion policy development and advocacy arenas will serve to dissolve the barriers that separate some of the existing disciplinary ghettos. When more health promoters and advocates will have been formally trained to use dialogue methodology appropriately, the likelihood of its misuse will be diminished.

Acknowledgements. The authors would like to extend their sincere thanks to Anne Bunde-Birouste and Spencer Hagard for their support, encouragement and useful comments in the development of this chapter. Anne Bunde-Birouste, as the designer and coordinator of the original European project, has made substantial contributions to the creativity and enthusiasm which drove the original project to successful fruition in partnership with many experts from around the world. Her management and supervision of this original process was a source of inspiration to the development and launching of the GPHPE. Spencer Hagard has been a steadfast and persistent leader in this field, providing guidance and direction as a participant in many of the IUHPE collaborative projects which have been constructed upon dialogue in some shape or form.

References

Brown, Juanita and Bennett, Sherrin. 1995. Mindshift: Strategic Dialogue for Breakthrough Thinking. In: S. Chawla and J. Renesch (eds) *Learning Organisations: Developing Cultures for Tomorrow's Workplace* Portland, OR: Productivity Press.

The Co-Intelligence Institute. 2007. Dialogue.
http://www.co-intelligence.org/P-dialogue.html Accessed January 6, 2007.

de Haas, Marco; Algera, Jen A.; van Tuijl, Harrie F.J.M. and Meulman, Jacqueline J. 2000. Macro and Micro Goal Setting: In Search of Coherence. *Applied Psychology: An International Review* 49 (3): 579–595.

Innes, Judith E. and Booher, David E. 2000. Collaborative Dialogue as a Policy Making Strategy. Institute of Urban and Regional Development Working Paper Series. Berkley: University of California. Available at http://repositories.cdlib.org/iurd/wps/WP-2000–05.

IUHPE. 1999. *The Evidence of Health Promotion Effectiveness: Shaping Public Health in a New Europe.* A report for the European Commission by the International Union for Health Promotion and Education, ECSC-EC-EAEC, Brussels – Luxembourg. Paris: Jouve Composition & Impression.

IUHPE. Scientific Activities: GPHPE – Promoting Health Promotion Effectiveness, the IUHPE blueprint.
http://www.iuhpe.org/?lang5en&page5projects_project2 Accessed: January 6, 2007.

Labonte, Ronald; Feather, Joan and Hills, Marcia. 1999. A Story/Dialogue Method for Health Promotion Knowledge Development and Evaluation. *Health Education Research* 14 (1): 39–50.

Ratner, Blake D. 2004. "Sustainability" as a Dialogue of Values: Challenges to the Sociology of Development. *Sociological Inquiry* 74 (1): 50–69.

Schatz, Mona; Furman, Rich and Jenkins, Lowell E. 2003. Space to Grow: Using Dialogue Techniques for Multinational, Multicultural Learning. *International Social Work* 46 (4): 481–494.

Shein, Edgar. 1998. *Process Consultation Revisited: Building the Helping Relationship.* Part of the Addison-Wesley series on Organizational Development. Boston: Addison-Wesley.

Sliska, Lyubov; Karelova, Galina Nikolaevna and Mitrofanova, Eleonora. 2003. Dialogue among Civilisations. Report from the International Expert Symposium on "A Culture of Innovation and the Building of Knowledge Societies". United Nations Educational, Scientific and Cultural Organisation and the Institute of Strategic Innovations, Moscow: November 9–11, 2003.

Steinberg, Shoshana and Bar-On, Dan. 2002. An Analysis of the Group Process in Encounters between Jews and Palestinians using a Typology for Discourse Classification. *International Journal of Intercultural Relations* 26: 199–214.

United Nations. 2001. A Survey of Good Practice in Public-private Sector Dialogue. Release from the United Nations Conference on Trade and Development. UNCTAD/ITE/TEB/4. Geneva.

VanWynsberghe, Rob; Moore, Janet; Tansey, James and Carmichael, Jeff. 2003. Towards Community Engagement: Six Steps to Expert Learning for Future Scenario Development. Futures 35: 203–219.

4
The Global Programme on Health Promotion Effectiveness
A Case Study of Global Partnership Functioning

J. HOPE CORBIN AND MAURICE B. MITTELMARK

Introduction

Building the case for effectiveness in health promotion cannot end with creating evidence, but must extend to assembling and disseminating the evidence in ways that communicate convincingly with people in positions to make a difference. In health promotion, there has been lively debate about the best methodology for these activities.

Some feel the traditional academic approach is best, in which scholars examine findings from empirical studies and publish reviews in peer-reviewed academic journals. Critics point out that this approach has limits, both in the selection of evidence and in the audience reached. Effective health promotion that is unpublished, or published in languages other than English, is usually omitted. Further, the results presented in these reviews have mostly to do with health effects and fail to explore political, social or economic implications of the science. Perhaps most limiting, the dissemination of such reviews hardly ever reaches beyond the scholarly community. There is no dependable mechanism to bring academia to policy makers. However, some scientists are effective lobbyists, showing that better connection between science and policy can result when scientists break with their traditional ways of assembling and communicating knowledge.

Academics working in the disciplines that feed health promotion have been increasingly concerned with these issues. If inappropriate methods produce weak findings, making the case for effective health promotion is a hopeless cause. This situation has prompted the emergence of alternative frameworks for evaluating and communicating health promotion's effectiveness, of which the Global Programme for Health Promotion Effectiveness (GPHPE) is an exemplar. As the first global partnership for health promotion effectiveness, the GPHPE has lessons to offer regarding what makes such a partnership function well, and what inhibits good functioning. This chapter's purpose is to examine the GPHPE, summarizing key results from a 2006 study of its work processes and functioning (Corbin, 2006). In turning the light of inspection inwards, to examine the GPHPE's functioning, our aim is to suggest ways in which the GPHPE and large-scale partnerships in health promotion in general, can be organized and managed for optimal functioning.

Specifically, the study used a systems theory framework – inputs, through-puts and outputs – to examine the GPHPE as a new way of addressing the effectiveness issue (Wandersman, Goodman & Butterfoss, 1997). How does a partnership model work when the aim is to review evidence of effectiveness and disseminate the results to decision-makers? What do the partners bring to the work, and what do they get back? In what ways does partnership create synergy? What aspects of a partnership have the potential to impede its func-tioning? Exploration of these questions can provide a basis for improvements in the GPHPE itself, but may also suggest guidelines for partnership develop-ment and management for other types of health promotion partnerships. This is highly relevant, because the field of health promotion places great value on the partnership model of collaboration, yet little research is available about how health promotion partnerships function.

The Global Programme for Health Promotion Effectiveness

The GPHPE is a worldwide partnership looking at health promotion effectiveness around the globe. The multi-partner initiative is coordinated by the International Union for Health Promotion and Education (IUHPE) in collaboration with the World Health Organization (WHO) and partners from national agencies and organizations in Kenya, Switzerland, England, The Netherlands, Canada, the United States and India, among others (GPHPE, 2005).[*]

The main aim of the GPHPE is to "raise the standards of health promoting pol-icy making and practice world-wide by: reviewing and building evidence in terms of health, social, economic and political impact; translating evidence to policy makers, teachers, practitioners, researchers; and stimulating debate on the nature of effectiveness" (GPHPE, 2005).

History

The GPHPE grew out of a similar initiative in Europe. In 1999, the IUHPE pub-lished the culmination of an evidence-gathering project funded by the European Commission and the US Center for Disease Control, in a set of books called *The Evidence of Health Promotion Effectiveness*. This project gathered the expertise of the IUHPE professional network, politicians, and media and communications spe-cialists to review the evidence for health promotion effectiveness with a special focus on practical outcomes. As recommended by the partnering policy makers, the books examine not only the health impacts of health promotion but also the economic, social and political impacts as well. The balance of scholarly evidence and practical utility of the books has made them "the most sought after references in the field (GPHPE, 2002, p. 1)."

---

[*] The complete list of partners is available in the Annex of this volume.

The popularity of the books, and the appeal of the methodology that spawned them, spread quickly beyond Europe, and many experts suggested that similar efforts in other parts of the world were needed. The IUHPE decided that, not only was there a need to contribute more evidence to the knowledge base, but that the bias excluding evidence in languages other than English also needed to be addressed and rectified. The GPHPE was initiated to address these issues. The planning began shortly after the publication of the books in 1999 and the first Global Steering Group meeting was held in Amsterdam in 2001 (GPHPE, 2002).

Originally, the plan for the GPHPE was for partners in the IUHPE's regional divisions around the world to move forward in parallel using the European work as a blueprint for their work. Initial assessments illuminated significant variations in health promotion's research capacities and accomplishments, both between and within the regions. Therefore, the GPHPE decided collectively to encourage the regions to undertake the effectiveness review and dissemination work at a pace and in a manner suited to the particular conditions and contexts of each region (GPHPE, 2004b).

Structure

The work of the GPHPE is conducted in seven regions: Africa, Europe, Latin America, North American, Northwest Asia, Southeast Asia and the Southwest Pacific. Each of these regions has a regional leader or in some cases, co-leaders and some regions also have a regional coordinator. At the global level, there is a global leader and a global coordinator. The work of the GPHPE is overseen by the Global Steering Group (GSG). The GSG is comprised of representatives from each regional program, donor organizations, some technical advisors and the global leader and coordinator. The GSG is the main decision making body of the global partnership (GPHPE, 2004a). So, the GPHPE is actually a global partnership comprised of multiple regional partnerships. The present study did not delve into the functioning of regional partnerships but focused on global functioning.

Products

One of the first tasks undertaken by the GPHPE was translating the original European Effectiveness books from English into other languages, including as of this writing French, Spanish, Russian, Chinese, Mongolian, Japanese and Korean.

In 2004, a special supplemental issue of the IUHPE journal, *Promotion & Education*, was dedicated to a summary of the proceedings of a one-day symposium held in Paris on the international debate on the effectiveness of health promotion. The event was arranged to raise awareness and provide a forum for exchange on the highly debated concepts of evaluation, evidence, effectiveness and how they relate to policy. This special issue was then launched at another conference concerned with these topics, held in Quebec in October 2004 (GPHPE, 2004b).

Also in 2004, members of the GPHPE organized and arranged a track on effectiveness at the 18th World Conference on Health Promotion and Health Education held in Melbourne, Australia. At the conference, the GPHPE was presented in "its integral entirety." A symposium offered an overview of GPHPE activities, and a number of regional symposia were held as well (GPHPE, 2004b).

In 2005, another special issue of *Promotion & Education* was published on the theme of effectiveness in mental health promotion. The monograph in which this chapter appears is the latest GPHPE product, and together with the other products illustrates how the partnership has utilized IUHPE communication channels for the dissemination aspects of the project.

Funding

The GPHPE is an ongoing programme of the IUHPE. Rather than operating like a project with specific funding for specific products, it is a continuous effort supported largely by voluntary efforts of IUHPE members. At times, certain regions have received funding from GPHPE partners while others have never received such support. Thus, distribution of the few financial resources available is uneven.

Partnership Research in the GPHPE

Here, selected findings from the 2006 study of the GPHPE are summarized, and some implications for global partnership for health promotion are considered. The analysis used a systems theory framework, as mentioned above, and the results are summarized using the systems elements inputs, throughputs and outputs.

Partnership Inputs

Three types of inputs were identified from the data, including one type of input whose significance might have been overlooked in a casual analysis. Partner resources (peoples' time and effort) and financial resources were expectedly referred to in many ways by the study respondents. In addition, the raison d'etre of the GPHPE's establishment, to raise the standards of health promoting policymaking and practice, lent an air of urgency to the enterprise that motivated partners to join and that helped to attract financial support. The three inputs – partners, finance and the problem – interacted in positive ways. The problem stimulated motivation to join, the partners mobilized financial resources, and these in turn enabled the partners to conduct work (e.g., meetings, publications) that would otherwise not have happened.

Throughputs: Partnership Processes

The throughput portion of the partnership system refers to partnership processes. Throughput can be enhanced and reinforced by positive cycles of interaction, or can be impeded and diminished by negative cycles of interaction. Here, both types of cycles are illustrated using examples having to do with GPHPE leadership and communication practices.

Leadership

Cycles of positive interaction were enabled by skilled leadership, which in the GPHPE created a positive partnership context. Data from the study revealed that leadership:

- fostered positive interaction,
- inspired confidence,
- focused partners on the tasks at hand,
- promoted a climate of openness, trust, autonomy and patience,
- resolved conflict, and
- modelled pragmatism.

At the same time, the study of the GPHPE revealed that leaders need to be alert to, and prevent if they can, partnership problems that can arise despite the best of intentions. In a complex globe-spanning partnership, the potential for inevitable misunderstandings to blossom into diminished trust, conflict, and dominance problems should be anticipated. Lowered trust can inhibit the partnership's ability to function by acting as a dividing force, fostering suspicion among some partners and draining motivation to invest in the partnership. Left unchecked, negative cycles may result in some partners withdrawing, others coming to dominate, and others feeling unappreciated. Managing negative tendencies is a particular challenge in a global partnership because people are dispersed and face-to-face contact is rare, and also because cultural and language differences add to the communication challenge.

Communication

Positive processes for communication include purposeful, frequent, and recognisable information exchanges. In the GPHPE, no mechanism for communication was more positive than occasional face-to-face meetings. Face-to-face meetings allow for immediate, unfettered exchange that is conducive to the production of synergy. This immediate interaction also facilitates joint decision-making and goal-setting. Face-to-face meetings also allow new partners to integrate into the ongoing dynamic of the partnership and feel included. This lesson from the GPHPE has important implications in the era of the Internet, in which email and teleconferencing are looked to as cost saving communications technology. It seems that the successful use of distance communications depends on interpersonal ties forged by periodic direct contact, and operating budgets need to be planned with this in mind.

On the other side of the coin, poor communication can negatively impact partnership functioning by leaving people feeling overwhelmed, or left out and confused. Poor communication can exacerbate problems of accountability, and can reduce a partnership's capacity for exchange and synergy. If mechanisms for efficient and dependable communication are not firmly in place, partners' perceptions of the collaboration can deteriorate and a climate of discouragement can take hold. Good communication ensures maximum transparency, important because without transparency, trust suffers. With too little information, partners can become discouraged. With too much information, people may feel guilty about not being able to keep up. Inadequate communication may lead to missed opportunities for collaboration by not keeping the partnership in the forefront of people's minds and by not creating forums for sharing.

Output

Three types of partnership output were identified in the case data of the GPHPE. These outputs were additive outcomes, synergistic outcomes and antagonistic outcomes.

Additive outcomes are outcomes that have not been affected by the interaction of the partnership. The mathematical description of this relationship would be $2 + 2 = 4$. The inputs bypass the throughput portion of the partnership and therefore the output remains unchanged. The partners produce what they would have produced on their own. The absence of partnership interaction leaves the partnership also unchanged by these outcomes.

Synergy is the integration of inputs in interaction that produces outcomes that could not have been produced by those inputs in isolation. Mathematically this would be represented as $2 + 2 = 5$. Synergy is produced through the functioning of the partnership. Examples of synergy provided from the case data suggest that positive interaction enhances the partnership's ability to produce synergistic results. The data also suggest that the creation of synergy, or partnership success, feeds back in to the partnership positively effecting functioning and thus enhancing the ability of the partnership to attract more partner input and financial resources. Synergistic outcomes may also have the potential to affect the partnership problem although that was not observed in this case.

Antagonistic outcomes occur when the partnership interaction has an overly taxing effect. Antagonistic output is actually less than what the inputs would have produced without the partnership process. Mathematically, antagony would be expressed as $2 + 2 = 3$. That is, through the partnership process something was lost. For example, partnership processes that waste partner time or financial resources by definition produce antagony. In the worst case, $2 + 2 = 0$, the case of a partnership that dissolves before meeting its aims. The data of the present case suggest that antagonistic output often appears to be no output at all. This wasting time and money can negatively affect functioning by contributing to cycles of negative interaction and by leading to withdrawal of partner and financial resources.

Summary

Here, we return to the questions asked in the introduction. How does a partnership model work, when the aim is to review evidence of effectiveness and disseminate the results to decision-makers? What do the partners bring to the work, and what do they get back? In what ways does partnership create synergy? What aspects of a partnership have the potential to impede its functioning?

The first point to be made is that the full potential to study the GPHPE as a model of partnership for reviewing and disseminating evidence will be realized in the future. The GPHPE is an ongoing process, not a time-defined project, so lessons from its functioning will emerge continuously. However, there are already some indications that the GPHPE is a workable model for managing and disseminating evidence of health promotion effectiveness. Most importantly, the GPHPE has published evidence summaries that incorporate evidence from cultures and arenas that would have been overlooked by traditional review approaches.

The results show that the GPHPE functions well in many ways. There are many committed partners willing to devote their time to the programme. The problem uniting these people is sufficiently urgent that it is able to inspire and motivate participation and production. While the data point out some instances of poor communication, distrust and unresolved conflict, overwhelmingly, the overall impression reported by GPHPE participants is of strong leadership and good communication.

The greatest obstacle for working in partnership as identified in the results of the GPHPE case study is a lack of financial resources. The GPHPE relies almost entirely on its volunteer base. Unfortunately, it can be quite difficult to hold volunteers strictly accountable to meet obligations and deadlines. Financial resources actually provide two mechanisms that address this issue. Financial resources often come with external accountability measures that can help ensure that promises are kept, and kept on time. Financial resources can also help facilitate travel for face-to-face meetings. As described earlier, this type of communication greatly improves relationships and exchange, thus increasing the likelihood of producing synergy.

The ultimate test of the partnership model for managing and disseminating evidence of health promotion's effectiveness, as represented by the GPHPE, will be its impact on policy-makers. That assessment is a task for the future, but the interim analysis summarized in this chapter shows that the GPHPE is functioning largely as planned, it is producing evidence reviews that include a widened range of evidence, and it is of sustained importance to its partners. It seems, therefore, that the conditions are in place needed to make the GPHPE a fair test of a new way of working in the evidence and effectiveness arena.

References

Corbin, J.H. (2006). Interactive Processes in Global Partnership: A Case Study of the Global Programme for Health Promotion Effectiveness. *IUHPE Research Report Series*. 1 (1), 1–70.

GPHPE. (2002). Brief Presentation of the Global Programme on Health Promotion Effectiveness: Global Programme on Health Promotion Effectiveness.

GPHPE. (2004a). Brief Presentation of the Global Programme on Health Promotion Effectiveness: Global Programme on Health Promotion Effectiveness.

GPHPE. (2004b). The Global Programme on Health Promotion Effectiveness. *Promotion and Education*, XI (3), 167–168.

GPHPE. (2005). The Global Programme on Health Promotion Effectiveness Leaflet (pp. 167–168): Global Programme on Health Promotion Effectiveness.

Wandersman, A., Goodman, R.M. & Butterfoss, F. (1997). Understanding Coalitions and How They Operate: An "Open Systems" Organizational Framework. In: M. Minkler (ed), *Community Organizing and Community Building for Health* (pp. 261–277). New Brunswick, N.J.: Rutgers University Press.

Section 2
Reports from the Field

5
Policies for Health
The Effectiveness of their Development, Adoption, and Implementation

Evelyne de Leeuw

Framing the Effectiveness of Policy for Health

There is a strong belief, and in many cases a strong evidence-base, that policy impacts on our collective shaping of individual, population and global parameters of life, in terms of operations of humanity, and of the natural world of which we are such an intricate and fragile part. Unfortunately, the same could be said of the absence of policy: a failure of governments to address, for instance, global climate change may have severe health, eco-systemic and social impacts.

In looking at the effects of policy on health we therefore have to specify what we are seeking to examine, and how we will assess impact. As policies have such a profound and sweeping impact, our assessment of the effectiveness of policies for health should therefore reach beyond efforts in health sectors. Yet, at other conceptual levels we will have to limit our analysis.

A first proxy is that we will be including deliberate policy action, with the added condition that deliberate inaction, in spite of its sometimes overwhelming impact on health, is not within the remit of this chapter. Secondly, we will have to look at policy that has been implemented. This statement merits some reflection on the conceptual nature of "policy". There are two extremes on a conceptual continuum: at the one end, there are those who believe a policy to be a rule or principle that guides decision-making. In many cases, such rules or principles might remain implicit. At the other extreme, policy has been defined as the explicit (and thus documented) formal decision by an executive agency to solve a certain problem through the deployment of specific resources, and the establishment of specific sets of goals and objectives to be met within a specific time frame. Legislation (with associated sanctions and incentives) could be regarded as ultimate policy statements. In this chapter we wish to look at deliberate decisions to solve (health) problems, and thus exclude "policy" that could be characterized as implicit general rules of principles for further decision-making. It is for this reason that we are interested not just in the decisions per se, but precisely in active implementation.

A third element that we will have to include is therefore a review of the implementation tools. Policy as an ambition needs to be translated into an operational

Box 5.1. HIV/AIDS prevention and the optimal intervention mix

Many studies have identified bars and discotheques as venues for high risk behaviour leading to infections with STDs, including HIV/AIDS. In many instances, health promotion agencies have endeavored to *communicate* these risks to the clientele, and advise options to limit them. One of these options would be to practice safe sex. This would involve the use of reliable condoms.

Access to such condoms could be *facilitated* by the installation of vending machines (or, as is common practice in some gay entertainment venues, free hand-outs).

Some local governments, after considering the impact of the communication-facilitation mix, have decided to *regulate* the compulsory presence and operation of these vending machines.

form if it is to be executed. These operational forms are known in the practice and academia of health promotion as "interventions". In the political sciences they are known as "policy instruments". Described by some as carrots, sticks and sermons, a more functional classification would distinguish between communicative, regulatory, and facilitative interventions/instruments. It is generally recognized that some optimal magical mix between the three would yield the highest policy effects. Thus, in this review we will also attempt to identify the types of health interventions/policy instruments that have been developed to implement policy.

It may be worthwhile to reiterate the fact that, in our view, "policy" is not simply equivalent to "intervention". Policies are higher order arrangements that, in our view, frame, order and define sets of interventions.

In terms of these arrangements, three policy types can be distinguished. Redistributive policies are policies that impose costs or provide incentives to encourage the adoption of certain types of individual and systems behaviors. These costs or incentives generally come in the form of taxations or subsidies. Regulatory policies impose restrictions or inducements on defined individual and systems behaviors. They specify sanctions, for instance fines. "Allocational" policies finally fund activities and strategies with the intent to produce longer-term health benefits for the population. The more specific the policy relates to behavioural outcomes, the easier it is to evaluate its effects. Redistributive and regulatory policies are thus easier to evaluate than allocational ones.

A policy can only be effective if its constituent parts are. Policies would be more effective if these constituent parts are developed, planned and implemented, preferably synergistically, from a solid evidence-, community and theoretical base. This is the core of the argument that follows, and we will return to this in the conclusion.

What is Health Policy?

Since Nancy Milio's landmark publication, *Promoting Health Through Public Policy* (1986), and the inclusion of its critical conceptualization of Healthy Public Policy in the Ottawa Charter and subsequent global conference statements on the role of policy in health promotion, policy development has become a legitimate concern of the health promotion community.

There is, however, considerable conceptual confusion around the various combinations of "health", "policy" and "public". If we are to review the evidence of effectiveness of policies on health, we need to develop an appropriate typology.

Policies can be developed by virtually any organized group in society with a substantial constituency. Public and private agencies have the legitimacy to formulate decisions to solve existing, emerging, or potential problems. *Health policy* is thus a generic term for any policy, public, private, or elsewhere (NGOs, QUANGOs – quasiautonomous non-governmental organizations), explicitly addressing health and/or quality of life issues.

Relating specifically to the level and type of governance, one can distinguish between public and corporate policies. Within the public policy domain, there should be an effort to develop *Healthy Public Policy*. Healthy public policy might these days be labeled a "whole of government approach to health", "joined-up government" or "Health in All Policies": some policy issues merit the attention of a range of government sectors. The Health Promotion Glossary (Nutbeam, 1998) states that *healthy public policy is characterized by an explicit concern for health and equity in all areas of policy, and by an accountability for health impact.*

Some of these issues frequently mentioned in the literature include "early-life interventions" (maternal and child health sector, education, social work, economic interventions, gender-specific policies, etc.) and indigenous quality of life issues (policy domains such as justice, social work, provision of essential health and social services, and possibly specific policy domains such as agriculture and fisheries, cultural affairs and education, etc.). Milio's recent glossary of policy terminology in the health field (2001) is further helpful in understanding the dynamics involved.

How does Policy Impact on Health?

Lasswell (1936) has defined policy succinctly as deciding who gets what, where and how. Apart from further philosophical academic reflections on the nature of (public) policy this definition demonstrates how policy impacts on health: with an increased understanding of the importance of social determinants of health it is obvious that policy regulates choices in every domain pertaining to such social determinants, be it housing, social assistance, environmental protection, employment and economic issues, agriculture or science and technology policy.

It is Milio's assertion that it would be governments' moral obligation to develop and sustain policies that are healthful or at least not detrimental to health. Ideally, the development and sustenance of such policies would be a

Box 5.2. Policy types – examples of innovation

public policy for health – a local government stimulating safe cycling by designing and building bicycle routes for work and leisure purposes.

corporate policy for health – a business regulating and facilitating the availability of healthy food choices in its canteen.

health policy – a partnership between government, business and NGO (Cancer Council) communicating, regulating and facilitating accessibility and affordability of sun protection measures – the Australian SunSmart programme.

healthy public policy – a government programme regulating, communicating and facilitating the primary production, processing and delivery of healthy food and nutrition across ministries of agriculture, economic affairs, taxation, health and social affairs – the Norwegian farm-food-nutrition policy.

public health policy – a government programme for mandatory vaccination packages.

health care policy – a government programme facilitating the establishment of 'transmural nursing', taking care of continuity of care between hospital and primary care settings.

purposeful endeavour at all levels of government. In some countries (such as Sweden and Finland) this focused development has a high policy priority. In others (such as The Netherlands and Australia) the national government requires local authorities to develop healthy public policy. This happens with varying degrees of success (Hoeijmakers, 2005).

When is Policy Effective?

This leads us to consider the question when policy is effective. Naively, one might assume that the mere adoption of a policy by its constituency is an indication of its effectiveness: it would establish the intent to solve an identified problem, and would thus suggest that appropriate interventions are in place to be implemented.

Although the formal adoption of policy is often a major accomplishment involving years of negotiation with stakeholders and the generation of knowledge suggesting appropriate policy directions (cf., for instance, the WHO Framework Convention for Tobacco Control, 2006) it does not solve the problem per se. On the contrary, there are policies that have no intent of solving a problem; they are merely generated for their symbolic value. For instance, in March, 2005, the European Union embarked, according to its own press releases, on an ambitious programme to combat smoking in its 25 member states. With a budget of 72,000,000 euros over a three-year period the campaign aims to reduce smoking among young adults through television campaigns, road shows, and advertorials (HELP, 2006).

There is very little evidence that this type of intervention effectively reduces smoking prevalence. Yet, it is apparently important to the EU (and thus its member states) to develop such a policy – it purports to show that the Union takes the smoking epidemic seriously. This would be in line with a decision to phase out agricultural subsidy programs for tobacco growing in 2001. Such subsidies continue to total nearly 1,000,000,000 euros annually. This policy seems to be symbolic rather than anything else: the subsidies continue, and a fraction of the amount is symbolically spent on tobacco control.

In our view, a policy can only be regarded effective if the problem it has defined has been reduced significantly, and if that reduction can be attributed unequivocally to changes that the policy has brought about. Policies that focus on relatively simple, discrete issues, would thus have a higher potential to be defined effective than policies that address complex issues involving intricate chains of proximal and distal determinants of health, such as for instance policies to reduce health inequities. A further complication for determining the effectiveness of such policy types are secular social trends and biases. For instance, governments that adopt policies to reduce inequities in health are likely to be the same governments that developed policies on social and environmental justice, equitable work conditions, et cetera.

A Meta-Review of Healthy Public Policies and Health Policies

Any policy, thus, has a potential impact on health. Milio (1986) has already adequately reviewed the extent to which this is the case. We would be interested, in this chapter, to review what health effects purpose-built policies have. To find out, we have reviewed a review.

The government of the United Kingdom has, over the last decade, endeavored to develop a wider health agenda (taking into account insights on social determinants of health) drawing on "hard" evidence of effectiveness. Focusing on the main scourges of public health, a White Paper proposed policy action on cancer, coronary heart disease and stroke, accidents, and mental health. A review of the effectiveness of the proposed policies and associated interventions was carried out by the National Health Service Centre for Reviews and Dissemination (Contributors, 2000). Materials were provided and analyzed by the Cochrane and Campbell Collaborations.

For the majority of the proposed policies evidence of effectiveness could be demonstrated, for the health sector predominantly on policies impacting on disease, and for non-health sectors on proximal and distal determinants of health. Surprisingly, though, there is a substantial number of policy options that does not seem to be effective. Also, some policy options impact neither on disease nor determinants, but seem to have synergy with other policy alternatives. A final 36 policy options could not be classified: they appeared to have some hypothesized, but no demonstrated effect.

It must further be observed that virtually all "policies" reviewed in fact are interventions; the health sector interventions impacting on disease parameters are all clinical interventions. Very few of the "policies" are such in the sense that policy and political science, politicians or decision-makers would define them.

This conceptual opacity limits not only our analysis of evidence of effectiveness, but is more importantly problematic in the discourse that would lead to the establishment of true policies for health: if (health) practitioners continue to believe that "policy" can be equalled with "intervention", then their effective input into the policy development process is limited.

In considering policy options, politicians and other decision-makers operate on the basis of sets of assumptions and implicit values. They generally generate, often implicit, policy ontologies, sometimes called "causal field models" (Milewa & de Leeuw, 1996). These map causal (cause-effect), final (intervention-outcome) and normative considerations, e.g. "Poverty causes ill health", "Income support reduces poverty", and "In our country we do not subsidize individuals". Whether these considerations are valid, just or equitable is no issue in policy development, unless governed by normative frameworks.

One type of causal relations often found in policy considerations can be called the hypothetical effect, or "hypo-effect". For instance: covering a perimeter around high-rise apartment buildings with heavy padding would minimise casualties in case of fire. Obviously there may be truth in such effectiveness arguments, but they do not take into account whether a real problem is tackled, and whether the intervention meets efficiency criteria.

Finally, in choosing between intervention options considerations of effectiveness or efficiency (greatest gain at least cost) are not dominant. Before anything else, the "least coercion rule" is applied (Van der Doelen, 1998): always choose the intervention first which is least intrusive/coercive into peoples' lives. This rule explains why governments generally prefer the communicative intervention (even when not supported by evidence of effectiveness) over other types.

Our analysis is moreover clouded by a phenomenon already identified by the Swedish government in the 1980s (Figure 5.1). It is very rare that there is a unique relation between one determinant and one disease (group): for instance, the physical work environment impacts on five out of six disease categories, whereas respiratory diseases are affected by seven out of ten determinant categories. This means that policy on diet and nutrition would affect much more than, say, nutrient deficiency syndromes alone. Referring to Table 5.1, there were policy types and associated interventions that had evidence of effectiveness related to one type of health issue, whereas the same package did not impact on another type of health issue, although it was theorized that it should. More often than not this difference could be attributed to an absence of effectiveness studies rather than the pure absence of evidence of effectiveness.

The UK review has one final drawback which has been highlighted most astutely by a US Institute of Medicine (IOM) review of the contributions of the social and behavioural sciences to the promotion of health (Smedley & Syme, 2000). This work identified that a multitude of intervention types at different levels of interaction (individual, group, community, system) for any segment of the population (gender, age, ethnicity, ability status, etc.) would yield synergistic effects far beyond the development and implementation of singular and isolated

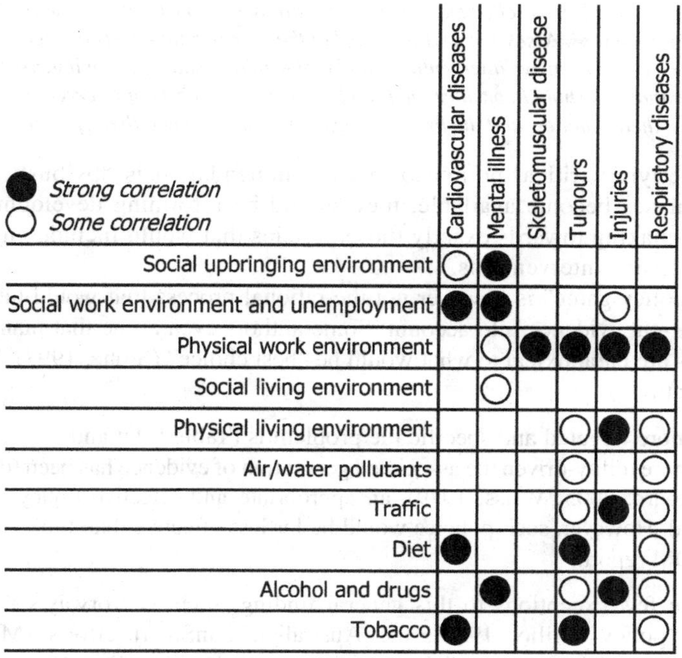

● *Strong correlation*
○ *Some correlation*

	Cardiovascular diseases	Mental illness	Skeletomuscular disease	Tumours	Injuries	Respiratory diseases
Social upbringing environment	○	●				
Social work environment and unemployment	●	●			○	
Physical work environment		○	●	●	●	●
Social living environment		○				
Physical living environment				○	●	○
Air/water pollutants				○		○
Traffic				○	●	○
Diet	●			●		○
Alcohol and drugs		●		○	●	○
Tobacco	●			●		○

FIGURE 5.1. Correlates between determinants and health states (HS90, 1984).

interventions, be they communicative, facilitative, or regulatory. At this stage in our argument this should come as no surprise, as such a finding is consistent with the complexity of the field. It is worth noting one of many recommendations the IOM report makes:

TABLE 5.1. Analysis of proposed policies' evidence of effectiveness (Contributors, 2000)

Impact of policy divided into evidenced impact direct on disease; on proximal/distal determinants of specific etiology; or as a synergy or prerequisite factor for other effective policy, and further into whether the policy could legitimately be considered as a planning and implementation remit of the health sector, or of other sectors. 36 policies are *hypo-effective* (cf. below).

	Evidence of effectiveness	No evidence of effectiveness	Evidence of synergy or support
Health			
On disease parameters	25	20	5
On determinants parameters	15	3	2
Non-Health			
On disease parameters	16	27	3
On determinants parameters	49	11	18

Recommendation 17: Cost-effectiveness analyses are necessary to assess the public health utility of interventions. Assessments are needed of the incremental effects of each component of multilevel, comprehensive interventions, and of the incremental effect of interventions over time. Such analyses should consider the broad influence and costs of interventions to target individuals, their families, and the broader social systems in which they operate.

The underlying critical notion to this recommendation is obviously that, as such analyses become available, they should be informing development and decision-making towards exactly those policies that would include multilevel, comprehensive interventions.

The "policy game" is however not the rational process that would take available clear-cut evidence into account. Some authors even argue that many policy decisions are paradoxical to what would be "best choice" (Stone, 1997). We have found that:

(a) the more targeted and specific the problem is (Table 5.1); and
(b) the more utility-driven the associated generation of evidence has been (de Leeuw & Skovgaard, 2005; Weiss, 1979), an appropriate and effective policy might be developed. However, such policies would be far less effective than those suggested by the IOM report.

There are few exceptions to this general finding, such as Norway's farm-food nutrition policy (Milio, 1981), the Australian SunSmart efforts (Montague, Borland & Sinclair, 2001), and the Swedish overall health policy (Hogstedt et al., 2004), all of which are comprehensive healthy public policy packages dealing with highly complex issues. As such, these are three examples of effective healthy public policies at the national level, albeit with very different perspectives, lead stakeholders, and to some extent different political ideologies. The success of these policies can be attributed to three factors:

- the strong resource-base on which the policy could draw;
- the long-range policy negotiation tradition, or the persistent policy push exerted by a committed agency, that enabled involvement of a broad domain of stakeholders; and
- strong political commitment to the preferred outcomes of the policy package.

There is also documented evidence of the factors that play a role in failures to develop national healthy public policy (de Leeuw, 1989b):

- competing policy agendas (where agendas with profound economic aspects will win);
- the drivers of policy (Kingdon (2003) calls them "policy entrepreneurs", but Skok (1995) found that others theorists have described similar roles under different names: "social entrepreneur," "issue initiator", "policy broker", "strategist", "fixer", "broker" or "caretaker") are found to be associated with one unique agency rather than the full policy domain;
- critical actors maintain a position of "benevolent inaction" which is misinterpreted as support for the suggested policy.

At the local level, the international Healthy Cities movement claims policy successes, though (de Leeuw, 2001; de Leeuw & Skovgaard, 2005; Awofeso, 2003). The integration of different policy domains (health and Local Agenda 21 initiatives, for example), the involvement of a range of "new" actors (NGOs, industry), the active engagement of communities, and a persistent focus on health inequities and social determinants are accomplishments that are rarely mirrored in other health policies. But again, there are very few demonstrations of the health impacts of (healthy public) policies developed in Healthy City contexts. An exception is a study from Curitiba that found that such policies are significantly more effective in the prevention of dental trauma (Moysés et al., 2006). Again, some "magical" mix of interventions is more effective and more synergistic than a series of disconnected singular interventions. An explicit comprehensive policy theory (that is, the set of assumptions underlying the policy ontology) would be helpful in structuring these different interventions into a policy package. In an evaluation of ten Healthy Cities in the European Union de Leeuw, Abbema & Commers (1998) found that there is strong commitment among city administrations to develop such broad policies, but Goumans & Springett (1997) do not necessarily view the "Healthy City" label as the crucial factor for such a position.

Multiple Case Studies: Examples from Canada[*]

In this section, we draw upon the experience of evaluating many of Canada's major public health initiatives over the past 20 years. In so doing, we fully recognize the limitations of such an approach – that lessons learned from the Canadian experience may not apply similarly elsewhere.

Compressed Time Frames

In Canada, a majority government has a maximum life-span of 5 years before standing for re-election. In the case of minority government, the period may be much shorter. As such, many of the major public health strategies have been introduced with a five year time frame. This leads to a succession of health strategies – some of which are renewed after the initial period – others, not. Among others, these have included the following:

• Canada's Health Promotion Strategy;
• Canada's Tobacco Strategy (Various versions);
• The Canadian Strategy to Reduce Impaired Driving;
• The Canadian Alcohol and Other Drugs Strategy;
• The Canadian Heart Health Strategy;

---

[*] This section provided by Reg Warren, Reg Warren Consulting Inc., Ottawa, Canada.

- The Canadian Breast Cancer Initiative;
- The Canadian Strategy on HIV/AIDS;
- The Canadian Diabetes Strategy.

Generally the first year of the Strategy involves the national government in preparing the infrastructure to implement the Strategy. By year two, key activities are being developed and community groups and intermediaries are being funded to deliver programs to the population. By year three, implementation has begun. In year four, full implementation is in progress; by the end of year four, most activity is devoted to project finalization (evaluation; renewal of funding proposals; looking for other employment; sources of funding).

Ultimately, in order to ensure continued funding, the Strategy is required to demonstrate reductions in morbidity and mortality accruing from this large investment of public funds (the objective of each of these strategies is to accomplish this – otherwise it likely would not receive funding).

Of course, in most cases this is impossible to demonstrate, and simply will not occur, given 1–2 years of full implementation. In fact, in many instances reported morbidity and mortality actually increase during the funding period – given increased public and institutional awareness; and improved detection and reporting systems.

The Impossibility/Implausibility of Control Groups

Simply stated, it is impossible (as well as politically, ethically and morally unfeasible) to exclude societal groups from the benefit of a health promoting public policy. Thus, threats to internal and external validity are virtually impossible to rule out – no matter the research design used, and requires the investigator to rely upon triangulation of multiple (frequently competing) sources of evidence. This is especially problematic, given that most major public health strategies tend to be information-driven. There is simply no way in the information age to exclude even non-participating sub-jurisdictions or the citizenry itself from the benefits of access to information. In fact, in a great many evaluations, populations effected by the policy have shown improvements – but so too have others – leading to highly equivocal conclusions regarding effectiveness.

Diffusion of Implementation

In large industrialized countries, like Canada, it is rare that national governments deliver public health programs directly to the citizenry. Generally, an "empowerment-of-intermediaries" approach tends to be adopted, with national governments supporting those civil societies, NGOs, other levels of government and other groups who are better positioned to deliver programs to the citizenry.

While this is an excellent delivery model, the difficulty – from an evaluation point of view – is that these intermediaries (particularly, other levels of government) tend to be extremely reluctant to have their activities evaluated by the federal government. And, this is entirely understandable given that they have their own constituencies and accountabilities – which may not always completely accord with those of the federal government.

Unfortunately, this renders the attribution issue functionally impossible to address – since the evaluation frequently ends with examining the role of the federal government in the empowerment of intermediaries.

Multiple Actors

There are a great many groups in Canada, including various levels of government involved in promoting public health. In fact, an examination of a recent federal public health strategy noted that the amount of money invested represented less that a 5% increase in the amounts of funding already devoted to the issue.

Policy = Politique = Politik

Whereas in English there is a clear semiotic distinction between "policy" and "politics", the French word for policy translates into politics. The same is true in German. And this is perhaps is the greatest barrier to the evaluation of national policies for health.

In Canada, most of the evaluations of major public health policy initiatives are funded and controlled by the federal bureaucrats in charge of those programs – compromising the independence of the evaluation exercise. And, indeed as far as we are aware, the plans tend to suggest increased controls on this information in the future.

Any results that could potentially be perceived as "negative" have the potential to compromise the Minister (policy) or the Department (implementation).

As such, insofar as we are aware, the vast majority of evaluations of national public health policies carried out over the past 20 years have neither been published, nor made available to the public or to partners/stakeholders – other than through rarely used "Access-to-Information" requests. This not only deprives the broader community from learning the lessons of major policy initiatives, but also to a lesser degree, calls into questions the credibility of the information that is made available though the many dissemination mechanisms available.

The Success of Healthy Public Policy

Whether or not the public sector is able to develop and implement healthy public policy depends on a range of factors. Some of these factors relate to the very substance of the policy, others on the context in which policy is developed (de Leeuw, 1989a, b). We have assessed these factors as follows:

TABLE 5.2. Overview of design complexities and parameters, including feasibility and effectiveness considerations (and their measurement aspects) of policy types

| Policy type | Indicator | | | |
	Synergy with other policy types	Population health impact assessment	Feasibility to implement at national and local levels	Complexity of policy design
Specific policy elements and isolated communicative, facilitative or communicative policy interventions	low	specific and relatively easy to assess	Nat: easy Loc: easy	relatively simple
Health Care Policy	low	specific, and believed to be assessed easily through, e.g., RCTs	Nat: moderate Loc: easy	relatively simple but much depends on ❶ degree of professional autonomy of stakeholders; and ❷ public/private financing mix
Public Health Policy	medium	Proper assessment should be multi-level, long-term, and multi-method: hard to assess	Nat: hard Loc: contextual (depends on national parameters and local culture)	complex, as it depends on the alignment of a range of public sector stakeholders
Healthy Public Policy	high	Potentially very high, but difficult to frame as few such policies are being developed purposefully	Nat: very hard Loc: contextual (depends on national parameters and local culture)	very complex, as it includes the range of stakeholders from Public Health Policy plus NGOs, community representation, etc.
Health Policy	very high	Potentially very high, but final attributions between cause and effect are hard to establish	Nat: extremely hard Loc: contextual (depends on national parameters, local culture, and corporate commitment)	extremely complex to establish one coherent health policy package as the range of stakeholders is at its extreme

Theory to the Rescue

In the above we have seen that a considerable number of policy options can be considered effective in the promotion of health. We have also seen, though, that a larger number of policy options claims unsubstantiated effectiveness. More, and new types of, research is required to demonstrate the effects of such policies. We have also seen that a range of intervention types is effective, whereas others are not, and that a mix of interventions addressing a variety of determinants of health will be more effective than the simple sum of isolated interventions. More studies are required to shed light on the developmental logic and evaluation of such intervention mixes. It is worth noting that most of the communicative and facilitative intervention types are subject to effectiveness inquiries and Cochrane and Campbell Collaboration reviews, and that the findings of such reviews in an ideal world should inform policy making. There is a lack of effectiveness studies on regulatory interventions for health. Most of these interventions, plus a substantial number of other intervention types and most policy packages, can be typified as hypo-effective. Finally, we have seen that the development of policy is not a rational process that draws on scientific insight alone.

To explain the realities of policy-making, and in order to interpret the findings of Table 5.2, it is helpful to apply current theoretical insights into the "policy game". Rather than viewing policy development as a relatively simple democratic process, these insights maintain that policy development takes place in highly complex and fluctuating policy domains (Kingdon, 1995). The range of stakeholders and interests involved in these domains depends on the framing of the policy issue (Stone, 1997). This framing is constantly adapted by both stakeholders as well as policy and social entrepreneurs, thus incessantly moving ownership of the policy issue between stakeholders (Gusfield, 1981). The final outcome of this networking process has so far been hard to predict. However, dynamic network modeling provides new insights into the purposeful manipulation of the domain and its components (Hoeijmakers, 2005).

There is another theoretical realm that closely relates to our question: the art and science of policy implementation. Not all policies seem to be implemented effectively. This failure might generally not be attributed to the policy itself, but rather to characteristics of the policy *environment:* one might have, for instance, formulated a policy in the area of counselling, but if no properly trained personnel would be available, or resources to develop counselling capacity, the policy is bound to fail. Regrettably, sometimes policy are designed to be ineffective. Weiss (1979) identifies six ways in which "knowledge" (or "evidence") is utilized for political purposes, one of which is to stall effective action. Combining these insights with, for instance, Mazmanian & Sabatier's (1989) policy implementation theory, it is clear that there is no "ideal world" where all available evidence can be translated into effective policy frameworks.

In the perspective of Mazmanian & Sabatier there are factors conducive to effective implementation of policy that fall within the remit of the implementing agency, factors in the socio-economic environment, and issues directly related to the nature of the problem the policy intends to resolve. This approach has been

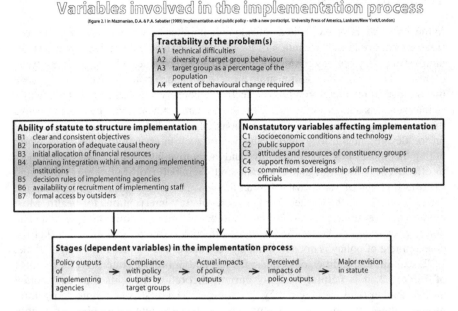

FIGURE 5.2. Variables involved in the implementation process (Source: Figure 2.1 in Mazmanian, D.A. & P.A. Sabatier (1989) Implementation and public policy – with a new postscript. University Press of America, Lanham/New York/London).

criticized as too top-down, focusing only at actions that can be taken by policy and decision makers (e.g., Hill & Hupe, 2002) whereas a more whole-of-systems approach would engage communities, their representatives, and practitioners in making implementation work (e.g. Lipsky's (1980) street-level bureaucracy as a critical force in effecting policy change). Much can be gained by the health promotion community in developing a more profound understanding of such implementation issues, as signalled for instance by Bartholomew et al. (2006).

Making Policies for Health more Effective

There are lessons to be learnt from the findings and propositions formulated above. If health policy issues are extremely clear-cut, mono-causal and impacting on very specific segments of the population (which should preferably be part of mainstream political consideration) effective policy programs can easily be developed, even more so at the local than at higher levels of government. However, most if not all public health problems do not fit this description. They are multi-dimensional (spatially, temporally, and cognitively) and generally "messy" or "wicked" problems (Mitroff & Mason, 1980). The populations that matter in health promotion (policy) are generally on the periphery of the decision-making radar scope and getting their health issues on the policy agenda is not easy. However, theoretical reflections on the policy process provide insights how this might very well happen.

One approach recognizes the importance of engaging "non-traditional" actors in the policy debate. Beyond the often mere symbolic acknowledgment of community interests, this engagement would include sectors such as social work, education and agencies involved in (fiscal and physical) infrastructures. These would, often surprisingly to the health promotion community, offer problem analyses similar to the health realm, but can present other problem-solving patterns and policy entry points than commonly used in health promotion.

In sum, some of the core qualities of the Ottawa Charter (enable, mediate, advocate) equip the health promotion community more than anything else to effectively engage in the policy-making enterprise and contribute further to its effectiveness.

References

Awofeso, N. (2003) The Healthy Cities approach – reflections on a framework for improving global health. *Bulletin of the World Health Organization*, 81(3), 222–223.

Bartholomew, K., G.S. Parcel, G. Kok & N.H. Gottlieb (2006) Planning Health Promotion Programs: Intervention Mapping, 2nd Edition. Jossey-Bass, San Francisco.

Contributors to the Cochrane Collaboration and the Campbell Collaboration (2000) Evidence from systematic reviews of research relevant to implementing the "wider public health" agenda. NHS Centre for Reviews and Dissemination, York. www.york.ac.uk/ inst/crd/wph.htm, last accessed 27 May 2006.

de Leeuw, E. (1989a) The Sane Revolution – Health Promotion: Backgrounds, scope, prospects. Van Gorcum, Assen/Maastricht.

de Leeuw, E. (1989b) Health Policy. An exploratory inquiry into the development of policy for the new public health in The Netherlands. Savannah Press, Maastricht, The Netherlands.

de Leeuw, E. (2001) Global and local (glocal) health: The WHO Healthy Cities Programme. *Global Change and Human Health*, 2(1), 34–53.

de Leeuw, E., E. Abbema & M. Commers (1998) *Healthy Cities Policy Evaluation – Final Report*. WHO Collaborating Centre for Research on Healthy Cities, Maastricht / EUDGV, Luxembourg.

de Leeuw, E. & T. Skovgaard (2005) Utility-driven evidence for healthy cities: Problems with evidence generation and application. *Social Science & Medicine*, (61), 1331–1341.

Goumans, M. & J. Springett (1997) From projects to policy: "Healthy Cities" as a mechanism for policy change for health? *Health Promotion International*, 12(4), 311–322.

Gusfield, J. (1981) The Culture of Public Problems: Drinking-Driving and the Symbolic Order. University of Chicago Press, Chicago.

HELP (2006) HELP – for a life without smoking. European Union DG Health and Consumer Protection. http://ec.europa.eu/health/ph_determinants/life_style/Tobacco/ help_en.htm, last accessed 4 October 2006.

Hill, M. & P. Hupe (2002) Implementing Public Policy. Sage Publications, London.

Hoeijmakers, M. (2005) Local health policy development processes. Health promotion and network perspectives on local health policy-making in The Netherlands. Maastricht, Maastricht University.

Hogstedt, C., B. Lundgren, H. Moberg, B. Pettersson, G. Ågren (2004) Foreword – Swedish Health Policy Special Supplement. *Scandinavian Journal of Public Health*, 32(Suppl 64), 1–64.

Kingdon, J.W. (2003) Agendas, Alternatives and Public Policies; 2nd edition. Harper Collins College Publishers, New York.

Lasswell, H. (1936) Politics: *Who gets what, when, how*. McGraw-Hill, New York.

Lipsky, M. (1980) Street-Level Bureaucracy: Dilemmas of the Individual in Public Services. Russell Sage Foundation, New York.

Mazmanian, D.A. & P.A. Sabatier (1989) Implementation and Public Policy. With a New Postscript. University Press of America, Lanham/London.

Milewa, T. & E. de Leeuw (1996) Reason, power and protest in the new urban public health movement: A basis for sociological analysis of political discourse in the "healthy city". *British Journal of Sociology*, 47(4), 657–670.

Milio, N. (1981) Promoting health through structural change: Analysis of the origins and implementation of Norway's farm-food-nutrition policy. *Social Science & Medicine*, 15(A), 721–734.

Milio, N. (1986) Promoting health through public policy. F.A Davis Co., Philadelphia.

Milio, N. (2001) Glossary: Healthy Public Policy. *Journal of Epidemiology and Community Health*, 55, 622–623.

Mitroff, I.I. & R. Mason (1980) Structuring ill-structured policy issues: Further explorations in a methodology for messy problems. *Strategic Management Journal*, 1(4), 331–342.

Montague, M., R. Borlan & C. Sinclair (2001) Slip! Slop! Slap! And SunSmart, 1980–2000: Skin cancer control and 20 years of population-based campaigning. *Health Education & Behaviour*, 28(3), 290–305.

Moysés, S.J., S.T. Moysés, M. McCarthy, A. Sheiham (2006) Intra-urban differentials in child dental trauma in relation to Healthy Cities policies in Curitiba, Brazil. Health & Place (2006) 48–64.

Nutbeam, D. (1998) Health Promotion Glossary. *Health Promotion International*, 13(4), 349–364.

Skok, J.E. (1995) Policy issue networks and the public policy cycle: A structural-functional framework for public administration. *Public Administration Review*, 55(4), 325–332.

Smedley, B.D. & S.L. Syme (2000) *Promoting Health. Intervention Strategies from Social and Behavioral Research*. Committee on Capitalizing on Social Science and Behavioral Research to Improve the Public's Health. Division of Health Promotion and Disease Prevention, Institute of Medicine, Washington DC.

Stone, D. (1997) Policy Paradox. The art of political decision making. W.W. Norton, New York/London.

Van der Doelen, F.C.J. (1998) The "Give-and-Take" Packaging of Policy Instruments: Optimizing Legitimacy and Effectiveness. Ch. 5, pp 129–148 In: Bemelmans-Videc, M.-L., R.C. Rist & E. Vedung (1998) Carrots, Sticks & Sermons. Policy Instruments & Their Evaluation. Transaction Publishers, New Brunswick/London.

Weiss, C.H. (1979) The many meanings of research utilization. *Public Administration Review*, Sep/Oct, 426–431.

WHO Framework Convention for Tobacco Control (2006) www.fctc.org, last accessed 4 October 2006.

6
Strengthening the Evidence Base for Mental Health Promotion

MARGARET M. BARRY, VIKRAM PATEL, EVA JANÉ-LLOPIS,
JOHN RAEBURN AND MAURICE B. MITTELMARK

Introduction

Mental health promotion is concerned with achieving positive mental health among the general population and addresses the needs of those at risk from, or experiencing mental health problems. The focus of this multidisciplinary area of practice is on enhancing the strengths, competencies and resources of individuals and communities, thereby promoting positive emotional and mental well-being. The underlying principle of this approach is that mental health is a positive concept, which is important in its own right and is an intrinsic component of the broader health promotion agenda. Building on the basic tenets of health promotion, (WHO, 1986) mental health promotion shifts the focus from an individual disease prevention approach towards the health actions and wider social determinants that keep people mentally healthy. Mental health promotion emphasizes that mental health is created where people live their lives and that the everyday contexts or settings, such as the home, school, workplace and community, is where mental health is created and promoted. Mental health promotion is moving onto the global political agenda and there is a momentum behind international and national developments in terms of policy, research and practice in many countries (Marshall-Williams, Saxena & McQueen, 2005). It is therefore critical that there is a strong evidence base to support best practice and policy in meeting the global challenge of promoting population level mental health (WHO World Report, 2001; WHO, 2002a; WHO, 2004a, b) and reducing the increasing burden of mental disorders worldwide (Murray & Lopez, 1996; WHO, 2003). This chapter considers how current progress in demonstrating the effectiveness of mental health promotion can be further strengthened in order to best support international practice and policy.

Evidence of the Effectiveness of Mental Health Promotion

There is a growing international body of evidence that mental health promotion works and there are effective interventions which can be implemented successfully with diverse population groups across a range of settings (Jané-Llopis, Barry,

67

Hosman & Patel, 2005; Hosman & Jané-Llopis, 2005; Barry & Jenkins, 2007). Clusters of known risk and protective factors for mental health have been identified and there is evidence that interventions can reduce these risk factors and enhance protective factors (Mrazek & Haggerty, 1994). The findings from systematic reviews and effectiveness studies confirm that programs promoting positive mental health can have long-lasting positive effects, not only on mental health but also on a range of social and behavioral health outcomes (Durlak & Wells, 1997; Tilford, Delaney & Vogels, 1997; Hosman & Jané-Llopis, 1999; Hosman & Jané-Llopis, 2005; Mentality, 2003). The evidence to date supports the view that competence-enhancing interventions carried out in collaboration with individuals, families, schools and wider communities, have the potential to impact on multiple positive outcomes across a number of health domains (Jané-Llopis & Barry, 2005). Most mental health promotion interventions have been found to have the dual effect of reducing mental health problems and disorders while also increasing competencies (Hosman & Jané-Llopis, 1999; Durlak & Wells, 1997).

An overview of effective mental health promotion programs across different settings and stages of the life span is presented by Jané-Llopis and colleagues (2005) and in other recent reviews (WHO, 2004a; WHO, 2004b). Jané-Llopis, Barry, Hosman and Patel (2005) draw on different sources of evidence, ranging from randomized control trials (RCTs) to case studies, and using the Ottawa Charter framework (WHO, 1986) review the evidence across key settings in terms of effectiveness in health, social and economic impacts. This overview illustrates that there is a large range of programs in settings such as the home, schools, workplace, community and health services that have demonstrated their effectiveness in promoting mental health. These initiatives include early years and home visiting programs for families at risk, parenting programs, pre-school and school-based programs for young people, comprehensive interventions in the workplace, and community and health service programs (see Barry and Jenkins 2007 for a more comprehensive account of these programs). While acknowledging gaps in the evidence base, Jané-Llopis, Barry, Hosman and Patel (2005) conclude that there is sufficient knowledge to move evidence into practice and provides recommendations for action in terms of addressing poverty, gender and mental health in a global society (Patel, 2005); improving the quality of program implementation (Barry, Domitrovich & Lara, 2005); and integrating mental health into the health promotion and public health agenda (Herrman & Jané-Llopis, 2005). Moodie and Jenkins (2005) point out that there is a persuasive case for governments to invest in mental health promotion as an effective strategy for creating health and social gain. As demonstrated by the systematic reviews in the area, effective mental health promotion strategies have the potential to contribute to a range of improved health and social outcomes in terms of educational achievement, employment, reduced crime and delinquency, improved sexual health, better family and social relationships and reduced inequalities. Marshall Williams, Saxena and McQueen (2005) call for evidence-based programs to be brought to scale, disseminated, adopted and implemented across countries and different cultural, social and economic contexts.

Demonstrating Mental Health Promotion Effectiveness: Theoretical and Methodological Perspectives

As a multidisciplinary area of practice, mental health promotion draws on a diverse range of disciplines and as such, different theoretical and methodological perspectives may be brought to bear in establishing a sound evidence base. Effective mental health promotion programs are underpinned by sound conceptual and theoretical frameworks of human, organizational and environmental functioning, which provide a coherent framework for designing, conducting and evaluating programs. The competence enhancement model, which underpins mental health promotion practice, focuses on enhancing strengths, competence, life skills and enabling a sense of efficacy in diverse life areas (Barry, 2001). The goal, therefore, becomes enhancing potential and promoting positive mental health and well-being rather than focusing on reducing mental disorders. Mental health promotion concepts are positive, dynamic and empowering and this approach builds on the theoretical base of areas such as lifespan developmental theory, community and health psychology, social and organizational theory and the overarching socio-ecological perspective of health promotion.

Ecological models of human development (Bronfenbrenner, 1979) highlight how individuals are influenced by multiple interacting systems, including the social context in which they live such as neighbourhoods, physical environments, culture and society. This socio-ecological perspective highlights the interdependencies among social systems operating at different levels and shifts the focus beyond an individualistic approach to consider the influence of broader social, economic and political forces and how these are mediated through local community settings, norms and values. The ecological model shifts the intervention point to policy and organizational change as well as individual change. For example, early years programs need to be able to influence in significant ways the enduring environment in which the individual child, family, group or community is functioning (Olds, 1997) and effective school programs are those which adopt a whole school approach strengthening capacity at the level of the individual, the classroom and the whole school as a mental health promoting setting for living, learning and working (Wells, Barlow & Stewart-Brown, 2003; Jané-Llopis et al., 2005; Rowling, Martin & Walker, 2002; Weare, 2000).

Demonstrating the effectiveness of an ecological, whole system approach in practice, presents a number of methodological challenges. As Dooris (2006) points out, there has been a tendency in health promotion to evaluate only discrete projects in settings, and thereby not adequately capture the synergistic impact and outcomes of interventions which are dynamic, multifaceted and operating at many levels in complex systems. To capture the added-value of an ecological whole-systems approach requires an evaluation framework capable of tracking and demonstrating the interrelationships and interdependencies between its component parts. The application of theory-driven evaluation methods (Chen, 1990; Chen, 1998) in this context calls for clear articulation not only of the "causative" theories underpinning the intervention but also of the "prescriptive" theories guiding the dynamic process of synergistic change. For example, community programs may be planned to occur across different levels of the social ecology and programs at each level may be in turn be composed of multiple programme elements. Such multicomponent programs require an implementation and evaluation model which will track the sequence of activities that are needed for effective processes and outcomes at each level (e.g. individual, family, group and community level) and the synergistic impacts and outcomes that are likely to occur across levels. As McQueen and Anderson (2001) point out, there is a need to bring the emerging theoretical perspectives on health promotion practice "which embrace its participation, context and dynamism," to evaluation design and the building of the evidence base. In this way we will ensure that the principles and theories of mental health promotion practice will inform the development of appropriate evaluation frameworks and research methodologies.

The Challenges of Evaluating Mental Health Promotion

Evaluation of mental health promotion is a critical issue (Herrman, Saxena & Moodie, 2005), as a large majority of implemented interventions do not provide scientific insight on their outcomes. This is illustrated for example, by a European study on "best practices" in mental health promotion for children up to 6 years (Mental Health Europe, 1999), where only 11% of the 197 gathered "best practices" across 17 European countries could offer some evidence on their efficacy. Evidence in that context was defined as interventions that had an outcome evaluation component in their implementation. The picture is not different across other areas of the world (WHO, 2006), where evaluation is unfortunately not always included when a decision for first time implementation is taken. This raises questions on how governments or NGO's could legitimate serious investments in large scale implementation of interventions for which there is no information on whether they work.

Issues around what constitutes legitimate evidence in health promotion and what composes sufficient quality of mental health promotion research have long been discussed without reaching consensus (Barry & McQueen, 2005; Mittelmark et al., 2005; Hosman & Jané-Llopis, 2007). However, convincing evidence depends on how evidence is categorized and described, and in most instances evidence of whether an intervention works is related to whether there is an evaluation of sufficient quality that can provide proof of efficacy or effectiveness of that given intervention.

Even in those cases where evaluation is undertaken, its quality might be queried, at times related to the outcome measures chosen, the research designs applied, or the strength of the evidence provided by the evaluations, in terms of outcomes and their clinical significance. The root of the problem may lay in that these criticisms are frequently related to the understanding of best evidence emphasized by the principles of evidence-based medicine (EBM), which take as the gold standard the RCT.

However, it is important to note that for mental health promotion interventions the RCT will not always be the most appropriate research design to evaluate social interventions. As advocated by the WHO European Working group on Health Promotion (WHO EURO, 1998) and Evidence Based Public Health (Rychetnik et al., 2002), public health interventions need a combination of evaluation methods, including quantitative and qualitative approaches (e.g., interviews or focus groups, action research or observational qualitative studies), that can capture the idiosyncrasies of complex health promotion interventions (Jané-Llopis, Katschnig, McDaid & Walhbeck, 2007).

There are many examples of well evaluated mental health promotion interventions, where a combination of methodologies, over a period of time, have provided the proof that the mental health of populations can be improved. The area that has most evidence for mental health promotion is school based programs with mental health outcomes (Stewart-Brown, 2006) although there are other areas, as outlined earlier, where growing evidence is also available (Jané-Llopis et al., 2005).

So what should be taken into account in the discourse of evidence for mental health promotion? At the core of designing, undertaking and appraising evaluation of mental health promotion action there are two main critical considerations: a) what is it that we want to know or assess and, linked to that, b) are the methods used to answer such questions appropriate and of high quality?

What do we want to Assess?

Undertaking research on mental health promotion should not be different from any other area in health promotion. Evaluation methods can be applied building on the advances of health promotion and public health intervention research. However, in mental health promotion research there seems to be a lack of clarity on what is meant by mental health, what type of outcome measures should be assessed, and what instruments are available to measure those chosen outcomes. The choice of positive mental health indicators as outcomes for the evaluation proves a challenge, as their availability is scarce and will vary across contexts. However, there are a vast majority of related measures, such as resilience, self esteem, sense of mastery, participation or community mobilization, (WHO, 2004a) that can be used in the evaluation of these interventions. In these cases it is crucial to underline the links between the chosen measures and positive mental health to clarify and strengthen the value of such outcomes.

The concept of mental health varies across cultures and it is crucial to define it before undertaking an evaluation (WHO, 2004a). Measuring mental health outcomes across cultures in a reliable and valid way poses particular methodological challenges. The evolution of our current methodological understanding of the diagnosis and measurement of psychopathology across cultures has been well documented (Dohrenwend, 1990; Patel, 2001). If diagnostic entities can vary across cultures, then what is the likelihood that we will be able to measure mental health, a much larger construct that is far more likely to be influenced by sociocultural contexts, across communities? A recent report defined the outcomes of mental health promotion to include constructs such as quality of life, increased coping skills and better psychological "adjustment" (WHO, 2002a). Research which examines the validity of such a construct of mental health across countries is needed. For example: What is meant by mental health? What are its component parts? How is it experienced? What value is placed on it? How is it perceived in relation to other aspects of a person's life? These questions also raise more fundamental issues about the distinctions drawn between the "physical", the "mental", the "spiritual" and the "social" and how these are influenced by cultural belief systems. The divisions between mental health and other desirable social values are to an extent arbitrary, and are informed by cultural perspectives on health, illness and well-being.

Defining outcomes should reflect a thorough analysis of what we want to assess and how that can be achieved. The distinction between intermediate and ultimate outcomes is crucial, as well as how the intervention can also have far reaching social and economic outcomes. For example, in a workplace mental health promotion intervention, improved mental well-being and reduced levels of stress could be assessed as intermediate outcomes, while the ultimate outcome could include increased productivity and decreased sick leave due to mental health problems. Clarification of the hierarchy or chain of outcomes is crucial when developing an evaluation plan, and will impact on how and what evidence is produced.

Finally, in selecting the types of outcome measures to use and the links between them, it is important that these outcomes are assessed using validated instruments that can be applied to different populations and are sensitive to detecting the desired changes. In mental health promotion this poses an important challenge, as validated measures or instruments of positive mental health are scarce and might be difficult to utilize across cultures as the understanding of mental health varies greatly in different parts of the world. A more systematic definition and validated instrument to assess positive mental health would support the development of the field (Stewart-Brown, 2002; Parkinson, 2006).

What Research Methods do we Need to Apply to Answer Our Questions?

There are many different types of research methodologies and study designs that can be applied for evaluation, each with their strengths and weakness, and each particularly useful for answering different questions (Jané-Llopis, Katschnig, McDaid & Walhbeck, 2007). The choice of study design is critical in terms of minimizing the risk of systematic bias and in the generalisability of findings to other settings and contexts. Although different stages of program development might require different types of evaluation designs, the highest quality of evaluation procedures that are possible in a given situation should be applied. In essence, one of the perceived weaknesses of mental health promotion is the lack of a comprehensive approach to evaluation that combines both quantitative and qualitative methodologies (WHO, 2004b). While questions such as "Can it work or will it work here" can only be answered by quantitative research methods, qualitative research will provide insight on for whom does it work under given contexts or conditions (Barry, 2002; Jané-Llopis et al., 2007).

It is important to note that quantitative evaluation should not be limited to randomized controlled trials, which in cases of complex community interventions for mental health promotion cannot be easily applied (WHO, 2004b). There are a range of mental health promotion interventions evaluated with high quality, using alternative designs such as group or community randomized trials, group randomized wait listed designs, or quasi-experimental designs including simple or multiple time series designs or cohort studies, which have been able to provide reliable outcomes on program efficacy (Jané-Llopis et al., 2005). In addition to quantitative methods, it is crucial that qualitative research complements quantitative evaluation, to understand questions related to the process of implementation (Barry et al., 2005), differences across participants, contexts or satisfaction (Patel, 2005), which give necessary complementary data on how and for whom the program is effective (Rootman et al., 2001). Qualitative evaluation can also support and provide further explanations on quantitative findings, as well as identifying key issues around implementation, dissemination and sustainability of interventions.

The field of mental health promotion can be strengthened by the appropriate combination of quantitative and qualitative techniques in evaluation, using approaches such as triangulation (WHO, 2004a) and matching the right type of methodology to the different questions we are aiming to answer (Petticrew & Roberts, 2003).

What else is Needed?

Along with evaluation on does it work, for whom and under which conditions, it is crucial to understand the benefits of the intervention in terms of its costs and long-term impact. To provide evidence for a given intervention, as it is done for other topic areas within public health and health promotion, it is crucial to include cost effectiveness analyses; sustained long term follow ups; involvement of stakeholders and, as already highlighted, a proper balance of both quantitative and qualitative approaches to evaluation.

Strengthening the Evidence Base for Mental Health Promotion

Progress to date in building the evidence base for mental health promotion has to a large extent focused on individual or group level interventions rather than population level approaches. The impact of macro level strategies such as policy interventions on population level mental health need to be more clearly established, as does the effectiveness of community level interventions. It is also notable that much of the existing evidence in mental health promotion is derived from high-income English-speaking countries (Barry & McQueen, 2005; McQueen, 2001) and there is a relative paucity of evidence on the effectiveness of programs in low-income countries (WHO, 2002a; WHO, 2004a). In strengthening the evidence base there is a need for a greater focus on macro and meso level interventions, and building and applying the evidence base in low-income countries and settings where the conditions for improving mental health are compromised by poverty.

Evaluating Upstream Policy Interventions

There are many plausible policy interventions, such as improved housing, welfare, education and employment which may be expected to directly or indirectly affect mental health, for which evidence appears to be absent (Petticrew, Chisholm, Thomson & Jané-Llopis, 2005). However, Petticrew et al. (2005) caution that the "absence of evidence" should not be mistaken for "evidence of absence" and that plausible interventions such as improved housing can be reasonably expected to generate mental health gains. For example, a systematic review by Thomson, Petticrew and Morrison (2001) found evidence of a consistent pattern of improvements in mental health linked to improved housing. Petticrew et al. (2005) argue that there is a clear potential for positive mental health to be promoted through non-health policies such as the building of new roads, new houses, area-based regeneration, and the assessment of the "spillover" effects of such policies will make an important contribution to the mental health evidence base. This requires the development of mental health impact assessment methods, which will monitor the mental health impacts, both positive and negative, of public policies. Petticrew et al. also highlight that we are still fishing for much of our evidence "downstream" rather than "upstream" where mental health is created. The need to generate better evidence of the benefits, harms and costs of "upstream" interventions, such as non-health sector policies and programs, remains a critical area for development.

Effective Community Mental Health Promotion

In health promotion and mental health promotion, processes variously labeled community development/organization and capacity-building are used to cultivate community connectedness, the aim being the building of social support/ cohesion/ inclusion/capital, either for its own sake, or as an infrastructure for achieving collective goals (e.g. Whiteford, Cullen & Baingana, 2005). Optimal community-building approaches for mental health promotion are deemed to be those which are bottom-up, participatory and empowering, involving values and principles such as community control, self-determination, capacity-building, an emphasis on equity, the honoring of diversity and so on (Raeburn, 2001).

What is the evidence that such community approaches work? At the *whole community* level, most evidence comes indirectly from thousands of grey literature case studies around the world, many from developing countries. These provide overwhelming evidence of the efficacy of this approach for health, wellbeing and quality of life (e.g. Durning, 1989; Mukhopadhyay, 2004). In addition, there is a smaller but nevertheless powerful academic literature involving evaluated demonstration projects, quasi-experimental approaches, etc. which support the positive impacts of this approach (e.g. Jackson et al., 2003; Herrman, Saxena & Moodie, 2005). At the *subcommunity* level of schools, workplaces, etc., there are proportionately many more academic studies, although not many of an RCT nature, and overall these clearly demonstrate the efficacy of such approaches (e.g. Pransky, 1991; Weare & Markham, 2005; Keleher & Armstrong, 2005). At the *interest/issue/demographic* community level, studies of younger people, older people, community action groups, indigenous groups, minorities, rural populations, refugee camps, and others are strongly supportive of this approach (e.g. Saxena & Garrison, 2004).

In considering what needs to be improved in this domain of evidence, it could be argued that the need is not more rigor, but rather the opening up of the academic rules of what constitutes legitimate evidence. Evaluation methods and outcome measures need to be able to capture the extent to which the self-determination of the issues and goals to be addressed by the community and the attainment of those goals by the community itself are enabled and achieved through community approaches. The evidence needs to accommodate real life measures which show irrefutable signs of improved mental health, ones which are supplied by the people themselves, rather than those imposed by outside experts.

Building the Evidence Base in Low Income Countries

Mental health promotion in developing countries faces two key challenges: first, the stigma associated with mental illness, and second, the poor infrastructure for health and social welfare (Patel et al., 2005). In addition, for a range of reasons, some of which have to do with a lack of resources and capacity in developing countries, far less research has been conducted in these contexts than in wealthier countries (Patel & Sumathipala, 2001). The evidence that does exist includes mainly narrative and case study material of specific programs and evidence from the domain of physical health promotion which may be extrapolated to mental health. These programs focus on three major areas of action: advocacy, empowerment and social support.

The aim of advocacy is to generate public demand for mental health, place mental health issues high up on the political and community agenda, and effectively convince all stakeholders to act in support of mental health. Advocacy may be directed to a variety of stakeholders, including politicians, religious leaders, professionals and community leaders. There are good examples of advocacy being used to reduce the burden of substance abuse. These include a community-based approach to combating alcoholism and promoting the mental health of families in rural India (Bang & Bang, 1991; Bang & Bang, 1995) and an unblinded matched community-based trial conducted in Yunnan, China, to investigate the effectiveness of a multifaceted community intervention to prevent drug abuse among youths (Wu, Detels, Zhang, Li & Li, 2002). These programs, which led to significant reductions in alcohol and drug misuse respectively, involved community participation and action, together with collaboration with multiple sectors and community leaders, and employed multiple intervention strategies including education and awareness building, advocacy to politicians, literacy improvement and employment opportunities. The application of such approaches in advocating for mental health promotion initiatives would appear to hold much potential.

There is low awareness regarding mental illness and the importance of mental health in many communities in developing countries. Raising this awareness may help improve understanding about the risks to mental health and methods of coping with these risks, and thus promote mental health in the community. A school-based program in Rawalpindi, Pakistan (Rahman, Mubbashar, Gater & Goldberg, 1998) succeeded in increasing understanding of common mental health problems and reducing stigma in a rural community. The program, which was comprised of lectures and discussion on mental health with secondary school students, was found to positively influence the knowledge and attitudes of the students compared to a control group (Rahman et al., 1998). More impressive was the finding that parents, friends and even neighbours of the students who participated in the program also showed significant improvements in knowledge and attitudes. This trial shows that the school can serve as a gateway to the local community, and that school-based programs can be effective in raising awareness in the wider community, particularly in areas of low literacy.

Empowerment is the process by which groups of people in the community who have been traditionally disadvantaged in ways that compromise their health can overcome these barriers and exercise their rights so they can lead a full, equal life in the best of health. Economic empowerment is illustrated through enabling access to low-cost loans for the poorest to tide them over difficult times. Radical community banks and loan facilities – such as those run by SEWA in India and the Grameen Bank in Bangladesh – have been involved in making loans available to poor people who formerly did not have access to such facilities and services. Some evidence of the ability of such banks to promote mental health is available. The Bangladesh Rural Advancement Committee (BRAC) is the world's largest NGO in terms of the scale and diversity of its interventions (Chowdhury & Bhuiya, 2001). Evaluation of its programs, which include health care provision, education and rural development programs, show that BRAC members have better nutritional status, better child survival, higher educational achievement, lower rates of domestic violence and improved well-being and psychological health (Chowdhury & Bhuiya, 2001).

Empowerment of women is a key activity to reduce gender disadvantage. Gender is a powerful social determinant of health, which interacts with other determinants such as age, family structure, income, education and social support (WHO, 2000). The link between domestic violence and mental health problems has been firmly established in numerous studies (Patel et al., 2006; Heise, Ellsberg & Gottemoeller, 1999; WHO, 2000; WHO, 2005). Violence reduction programs are being implemented in many developing countries. Some of these, such as the Stepping Stones programme, have been shown to be effective in reducing violence (WHO, 2002b) and, given the linkages between domestic violence and common mental disorders in women, it is likely that such programs will have a powerful impact on mental health as well.

With regards to social support for health programs, there is evidence that supportive interventions and counselling during the antenatal period improves maternal and child health outcomes. For example, a trial from Zambia demonstrated that mothers who received such support took more action to solve infant health problems, an indirect measure of maternal empowerment and problem-solving abilities (Ranjso-Arvidson, Chintu & Ng'andu N, 1998). Women-to-women programs have increased maternal self-esteem and empowerment in Peru (Lanata, 2001).

Several interventions which target malnutrition as a risk factor, not only for physical health problems but also for poor psychosocial development, have been implemented in developing countries. Notable ones include the Integrated Child Development Scheme in India, the PANDAI (Child Development and Mother's Care) Project in Indonesia, the PRONOEI Programme in Peru, the PROAPE Programme in Brazil, the Integrated Programme for Child and Family Development in Thailand and the Hogares Comunitarios de Bienestar Programme in Columbia.

Older people face a triple burden in developing countries: a rising tide of non-communicable and degenerative disorders associated with aging, falling levels of family support systems and lack of adequate social welfare systems (Patel & Prince, 2001). There is some documentation of programs aimed at improving the quality of life of elders in developing countries (Tout, 1989). All of these examples target three risk factors for poor mental health in the elderly – financial difficulties, social isolation and poor physical health – and all are likely to have an important impact on the promotion of mental health.

Communicating Clear Messages About What Works in Mental Health Promotion

Scientific evidence about the effectiveness of mental health promotion can be used in several ways:

- To build the scholarly knowledge base and contribute to the development of theory in the disciplines which contribute to academic mental health promotion
- To inform mental health promotion practitioners on evidence of best practice
- To educate health professionals at all levels from introductory to continuing education
- To inform citizens about mental health promotion and prevention programs available in the community
- To provide arguments for mental health advocacy groups
- To influence policy-makers and policy processes who in turn can direct resources to improve mental health promotion capacity and quality at all levels from local to international.

The mental health knowledge base in the scientific literature is socially shaped by people with different interests, skills and resources, and knowledge travels via complex pathways and selective filters. Academic and health professionals have well-established communication methods to disseminate knowledge and they share venues, professional language, and other resources that promote good communication. Nevertheless, professional divisions continue to hinder full collaboration. The academic approach to generating, reviewing evidence, and summarising evidence from research has grown in sophistication in recent years, with regard to systems for managing evidence (e.g., the Cochrane Collaboration) and statistical techniques for combining information across studies (e.g., meta-analysis). Trickling down, the information available to citizens through media, family and acquaintances, non-governmental organisations and health professionals is filtered by print and broadcast media specialists, who try to bridge the professional worlds of academia and the practical world of peoples' everyday lives. The internet provides access to seemingly unlimited quantities of information, but web sites dedicated to managing information on specific topics like mental health promotion are growing in number. The result is a plethora of special interests groups, all hard at work communicating agendas that may be more or less complimentary or in conflict.

How then, to develop a communications strategy so that policy-makers and others can pick up the "right" signal out of all the noise? One answer comes from experience in Europe in the mid- to late 1990's, in the project "The Evidence of Health Promotion Effectiveness: Shaping Public Health in a new Europe", managed on behalf of a broad-based partnership by the International Union for Health Promotion and Education – IUHPE (IUHPE, 1999). The project had two aims: summarize twenty years of evidence on health promotion's effectiveness (including mental health), and communicate the information directly to policy-makers in Europe. This initiative brought experts and decision makers together in order to bridge the gaps of understanding in terms of language, needs, and priorities. Such an approach lays the foundation for sustained dialogue with decision-makers, using the evidence of effectiveness as the foundation for discussion, debate and ultimately more effective mental health policies.

Communicating Evidence for Policy Making

The implementation of mental health promotion requires support, as highlighted in a recent review of prevention and promotion action in 31 European countries, where the most important barrier identified was the lack of access to evidence-based knowledge (Jané-Llopis & Anderson, 2006). To support policy and decision makers for implementation, it is crucial that, in providing the evidence, the language used to communicate findings makes sense to the intended audience and, that the assessment of the evidence goes beyond the study design or given outcomes, to also include the policy relevant implications of the study findings.

Firstly, the decision making process and the implementation of mental health promotion programs and policies will require, among others, good evidence on feasibility, efficacy, effectiveness, and cost effectiveness, including assessing the appropriateness of using a specific study design, susceptibility to bias, the magnitude of effectiveness, (how important or clinically significant a result is in its context), how complete a study is (does it include outcomes of relevance to all stakeholders), or the transferability of the study to a similar given situation (Rychetnik et al., 2002). However, this will not suffice to support decision makers in drawing implementation action. Decisions will also have to be informed by other factors such as the acceptability of a policy or program to a target population, the ethical and political considerations linked to a given intervention, the strength and relevance of the evidence in relation to other population measures and priorities, or the expected impacts on social or economic gains in addition to the primarily expected outcomes (Jané-Llopis et al., 2007).

However, the three crucial aspects that will be most determining for policy makers to use of any evidence include: accessibility, comprehensibility, and relevance of the information provided. Firstly, for this it is crucial that the information is described using measures, indicators and language that make sense to decision makers, providing a synthesis of relevant aspects that need to be taken into account, providing a conclusive statement on the strength of the evidence and in which direction it points, and combining it with a conclusive remark on the limitations and implications of a given action. Secondly, it is crucial to make this evidence available and accessible in reader friendly formats. Thirdly, all relevant aspects to policy making and related stakeholders should be taken into account, for which at times, it is best to engage them in consultation from the beginning, to make sure those questions that are of relevance for them are addressed.

Only if the policy and decision makers can have access, read, understand and be provided with conclusive statements, regardless of the inevitable uncertainty always linked to any form of evidence, it is more likely that the evidence for mental health promotion will be translated into policy.

Communicating Evidence for Best Practice

An important challenge is disseminating and translating the evidence base so that it serves the needs of practitioners concerned with the practicality of implementing successful programs that are relevant to the needs of the populations they serve. This calls for the active dissemination of validated programs and guidelines on best practice based on efficacy, effectiveness and dissemination studies. User-friendly information systems and databases are being developed in order to make the evidence base accessible to practitioners. Targeted evidence briefings, which consist of summaries and syntheses of existing systematic reviews on a range of topics, have an important part to play in influencing policy and encouraging good practice. However, databases and reviews are more of a passive than active form of dissemination and there have been a number of initiatives to explore more active ways of disseminating and translating the evidence base into practice. Initiatives such as the IUHPE Global Programme on Health Promotion Effectiveness (GPHPE) aim to translate evidence to policy makers and practitioners and thereby raise the standard of policy making and practice worldwide (IUHPE, 2006). As noted by Kelly, Speller and Meyrick (2004), for evidence to be applicable in the field, the evidence needs to be accessible, contextualised and usable by practitioners. This requires an understanding of local contexts and circumstances, of local professionals' knowledge bases and resources, commitment, and engagement, and detailed assessment of the particular population for whom the intervention is intended (Speller, Wimbush & Morgan, 2005; Barry, 2005). Active strategies are required for disseminating the evidence base across diverse settings and countries and providing technical assistance and capacity-building resources for evidence-based mental health promotion practice, especially in low-income countries and settings.

This calls for a clearer focus on translational research in order to ensure the effective application of research evidence into practice and the documentation and evaluation of best practice for inclusion in the evidence base. Building the evidence base will then become a two way process in terms of innovation, adaptation and dissemination of promising programs and creative practice. The ultimate test is making the evidence base accessible so that it can be effectively used to inform practice that will reduce inequalities and bring about improved mental health, especially in disadvantaged communities and settings.

Communicating the Evidence to the Public

There is an onus on the "experts" in mental health promotion to communicate with the public about what mental health promotion can contribute to a global and national mental health problems such as depression, stress, suicide, violence and adaptation in a very demanding and catastrophe-prone world. A major consideration in this respect is tackling public perceptions of stigma related to mental disorder and by proxy to any initiative labeled mental health. Mass-media campaigns have an important role to play in addressing destigmatization (Vaughan & Hansen, 2004), and raising public awareness (Devault, 2000). However, to bring about meaningful change in whole populations, much more is needed than this. There is a need to start by attempting to de-stigmatize the concept of mental health itself, and to present what we know in a language that is friendly and appropriate to those with whom we are attempting to communicate. We need to transform mental health concerns from feared concepts to noble and desirable ones. The positive language of strengths or capacity, rather than pathology, is a good start here (Williams, 2002).

There is a need to consider how we as experts interact with "the public." Rather than regarding "them" as passive recipients of expert knowledge and "evidence," we need to consider how we can better partner and participate on a more equal basis with the public at different levels of society. This could include the development with interested groups of people-relevant policy at the global and national level, the provision of resources to support empowering collective action at the *community level*, and facilitation of access to tools for life skills and emotional/cognitive development for people to use for themselves at the family and individual level.

Only when we stop being "experts," and recognise that we and "the public" are one and the same, talking the same language and having the same human concerns, will we progress with sharing our mental health promotion knowledge and expertise with the world in a beneficial way.

Conclusions

Reviews of the evidence base for mental health promotion clearly show that there are many examples of high quality programs and initiatives, which lead to a range of positive health and social outcomes. However, it is also clear that best practice programs need to be at a coverage, scope and intensity to make a critical difference. Programs need to be brought to scale, disseminated and implemented across different cultural settings, especially in low-income countries. To support the translation of the evidence into best practice and policy, the evidence base needs to be made accessible, comprehensible and relevant for different target audiences. The active translation of evidence needs to be accompanied by the technical resources to make the evidence usable in the local context. This requires an increased focus on developing both the research and infrastructural mechanisms for high quality implementation of effective and sustainable interventions and the evaluation of mental health promotion practice. Partnerships between research institutions and those involved in delivery across all sectors could contribute centrally to strengthening and expanding the evidence base. Dissemination research and further systematic studies of program implementation, adoption and adaptation across cultures are needed so that evidence-informed practice and practice-based theory may be generated, which will guide the building of capacity for effective program delivery.

Political commitment to evidence-based policy and practice needs to be mobilized so that investment in mental health promotion research and evaluation is given greater priority. The research base needs to be strengthened in order to provide a strong foundation for evidence-based mental health promotion practice globally, including the costs and benefits of interventions, the public health relevance of mental health promotion outcomes and the potential gains at other health and social levels.

References

Bang, A. & Bang, R. (1991). Community participation in research and action against alcoholism. *World Health Forum, 12*, 104–109.

Bang, A. & Bang, R. (1995). Action against alcoholism. *Health Action, Dec 1994–Feb 1995(11)*, 2.

Barry, M.M. (2001). Promoting positive mental health: Theoretical frameworks for practice. *International Journal of Mental Health Promotion, 3(1)*, 25–43.

Barry, M.M. (2002). Challenges and opportunities in strengthening the evidence base for mental health promotion. *Promotion & Education, 9(2)*, 44–48.

Barry, M.M. (2005). The art, science and politics of creating a mentally healthy society: Lessons from a cross border rural mental health project in Ireland. *Journal of Public Mental Health, 4(1)*, 30–34.

Barry, M.M., Domitrovich, C. & Lara, M.A. (2005). The implementation of mental health promotion programmes. In: E. Jané-Llopis, M. Barry, C. Hosman & V. Patel (eds) The evidence of mental health promotion effectiveness: Strategies for action. *Promotion & Education, suppl 2*, 30–36.

Barry, M.M. & McQueen, D. (2005). The nature of evidence and its use in mental health promotion. In: H. Herrman, S. Saxena & R. Moodie (eds) *Promoting mental health: Concepts, emerging evidence, practice* (pp. 108–119). A WHO Report in collaboration with the Victorian Health Promotion Foundation and the University of Melbourne. Geneva: World Health Organization.
http://www.who.int/mental_health/evidence/ MH_Promotion_Book.pdf (2 October, 2006).

Barry, M.M. & Jenkins, R. (2007). *Implementing Mental Health Promotion*. Oxford: Elsevier.

Bronfenbrenner, U. (1979). *The Ecology of human development: Experiments by nature and design*. Cambridge, Massachusetts: Harvard University Press.

Chen, H. (1998). Theory-driven evaluations. *Advances in Educational Productivity, 7*, 15–34.

Chen, H.T. (1990). *Theory-driven Evaluations*. Newbury Park, CA: Sage.

Chowdhury, A., Bhuiya, A. (2001). Do poverty alleviation programs reduce inequities in health? The Bangladesh experience. In: D. Leon & G. Walt (eds) *Poverty, Inequality and Health*. Oxford: Oxford University Press, 312–332.

Devault, A. (2000). L'utilisation efficace des médias de masse dans des programmes de prévention et de promotion de la santé mentale. [The effective use of mass media in prevention and mental health promotion programmes]. *Canadian Journal of Community Mental Health, 19(1)*, 21–35.

Dohrenwend, B.P. (1990). "The problem of validity in field studies of psychological disorders" revisited. *Psychological Medicine, 20*, 195–208.

Dooris, M. (2006). Healthy settings: Challenges to generating evidence of effectiveness. *Health Promotion International, 21*, 55–65.

Durlak, J.A. & Wells, A.M. (1997). Primary prevention mental health programs for children and adolescents: A meta-analytic review. *American Journal of Community Psychology, 25(2)*, 115–152.

Durning, A.B. (1989). Grass-roots groups are our best hope for global prosperity and ecology. *Utne Reader, 34*, 40–49.

Heise, L., Ellsberg, M. & Gottemoeller, M. (1999). *Ending Violence Against Women*. Baltimore: Johns Hopkins University School of Public Health, Population Information Program.

Herrman, H. & Jané-Llopis, E. (2005). Mental health promotion in public health. *Promotion & Education, suppl 2*, 42–47.

Herrman, H.S., Saxena, S. & Moodie, R. (eds) (2005). *Promoting mental health: Concepts, emerging evidence, practice*. A WHO Report in collaboration with the Victorian Health Promotion Foundation and the University of Melbourne. Geneva: World Health Organization.
http://www.who.int/mental_health/evidence/MH_Promotion_Book.pdf (2 October, 2006).

Hosman, C. & Jané-Llopis, E. (1999). Political Challenges 2: Mental health. Chapter 3. In *The evidence of health promotion effectiveness: Shaping public health in a new Europe* (pp. 29–41). A Report for the European Commission. International Union for Health Promotion and Education, IUHPE, Paris: Jouve Composition & Impression.

Hosman, C. & Jané-Llopis, E. (2005). The evidence of effective interventions for mental health promotion. In: H. Herrman, S. Saxena & R. Moodie (eds.) *Promoting mental health: Concepts, emerging evidence, practice* (pp. 169–188). A WHO Report in collaboration with the Victorian Health Promotion Foundation and the University of Melbourne. Geneva: World Health Organization.
http://www.who.int/mental_health/evidence/ MH_Promotion_Book.pdf (2 October, 2006).

Hosman, C. & Jané-Llopis, E. (2007). The concepts of evidence in mental health promotion and mental disorder prevention. In: C. Hosman, E. Jané-Llopis & S. Saxena (eds) *Prevention of mental disorders: Effective interventions and policy options*. A report of the World Health Organization, Department of Mental Health and Substance Abuse in collaboration with the Prevention Research Centre of the Universities of Nijmegen and Maastricht. Oxford: Oxford University Press.

International Union of Health Promotion and Education (IUHPE) (1999). *The evidence of health promotion effectiveness: Shaping public health in a new Europe*. A Report for the European Commission. International Union for Health Promotion and Education, IUHPE, Paris: Jouve Composition & Impression.

International Union of Health Promotion and Education (IUHPE) *Global programme on health promotion effectiveness*. A multi-partner project co-ordinated by the International Union for Health Promotion and Education in collaboration with the World Healtlh Organization. Online. Available
http://www.iuhpe.org (3 October 2006).

Jackson, S.F., Cleverly, S., Poland, B., Burman, D., Edwards, R.K. & Robertson, A. (2003). Working with Toronto neighbourhoods toward developing indicators of community capacity. *Health Promotion International, 18*, 339–350.

Jané-Llopis, E. & Anderson, P. (eds) (2006). *Mental health promotion and mental disorder prevention across European Member States: A collection of country stories*. Luxembourg: European Communities. http://www.imhpa.net.

Jané-Llopis, E. & Barry, M.M. (2005). What makes mental health promotion effective? *Promotion & Education, suppl 2*, 47–55.

Jané-Llopis, E., Barry, M., Hosman, C. & Patel, V. (2005). Mental health promotion works: A review. In: E. Jané-Llopis, M.M. Barry, C. Hosman & V. Patel (eds) The evidence of mental health promotion effectiveness: Strategies for action. *Promotion & Education, suppl 2*, 9–25.

Jané-Llopis, E., Katschnig, H., McDaid, D. & Walhbeck, K. (2007). *Making use of evidence on mental health promotion and mental disorder prevention: An everyday primer*. A report of the EC Mental Health Working Party Taskforce on Evidence. Luxembourg: European Communities.

Keleher, H. & Armstrong, R. (2005). *Evidence-based mental health promotion resource*. Melbourne: Department of Human Services.

Lanata, C. (2001). Children's health in developing countries: Issues of coping, child neglect and marginalization. In: D. Leon & G. Walt (eds) *Poverty, Inequality & Health* (pp. 137–158). Oxford: Oxford University Press.

Marshall-Williams, S., Saxena, S. & McQueen, D.V. (2005). The momentum for mental health promotion. *Promotion & Education, suppl 2*, 6–9.

McQueen, D. (2001). Strengthening the evidence base for health promotion. *Health Promotion International, 16(3)*, 261–268.

McQueen, D.V. & Anderson, L.M. (2001). What counts as evidence: Issues and debates. In: I. Rootman, M. Goodstadt, B. Hyndman et al. (eds) *Evaluation in health promotion: Principles and perspectives*. Copenhagen: World Health Organization Regional Publications, European Series, No. 92.

Mental Health Europe (1999). *Mental health promotion for children up to 6 years. Directory of projects in the European Union*. Brussels.

Mentality (2003). *Making it effective: A guide to evidence based mental health promotion*. Radical mentalities-briefing paper 1. London: Mentality.

Mittelmark, M. B., Puska, P., O'Byrne, D. & Tang, K-C. (2005). Health Promotion: A sketch of the landscape. In: H. Herrman, S. Saxena & R. Moodie (eds) *Promoting mental health: Concepts, emerging evidence, practice* (pp. 18–34). A WHO Report in collaboration with the Victorian Health Promotion Foundation and the University of Melbourne. Geneva: World Health Organization.
http://www.who.int/mental_health/evidence/ MH_Promotion_Book.pdf (2 October, 2006).

Moodie, R. & Jenkins, R. (2005). "I'm from the government and you want me to invest in mental health promotion. Well why should I?" *Promotion & Education, suppl 2*, 37–41.

Mrazek, P.J. & Haggerty, R.J. (eds) (1994). *Reducing risks for mental disorders: Frontiers for preventive intervention research*. Washington DC: National Academy Press.

Mukhopadhyay, A. (2004). Khoj: *A search for innovations and sustainability in community health and development*. New Delhi: Voluntary Health Association of India.

Murray, C.J. & Lopez, A.D. (1996). The global burden of disease. *Harvard School of Public Health*. Boston: World Health Organization, World Bank.

Olds, D.L. (1997). The prenatal/early infancy project: Fifteen years later. In: G.W. Albee & T.P. Gullotta (eds) *Primary prevention works, Vol. 6: Issues in children's and families lives* (pp. 41–67). Sage: London.

Parkinson, J. (2006). Establishing national mental health and well-being indicators for Scotland. *Journal of Public Mental Health, 5(1)*, 42–48.

Patel, V. (2001). Cultural factors and international epidemiology. *British Medical Bulletin, 57*, 33–46.

Patel, V. (2005). Poverty, gender and mental health promotion in a global society. In: E. Jané-Llopis, M.M. Barry, C. Hosman & V. Patel (eds) The evidence of mental health promotion effectiveness: Strategies for action. *Promotion & Education, suppl 2*, 26–29.

Patel, V. & Prince, M. (2001). Ageing and mental health in developing countries: Who cares? Qualitative Studies from Goa, India. *Psychological Medicine, 31*, 29–38.

Patel, V., Sumathipala, A. (2001). International representation in psychiatric journals: A survey of 6 leading journals. *British Journal of Psychiatry, 178*, 406–409.

Patel, V., Swartz, L. & Cohen, A. (2005). The evidence for mental health promotion in developing countries. In: H. Herrman, S. Saxena & R. Moodie (eds) *Promoting mental health: Concepts, emerging evidence, practice* (pp. 189–202). A WHO Report in collaboration with the Victorian Health Promotion Foundation and the University of Melbourne. Geneva: World Health Organization.
http://www.who.int/mental_health/evidence/MH_Promotion_Book.pdf (2 October, 2006).

Patel, V., Kirkwood, B.R., Pednekar, S. et al. (2006). Gender disadvantage and reproductive health risk factors for common mental disorders in women: A community survey in India. *Archives of Geeraln Psychiatry, 63(4)*, 404–413.

Petticrew, M. & Roberts, H. (2003). Evidence, hierarchies, and typologies: Horses for courses. *Journal of Epidemiology and Community Health, 57*, 527–529.

Petticrew, M., Chisholm, D., Thomson, H. & Jané-Llopis, E. (2005). Evidence: The way forward. In: H. Herrman, S. Saxena & R. Moodie (eds) *Promoting mental health: Concepts, emerging evidence, practice* (pp. 203–214). A WHO Report in collaboration with the Victorian Health Promotion Foundation and the University of Melbourne. Geneva: World Health Organization.
http://www.who.int/mental_health/evidence/ MH_Promotion_Book.pdf (2 October, 2006).

Pransky, J. (1991). *Prevention: The critical need*. Springfield, MO: Burrell Foundation & Paradigm Press.

Raeburn, J. (2001). Community approaches to mental health promotion. *International Journal of Mental Health Promotion, 3*, 13–19.

Rahman, A., Mubbashar, M., Gater, R., Goldberg, D. (1998). Randomised Trial Impact of School Mental-Health Programme in Rural Rawalpindi, Pakistan. *Lancet, 352*, 1022–1026.

Ranjso-Arvidson, A.B., Chintu, K. & Ng'andu N et al. (1998). Maternal and infant health problems after normal childbirth: A randomised controlled study in Zambia. *Journal of Epidemiology & Community Health, 52(385)*, 391.

Rootman, I., Goodstadt, M., Potvin, L. & Springett, J. (2001). A framework for health promotion evaluation. In: I. Rootman, M. Goodstadt, B. Hyndman, D. McQueen, L. Potvin, J. Springett & E. Ziglio (eds) *Evaluation in health promotion: Principles and Perspectives*. Copenhagen: WHO Regional Office for Europe.

Rowling, L., Martin, G. & Walker, L. (2002). *Mental health promotion and young people: Concepts and practice*. Sydney: McGraw Hill.

Rychetnik, L., Frommer, M., Hawe, P. & Shiell, A. (2002). Criteria for evaluating evidence on public health interventions. *Journal of Epidemiology and Community Health, 56*, 119–127.

Saxena, S. & Garrison, P. (eds), (2004). M*ental health promotion: Case studies from countries*. A joint publication of the World Federation for Mental Health and World Health Organization. Geneva: WHO.

Speller, V., Winbush, E. & Morgan, A. (2005). Evidence-based health promotion practice: how to make it work. *Promotion & Education*, Suppl 1, 15–20.

Stewart-Brown, S. (2002). Measuring the parts most measures do not reach: A necessity for evaluation in mental health promotion. *Journal of Mental Health Promotion, 1(2)*, 4–9.

Stewart-Brown, S. (2006). *What is the evidence on school health promotion in improving health or preventing disease and, specifically what is the effectiveness of the health promoting schools approach*. Copenhagen: WHO Regional Office for Europe (Health Evidence Network Report).
http://www.euro.who.int/document/e88185.pdf accessed March 2006).

Tilford, S., Delaney, F. & Vogels, M. (1997). *Effectiveness of mental health promotion interventions: A review*. London: Health Education Authority.

Tout, K. (1989). *Ageing in developing countries*. Oxford: Oxford University Press.

Vaughan, G. & Hansen, C. (2004). "Like Minds, Like Mine": A New Zealand project to counter the stigma and discrimination associated with mental illness. *Australian Psychiatry, 12(2)*, 113–117.

Weare, K. (2000). *Promoting mental, emotional and social health: A whole school approach*. London: Routledge.

Weare, K. & Markham, W. (2005). What do we know about promoting mental health through schools? *Promotion & Education, XII(3–4)*, 14–18.

Wells, J., Barlow, J. & Stewart-Brown, S. (2003). A systematic review of universal approaches to mental health promotion in schools. *Health Education, 103(4)*, 197–220.

Whiteford, H., Cullen, M. & Baingana, F. (2005). Social capital and mental health. In: H. Herrman, S. Saxena & R. Moodie (eds) *Promoting mental health: Concepts, emerging evidence, practice* (pp. 70–80). A WHO Report in collaboration with the Victorian Health Promotion Foundation and the University of Melbourne. Geneva: World Health Organization. http://www.who.int/mental_health/evidence/MH_Promotion_Book.pdf (2 October, 2006).

Williams, N. (2002). *Building on strengths: A new approach to promoting mental health in New Zealand/Aotearoa.* Wellington: Ministry of Health.

World Health Organisation (1986). *Ottawa Charter for Health Promotion.* Copenhagen: World Health Organisation.

World Health Organization, EURO (1998). *Health promotion evaluation: Recommendations to policymakers.* Copenhagen: World Health Organization.

World Health Organization. (2000). *Women's Mental Health: An evidence based review.* Geneva: World Health Organization.

World Health Organization (2001). Mental health: New understanding, new hope. *The World Health Report.* Geneva: World Health Organization.

World Health Organization (2002a). *Prevention and Promotion in Mental Health.* Geneva: World Health Organization.

World Health Organization. (2002b). *World Report on Violence and Health: Summary.* Geneva: World Health Organization.

World Health Organization (2003). *Investing in mental health. Department of Mental Health and Substance Dependence, Non-communicable Diseases and Mental Health,* Geneva: World Health Organization.

World Health Organization (2004a). *Promoting mental health: Concepts, emerging evidence, practice.* Summary Report. A report of the World Health Organization, Department of Mental Health and Substance Abuse in collaboration with the Victorian Health Promotion Foundation and the University of Melbourne. Geneva: World Health Organization. www.who.int/mental_health/evidence/en/promoting_mhh.pdf.

World Health Organization (2004b). *Prevention of mental disorders: Effective interventions and policy options.* Summary Report. A report of the World Health Organization Department of Mental Health and Substance Abuse in collaboration with the Prevention Research Centre of the Universities of Nijmegen and Maastricht. Geneva: WHO. http://www.who.int/mental_health/evidence/en/prevention_of_mental_disorders_sr.pdf.

World Health Organization. (2005). WHO Multi-country Study on Women's *Health and Domestic Violence: Initial results on prevalence, health outcomes and women's responses.* Geneva: World Health Organization.

World Health Organization (2006). *Mental Health Promotion: Case Studies from Countries.* In: S. Saxena & P. Garrison (eds) Geneva: World Health Organization. http://www.who.int/mental_health/evidence/en/country_case_studies.pdf.

Wu, Z., Detels, R., Zhang, J., Li, V., Li, J. (2002). Community base trial to prevent drug use amongst youth in Yunnan, China. *American Journal of Public Health, 92,* 1952–1957.

7
Effectiveness and Challenges for Promoting Physical Activity Globally

Trevor Shilton, Adrian Bauman, Fiona Bull and Olga Sarmiento

Introduction

How do we know how to make a difference, and if we are making a difference? This is one of the central questions and challenges in determining the effectiveness of health promotion efforts aimed at increasing levels of participation in physical activity at the population level. Despite significant interest since the 1996 Surgeon General's Report on Physical Activity and Health, health promotion efforts aimed at physical activity remains a relatively new field. As such, this is one of many areas of research and practice where the evidence of health promotion effectiveness remains poor or at least insufficient.

Much of the evidence on physical activity interventions that exists, for example from systematic reviews, is derived from controlled studies with experimental or quasi-experimental research designs and using volunteer samples. Whilst these reviews are useful for generating one level of scientific evidence, it may not always provide the kind of field-based evidence required for population-level interventions carried out by health promotion practitioners.

One reason for this is that the scope of health-enhancing physical activity (often referred to as HEPA) interventions has broadened, to extend beyond the focus on only leisure-time physical activity outcomes. This is particularly true in developing countries, where effective interventions might focus on more prevalent domains such as the promotion of active transportation (such as walking or cycling for all or part of trips to destinations), and interventions to maintain active participation in cultural activities and settings. This increased range of settings for promotion of HEPA and related interventions also extends beyond simply working within the health sector; other agencies and partnerships need to be developed, including links to education, transport, urban planning and sport/recreation sectors.

Available physical activity data has mostly reported leisure-time physical activity, and points to generally flat trends, suggesting that in recent years the net sum of health promotion efforts has not made a notable impact on population-levels of leisure-time physical activity. Other domains of physical activity are infrequently measured in surveillance systems, but it is likely that total energy expenditure has declined due to reduced energy expended as part of daily living.

Since total physical activity in all forms, and sometimes total energy expenditure, is of interest, especially for obesity prevention, measurement and monitoring of physical activity remains a major challenge for health promotion. It also poses the challenge for developing broad-based interventions, to address HEPA in more than just the leisure time domain.

This article summarizes the history of efforts to promote physical activity and their effectiveness. It focuses on how the evidence base has developed around physical activity programs, and identifies the remaining challenges for achieving effective physical activity promotion globally.

Assessing the Effectiveness in Physical Activity Promotion

Health promotion has been defined as a combination of processes, including educational, organizational, economic and political actions, designed to affect changes in knowledge, attitude, behaviour and the environment that support and promote health. In addition optimal health promotion includes consumer and stakeholder participation, to enable individuals and communities to exert control over these processes and the determinants of health (WHO, 1986; WHO, 1997).

There are different approaches to identifying "best practice" in assessing health promotion effectiveness. These include rating evidence based on a scientific paradigm, that is the best research design, using the most reliable and valid exposure and outcome measurement and appropriate methods to minimize bias. Effectiveness is considered in the light of a methodological critical appraisal of the intervention: for example, was an experimental design used; was physical activity measured using objective measures; and will the results be generalisable to the source population? Another approach to effectiveness is "best practice" based on health promotion principles and values, which considers questions such as whether the intervention reached the desired population groups, [especially when these are marginalized or disadvantaged and in the case of physical activity interventions the "inactive" population] and whether the intervention is consistent with a health promotion approach. This approach is an appraisal of "best practice" and attempts to assess the potential effectiveness of interventions in achieving population- or community-wide measurable outcomes (Kahan & Goodstadt, 2002).

In the context of physical activity, health promotion interventions seek to increase population levels of physical activity by influencing personal, educational, social and environmental factors that contribute to physical activity behaviour. The determinants and antecedents of physical activity are diverse, and include awareness of the physical activity message and its benefits, attitudes and intentions towards being active, as well as supra-individual factors such as policies, environments and cultural norms that facilitate physical activity. To date, few studies have evaluated true multi-level and multi-strategy interventions using broader socio-ecological theoretical principles. In reality, much of the published research on interventions has been more narrowly focused, using selected (often single) intervention approaches, in defined settings with volunteer samples. Even the most recent distillations of "evidence" (e.g., Kahn et al., 2002) have reported on the body of scientific evidence, and hence recommendations emanate from a review of published (peer reviewed) papers only, around interventions based on mostly educational approaches sometimes using mediated materials (such as telephone, internet or written delivery systems) and often theoretically grounded in individual-based behaviour change models and theories. This body of evidence has been evaluated to assess the overall effectiveness at changing behavior at the individual level but such reviews provide less insight into the effectiveness of implementation and dissemination at the community-wide, population level. And yet it is this question that challenges health promotion practitioners and decision makers on a daily basis!

In addition to reviews of the peer-reviewed scientific literature, there are numerous similar reports in the "grey literature" conducted by Government and non-Government organizations, often conducted by governments who want to know "what works" (Bull et al., 2004; Gebel et al., 2005). The World Health Organisation (WHO, 2006) has developed an implementation framework for the Global Strategy on Diet, Physical Activity and Health (DPAS) and this also provides principles to assess progress towards the implementation of DPAS. One of the key principles that emanates from DPAS is the need for population-level interventions, and the need to move beyond high-risk screening, detection of risk and brief advice; such approaches are not effective in the long term to promote physical activity, and reach only a selected few in the community (Bauman & Craig, 2005).

In the last decade there has been a rapidly evolving body of knowledge and evidence that has shifted in focus from "exercise science" to "health promotion" effectiveness Early research focused on the necessary dose of activity required to gain health benefits, but more recently there is a keen interest in applied research with a focus on testing and developing an evidence base on intervention effectiveness. This has led to a rapid increase in the number of reviews of the literature. One attempt to distill an evidence base was developed by the U.S. Taskforce on Community Preventive Services, and the interventions reviewed were recommended for implementation based on the level and quality of evidence available. Eight categories of interventions have been classified in recent years as having a "strong" or "sufficient" evidence of effectiveness ad these are shown in Table 7.1. The US Centers for Disease Control (CDC) Community Guide provides a useful systematic review and recommendations based on evidence of tested interventions that promote physical activity. These recommendations are a starting point for interventions in developed and developing countries while accounting for their local needs and capabilities (Kahn et al., 2002; Heath et al., 2006; www.thecommunityguide.org/pa/).

One of the clear limitations of the current evidence base is the limited transferability of findings to developing countries. It is only more recently that attempts have been made to specifically identify and integrate evidence from developing countries and consider the transferability of findings. For example, recent efforts in 2005 have developed a framework to describe "good examples"

TABLE 7.1. Summary of recommendations for effective population-based interventions from the U.S. guide to community preventive services

Intervention	Recommendation
Informational approaches	
• Community-wide campaigns	Recommended (strong evidence)
• Point of decision prompts	Recommended (Sufficient evidence)
Behavioral and social approaches to increasing physical activity	
• School-based physical education	Recommended (strong evidence)
• Non-family social support	Recommended (strong evidence)
• Individually adapted health behaviour change	Recommended (strong evidence)
Environmental and policy approaches to increasing physical activity	
• Creation and/or enhanced access to places for physical activity combined with informational outreach activities	Recommended (strong evidence)

Subsequent to the Community Guide, Health and colleagues (2006) examined studies investigating the influence of urban design and land use policies, and concluded two further areas where there was evidence of effectiveness.

• Community-scale urban design and land use policies and practices (zoning regulations, street connectivity, residential and employment density)	Recommended (strong evidence)
• Street-scale design and land use policies and practices (lighting, ease and safety of crossing streets, continuity of footpaths, traffic calming measures and aesthetic enhancements).	Recommended (strong evidence)

of physical activity health promotion, describing principles for assessing the effectiveness of national level programs (WHO, 2005). The evaluation of physical activity programs in developing countries needs to take account of differences in the physical activity domains, the socio-economic and socio-cultural characteristics, and different issues related to the built environment infrastructure and climate, and their impact on everyday "active living" (Gomez et al., 2005; Hallal et al., 2003). The rapid urbanization in developing country cities provides a unique opportunity to evaluate the effects of "natural experiments" in these environments, such as evaluating physical activity impacts of transportation policy changes (Parra et al., 2006).

For example, in developing countries, interventions could have a larger impact if transport-related physical activity is prioritized compared with the focus on leisure-time or recreational physical activity because, in at least some developing countries, physical activity in the transportation domain is more prevalent than leisure-time physical activity (Gomez et al., 2005). Furthermore, it has been observed in developing countries that when socioeconomic conditions improve, the prevalence of car usage increases and physical activity as part of transportation (cycling and walking) will decrease (Bell et al., 2002). Within this context, interventions in developing countries that reinforce benefits of active forms of transport and the maintenance of cultural forms of expression that involve physical activity are likely to be effective ways of maintaining physical activity levels.

It is unlikely that country-or even region-specific systematic reviews will be possible in the near future, or that sufficient evidence exists to develop formal research syntheses at a such levels; thus adapting work carried out through the Community Guide and other organisations (WHO, 2005) through the developing country schemata are the best currently available frameworks. Nonetheless, compiling even a few interventions from different countries and conducting analyses that account for their effects and describe their differences could help in developing the evidence base in the developing world.

One approach to an evidence base, in both developed and developing countries is to use established criteria for effective public health programs and policies, and apply them to physical activity programs. These are suggested as necessary for at least "good practice" in promoting physical activity [adapted from Bull et al., 2004].

Eleven Criteria for Good Practice in Physical Activity Promotion

1. *Consultation* with relevant stakeholders during development of physical activity policy and action plans
2. Adoption of a comprehensive approach to physical activity promotion using *multiple strategies* (e.g., individual-oriented as well as environmental focused interventions) targeting different population groups (e.g. children, adolescents, women, older adults, disabled people, indiginous people)
3. Working at *different levels* (local, state and national as well as individual, whole community and physical environmental level)
4. Development and implementation of the policy and action plan across multiple agencies and settings by *working through coalitions, alliances and partnerships* (e.g. involving cross government, non government as well as relevant private sector partners)
5. *Integration* of physical activity policy within other health and non-health related agendas (e.g. in the field of health, nutrition, transport, environment)
6. *Stable base of support* and resources to implement the policy and action plan (e.g. from politicians and government with or without support from other supporting organisations)
7. Development of an *Identity* for the physical activity program by means of a logo, branding and/or slogan. This may include identifying and cultivating a spokesperson or "champion" for the initiatives as well as an advocacy / communication plan;
8. A clear statement of the *Timeframe* for implementation of the physical activity plan;
9. Specific plans and resources for *Evaluation* of the efforts to promote physical activity

10. Development and/or maintenance of physical activity *Surveillance or Monitoring Systems* which includes suitable population-level measures of levels of physical (in)activity and related factors;

11. Statement of recognition of existing *National guidelines / recommendations on physical activity* or intent to develop them.

One of the difficulties in establishing an evidence base around physical activity interventions has been the issue of measurement of physical activity. This is an ongoing source of debate and academic discourse globally because the measurement of activity is complicated by the multidisciplinary nature of the behaviour and the multiple dimensions and related environments in which activity can occur. A recent review of physical activity measurement for health promotion may assist in the identification of commonly used physical activity and related measures (Bauman et al., 2006a).

The physical activity field has been limited by relatively imprecise measures of the behaviour, predominantly self-reports, and by studies that are mostly cross-sectional in nature. Although self-report measures are reasonably reliable and show "moderate" levels of agreement with objective measurements, self-report measures may overestimate levels of physical activity. In addition, cultural and educational differences make comparisons within and between regions difficult. Effectiveness will be more accurately established when interventions can be assessed by agreed and possibly objective measurement techniques and tools.

There are a vast range of outcomes that might reflect effectiveness as shown in Figure 7.1. This shows a hierarchy of health promotion outcomes. Many of the health outcomes such as mortality, chronic disease incidence and risk factor changes are long-term associations, and may be far removed from physical activity

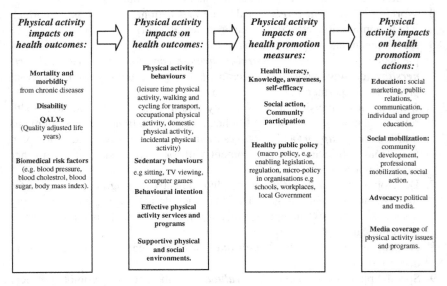

FIGURE 7.1. Hierarchy of indicators of physical activity effectiveness (Adapted from Nutbeam & Bauman, 2006).

```
┌─────────────────────────────────────────────────┐
│                   Formative                      │
│        Was the program developed with due        │
│              attention to the needs              │
│              of the target audience              │
└─────────────────────────────────────────────────┘
```

⇓

```
┌─────────────────────────────────────────────────┐
│                    Process                       │
│   Health promotion intervention processes. Was   │
│   the program implemented as planned? What were  │
│   the effective elements of the dissemination    │
│   and implementation of the intervention? Who    │
│   was engaged? How were they engaged and         │
│   retained in the intervention?                  │
└─────────────────────────────────────────────────┘
```

⇓

```
┌─────────────────────────────────────────────────┐
│             Outcomes (as in Figure 1)            │
│                                                  │
│                 Health outcomes                  │
│       Health promotion impacts and actions       │
└─────────────────────────────────────────────────┘
```

FIGURE 7.2. Formative, process and impact measures of effectiveness.

promotion interventions. Intermediate outcomes such as physiologic measures and fitness may also be measures that could provide challenges for attributing changes to health promotion interventions. Yet a more appropriate evidence framework for physical activity effectiveness would include demonstration of changes in proximal health promotion impacts and outcomes, such as individual, social and environmental attributes that relate directly to the intervention and modifiable determinants for physical activity intervention (Kahn et al., 2002).

In addition to careful measurement, attention should always be paid to implementing appropriate program evaluation in order to generate the best information possible about program development [formative evaluation], program implementation and reach [process evaluation] and short term program impact and effects. These are illustrated in Figure 7.2, and the principles underpinning good evaluation in health promotion practice are described elsewhere (Nutbeam & Bauman, 2006).

Chronology of Physical Activity Practice and Health Promotion

The Emergence of Inactivity as an Important Risk Factor for Health

The Global Burden of Disease is now dominated by the common chronic diseases, notably heart disease, stroke, cancers, type 2 diabetes and mental health.

(WHO, 2004) Physical activity is a central risk factor for many of these conditions, alongside hypertension, lipid levels and tobacco usage. Physical inactivity is both an independent risk factor for these health outcomes and an important contributor to hypertension, blood cholesterol and obesity (Bouchard et al., 2006). For most of these conditions, accumulating half an hour of at least moderate-intensity physical activity on most days of the week is sufficient to achieve these preventive benefits (US DHHS, 1996). Therefore, increasing physical activity and reducing sedentariness has significant potential to deliver substantial health benefits. Physical activity can also reduce the risk of depression, deliver social support to participants and prevent falls in the elderly, and may enhance cognitive function, delay the onset of dementia and improve academic performance in children (Katzmarzyk & Janssen, 2004).

The overall impact of physical inactivity on disease burden is accentuated by its high and increasing prevalence – it is the most prevalent among risk factors in the population, leading to physical activity contributing the largest share of population-attributable risk for chronic disease (Bauman & Miller, 2004). Although much of the current evidence on the benefits of physical activity was in place by 1990, [as we learned from tobacco control] it can take decades to translate an evidence base into public health policy. Physical activity promotion is still in its early development and remains to be developed as a major priority area for health promotion policy action.

The "health case" for Governments and community agencies to give greater priority to increasing physical activity is compelling. However, physical inactivity is not just a health sector issue. Increasing physical activity can also provide benefits by reducing health costs, stimulating economic growth in the sport and recreation sectors, and improving social capital, community safety and cohesion. In these ways, physical activity can contribute to individual and community levels of wellbeing and quality of life. Furthermore, the promotion of different types of physical activities in different settings, particularly for example walking and cycling, can link with other agendas such as cleaner air and reduction in traffic.

The Relationship between Changing Scientific Evidence and Health Promotion Policy and Practice

Before the 1996 US Surgeon General's Report on Physical Activity (USSG, 1996), the primary focus of physical activity promotion emphasized twenty minutes of vigorous-intensity exercise on three days per week to offer health benefits (ACSM, 1978). This more intensive recommendation was grounded in leisure-time physical activity, and offered little chance of adoption by completely sedentary or older adults. However, the evidence was re-appraised during the 1990s, and revised recommendations indicated that "at least half an hour of any form of moderate-intensity physical activity, on most days of the week was sufficient to accrue health benefits" (USSG, 1996). These revised "moderate-intensity" guidelines enabled governments, including agencies other than health and sport sectors, to engage with a component of the physical activity promotion agenda. Examples of this broader approach include programs and campaigns that promoted walking in multiple settings, such as for short transport trips; the promotion of physical activity as part of everyday activities, often referred to as "active living"; and the recommendation of accumulating even short bouts of incidental physical activity, such as using the stairs instead of the elevator.

A transformation in the global burden of disease to a state where chronic diseases dominate has heightened interest in effective methods for chronic disease prevention. Similarly, the emergence of physical inactivity as a central risk factor for chronic disease and a developing science about health-enhancing physical activity has impacted on approaches taken to promote population physical activity. In parallel, the emerging science of health promotion has led to new paradigms of thinking about and approaching chronic disease prevention.

Overall, contemporary efforts around the promotion of physical activity are more consistent with the original intent of the 1986 Ottawa Charter, namely the focus of interventions has shifted emphasis to a balance of approaches recognizing the behavioral, policy, environment and structural determinants of health behavior (WHO, 1986). Moreover, the promotion of physical activity is a particularly good example of the need for developing interagency partnerships as outlined in the Jakarta health promotion conference (Jakarta Declaration WHO, 1997). The chronology of the events described above are summarised in Table 7.2.

Translation of Evidence, Dissemination and Workforce Development and Training

In recent years there has been an increase in the avenues for dissemination of research findings of effective practices in physical activity. In particular, there has been an increase in published research in peer reviewed journals including dissemination of examples of evaluated programs. There has also been the development of publications dedicated to the topic such as the *Journal of Physical Activity and Health*, which publishes original research and review papers examining the relationship between physical activity and health, as well as the *International Journal of Behavioural Nutrition and Physical Activity*. In addition other journals have dedicated special Issues to focus on physical activity; these include the *American Journal of Health Promotion*, the *American Journal of Preventive Medicine*, and the IUHPE Journal *Promotion & Education*.

Until recent times there have been few conferences, or training opportunities directed at the physical activity workforce. However, with the increase in interest in physical activity there has been a renewed interest in providing training and professional development for those working in the field. There have been several efforts at capacity building through the development of international training courses in Physical Activity and Public Health (PAPH). These started with annual PAPH courses in the USA (hosted by the University of South Carolina and the CDC since 1995) and has developed into short courses being conducted in developed and developing countries, including Australia, Brazil,

TABLE 7.2. Chronology of physical activity practice and health promotion

Physical activity scientific development	Key physical activity scientific papers and documents	Year	Physical activity Health Promotion development	Key physical activity health promotion documents
First published evidence of health benefits of physical activity	Morris 1953	Pre 1980	Health education. Individual behaviour focus. Exercise focus. Focus on fitness change.	
American College of Sports Medicine recommendations 1978 that 'aerobic and vigorous' exercise is required for health	ACSM, 1978			
Landmark research indicates the health benefits of moderate intensity PA	Paffenbarger Blair 1989	1980s	Focus on health promotion models started but not well developed for PA until later	1986 Ottawa Charter on Health promotion
Continued research confirms benefits of moderate-intensity PA, walking		1990–1995	Evidence for the Health benefits of physical activity 'conclusive'	1993, AHA Statement elevates PA as a risk factor
Shift towards recognizing community based approaches as well as previously, where 'exercise training in clinical settings' was the norm.	1996 US Surgeon Generals Report on Physical Activity and Health	1995–1999	Acknowledgement of individual, environmental and policy influences on physical activity	1997, Jakarta Declaration on Health Promotion
			Growing interest in ecological models of physical activity	1997, AHA Plan for a strategic approach to PA
			Growing partnerships with sectors outside health	
Growing Research focus on the physical and built environments and their relationship to physical activity in leisure time, in active transport and in other settings	Active Living Research	2000–2005	Formation of Regional and International Physical activity networks	CDC Community Guide published to summarize program effectiveness [2002]
	Special issues of AJHP Special issue on AJPH Several issues of AJPM		Risk of obesity distracting from the physical activity focus and medicalizing it.	Formation of RAFA/PANA, HEPA and AP-PAN networks
Obesity epidemic gives new impetus to the PA movement and a new focus for research and advocacy	2004, WHO Global Strategy on Diet, Physical Activity and Health			Agita Mundo (Move for Health) movement
Increased focus on PA and environments				Joint statement of AHA, ACS, and DA on PA
Focus on upstream thinking and underlying determinants.				

	First International Congress on Physical Activity and Public Health	2006	First International Congress on Physical Activity and Public Health, Atlanta formation of the Global Alliance for Physical Activity (GAPA)

Likely future directions in physical activity scientific development.

The future — Likely future directions in physical activity health Promotion development.

Understanding measurement and impacts of:
- Inactivity (sitting less)
- Socio-demographic variations
- Physical activity variations among and within countries from the developed and developing world
- Economic impacts
- Environments and perceptions
- Advocacy processes
- Policy change
- Cultural norms
- Relationship of PA to cognitive function and decline.
- How to balance physical activity for transport and for leisure in rapidly urbanizing populations of the developing world.

Increased focus on
- Global Network development
- Implement Global and national Physical activity Plans around the global strategy on Diet, Physical Activity and Health (WHO 2004)
- Develop Cross sector development and partnerships, especially with transport, urban planning and Education sectors
- Interventions that address inequity and diversity
- Continued focus on developing evidence base through trialing interventions that influence physical and social environments
- Increased focus on advocacy and policy focused interventions
- Advocacy for recognition of physical activity as a whole-of-Government policy priority
- Prioritizing physical activity within over-weight and obesity programs, and independently of them
- Interventions to reduce the adverse effects on transport-related physical activity as car ownership increases and walkability decreases in developing countries.

Canada, Chile, Colombia, Costa Rica, Mexico and Scotland. Most recently a course has been implemented in the Asia-Pacific region (Malaysia) and others are planned for the African region and elsewhere in Latin America, Europe and the Asia-Pacific.

In addition, in 2006, the CDC auspiced the first International Congress on Physical Activity and Public Health held in Atlanta. This congress celebrated 10 years of progress since the US Surgeon General's Report on Physical Activity and Health in 1996. The congress was attended by over 900 delegates representing 44 countries. There has also been an increase in physical activity content of international health promotion conferences such as those conducted by the IUHPE in 2004 and 2007.

A further development that can assist in communicating and disseminating best practice is the development of international, trans-national and national movements to promote physical activity. Global and regional network development has occurred through the WHO's *Move for Health*, the *Agita Mundo* movement in South America, RAFA/PANA in Latin America (RAFA, 2006), regional networks for physical activity promotion in Europe (http://www.euro.who.int/hepa) and in the Asia-Pacific region (http://www.ap-pan.org). In addition, the Global Alliance for Physical Activity (GAPA) is providing a coordinating and linkage function across global efforts to promote physical activity. Communication networks have also been established at the country level in both developed and developing countries. For example, in Colombia, the Colombian Physical Activity Network has been established (or REDCOLAF: *In Spanish* Red Columbiana de Actividad Fisica) (REDCOLAF, 2006). A further development in Australia is the establishment of a national web and e-communication-based information dissemination network *The Australian Physical Activity Network (or AusPAnet)*. These initiatives hold promise for the increased dissemination and implementation of best practices and may facilitate the replication and in some cases institutionalization of effective health promotion practices. This would improve the current situation where the dissemination of good practice physical activity programs has been haphazard, little studied or understood, and often driven by factors other than evidence (Bauman et al., 2006b).

Case Studies of National-Level / Regional-Level Interventions

Emerging from the physical activity literature are examples of programs that show promise. Table 7.3 presents case studies from developed and developing countries of key programs, and demonstrates their setting and their effective components. It should be noted that the evidence to promote physical activity sometimes emanates from cross-sectional studies which really do not provide strong evidence of "effectiveness". Therefore much of the current evidence might be regarded as weak from a scientific "methodological" perspective, and the need to build better research designs into these projects is a critical aspect for the future evidence base.

TABLE 7.3. Examples of national-level and regional level interventions that show promise

Program	Description	Effective elements	How demonstrated
Ciclovia and Recreovia program. Bogotá Colombia. (Gomez et al., 2004; Gómez et al., 2006)	Ciclovia: 117 kilometers of main avenues are dedicated exclusively to recreational and sports activities on Sundays and Holidays from 7 am to 2 pm. On average about 1.4 million people participate per month. Cost for year 2006 was 1.5 million US dollars. Recreovia: Aerobic classes in 20 points of the Ciclovia	- Women who frequently participate in the Ciclovia are more likely to meet CDC recommendations (Gomez et al. 2004) - 20% of Ciclovia participants meet CDC recommendations during leisure time - Adults who use the Ciclovia are more likely to report biking as a means of transport. - 2005 creation of the Bicycle Network of the Americas (In Spanish: Ciclovias Unidas de las Américas) including 9 countries and 14 cities. (http://www.ciudadhumana.org/cicloviasunidas/red.htm)	Case studies and cross-sectional studies
Active transport in Bogotá, Colombia	Transmilenio: The new bus rapid transit system with fixed stations Ciclo-Rutas: Network of 320 km of bike paths	- Adults who live in blocks near Transmilenio stations are more likely to walk as a means of transport - Men who perceived that Ciclorutas were closer were more likely to use bicycles as a means of transport	cross-sectional studies
Community mobilization in Agita Sao Paulo	Multilevel intervention to promote physical activity in Sao Paulo. Since 1996 – present	Mass awareness raising through clear identified program logo and brand, developed multi-channel social marketing, and mass interventions targeting multiple sectors and populations, especially in Sao Paulo city; the development of regional plans and networks, and a Manifesto written for PA. (Matsudo SM et al: 2006b)	Various designs for different elements, including qualitative and quantitative research methods; serial cross section population based surveys, cohorts, and clinical exercise measures in small sub-samples

(Continued)

TABLE 7.3. (Continued)

Program	Description	Effective elements	How demonstrated
Cross Government PA Taskforces in Australia	Examples include the state based intersectoral taskforces around physical activity established in New South Wales [1996–2004] and in Western Australia [2001 onwards]	Clear mandate for inter-agency partnership to promote physical activity; these coalitions mainly of government agencies, but partners including NGOs such as the Heart Foundation, physicians societies, and the private sector	Demonstrated initially through process evaluation, with clear work plans, accountable agencies, and monitoring of the implementation of state level PA plans; overarching monitoring through PA surveillance as part of state health surveys
Active living programs funded by the RWJ Foundation in the USA	Programs of research and practice around active communities, ageing and physical activity, and the environment and PA funded through the philanthropic group, Robert Wood Johnson Foundation	Building through careful research and practice, the evidence base for measurement, action and policy in these areas, especially the physical environment and PA; three groups funded to lead this program of work	Better evidence base; optimal methods used for each funded project

The programs in Table 7.3 are diverse however there are a number of characteristics that have added to their effectiveness. These include:

• Theoretical underpinning of program design, with clearly articulated logic models
• Scientific underpinning of moderate intensity physical activity, with a population focus for promotion
• Well defined and feasible program goals
• Partnerships and inter-agency collaboration well defined and developed, with clear partner accountabilities
• Comprehensive methodology employed using multiple strategies
• Well evaluated, with measures of success well matched to goals and intervention.

Remaining Challenges in Demonstrating Physical Activity Effectiveness

Despite significant progress, physical activity promotion remains a "new" field. It is still dominated and dwarfed by other areas, including traditional ones [tobacco control], and new areas, such as obesity prevention, where the evidence and population burden may be smaller than that attributed to physical inactivity, but the funding and political interest is much larger. There are many areas of physical activity research and practice where the evidence of effectiveness is insufficient, or can only at best be described as "promising". In this last section we discuss remaining challenges for physical activity promotion. These challenges reduce the capacity for physical activity to be promoted in countries and regions, act as barriers to health promotion action and have inhibited political interest in physical activity. First, physical activity is not resourced commensurate with its potential to promote health. This requires ongoing advocacy to foster political commitment and policy development. Optimal physical activity promotion works within and outside the health sector, and interagency partnerships, co-funding and joint planning are needed, but slow to establish. These issues are particularly difficult in developing and rapidly urbanizing countries. Those who plan and build our built environments and transport systems are critical future partners in addressing physical inactivity. So too, policy makers in key settings such as schools, workplaces and local Government preside over policy decisions with significant impact on physical activity. The cross-disciplinary nature of the field also presents methodological challenges, including engaging with researchers, policy makers and practitioners outside the health sector. This will require working in different ways and in entirely different paradigms.

Our understanding of "inactivity" or "sedentariness" is limited. The changing workplace and economies, transport systems and lifestyles have lead to increased hours of inactivity and sitting time, both at work and at home. In this area, we have little understanding of effective health promotion approaches to encourage people to "sit less and move more". Given the increasing cultural predilection for sedentary recreation and occupations, it is likely that influencing sedentariness will require well-funded social marketing campaigns, to re-frame "active living" and persuade populations to spend less time sitting.

Physical activity needs differ throughout the life cycle. Our understanding of the specific elements of effective practices that work with different age groups and sub populations is not well developed. In addition, socio-demographic inequalities are important drivers of ill-health and chronic disease. A disproportionate burden of inactivity is experienced in poorer and less educated populations. Despite this, evidence is limited regarding effective physical activity interventions for targeting minorities, low socio-economic status (SES) groups and marginalized sub-populations at highest risk.

Predominant technology and social changes in recent decades have been to the detriment of physical activity. We have engineered physical activity out of our lives and out of our culture. How do we reverse this process? How do we better understand the successful cases of "bucking the trend", e.g. continued prevalence and cultural norm of cycling in The Netherlands, and the success of the *Ciclovia* (Montezuma et al., 2006) in Bogotá in reclaiming the streets.

Economic analyses of the cost of physical inactivity, cost effectiveness of interventions and cost benefits of increasing physical activity is an important driver of policy decisions by Governments. Therefore developing a better understanding of the economics of inactivity is likely to be a powerful political advocacy lever. Economic justifications for investing in physical activity interventions are poorly developed (Pratt et al., 2004; Sturm, 2005).

Despite the increased profile of physical activity, most national Governments still do not have a formal and specific National Physical Activity Plan. Currently, physical activity doesn't exist in health plans, or is subsumed under obesity or non-communicable disease prevention plans. Since many of the effector arms and partnerships around promoting physical activity are outside the health sector, then whole of Government integrated physical activity plans are required. Such formal plans can increase the profile and visibility of physical activity, and act as a rallying point for action. When Governments take the lead on developing such plans, this will allow non-Government agencies to focus their attention on disease-specific, or strategy specific interventions.

National plans and polices have the potential to have cross-community population impact, and relative to individual behavioral approaches have greater opportunity to be sustained over time. Policy approaches are frequently inexpensive as they may apply existing resources. An example of a policy approach would be to ensure that the education sector to provide all children with increased time (30 mins/day) and increased quality of physical education classes throughout their schooling.

For all of the above challenges, physical activity needs to be better positioned and therefore, physical activity advocacy should be a priority strategy. A continued lack of high priority afforded to physical activity by national governments has attenuated health promotion efforts to promote physical activity, and despite the WHO's Global Strategy on Diet, Physical Activity and Health (2004), physical activity has become subservient to the obesity and nutrition agendas.

TABLE 7.4. Recommended advocacy approaches to better position physical activity in relation to government, media and community agendas

Community issues	Advocacy opportunities for physical activity
Economy	Articulate the economic burden of inactivity and benefits of increased physical activity
Environment	Relate physical activity targets to clean air, decongested roads and livable communities as well as health benefits
Crime and safety	Position physical activity, especially increased walking in neighborhoods, as a strategy to increase community safety and lower crime
Fuel	Position walking and cycling as 'solutions', healthy, green and inexpensive transport modes
Children	Inactivity threatens the health of our next generation, with dire consequences for health, productivity, economy and even national security. Our children are our future
Grass roots culture	Link physical activity to local political issues and target local representatives accordingly

Physical activity professionals need to better understand the science and the art of advocacy and apply these talents more effectively. This will require better articulation of the evidence arguments, a better articulated physical activity agenda (best buys) and a strategic approach to advocacy (Shilton, 2006). These approaches need to be applied to elevate the political status of physical activity. The status of physical activity can be advanced by advocacy around the health issues and benefits. However, in addition opportunities exist for advocates to align physical activity with the "big issues" that capture political, public and media spotlight. Examples of this are outlined in Table 7.4.

Conclusion

We have examined the meaning of effectiveness in the context of physical activity and described the advances that have resulted in physical activity effectiveness being demonstrated. In addition we have identified some of the recent approaches to disseminating effective practice and developing and distributing evidence-based recommendations to the field. Physical activity has become better recognised in recent years, but there is much that we still don't understand. Remaining challenges include understanding effective practice in developing countries and in sub-populations with increased needs. While the epidemiological evidence for the health of physical activity are strong, this has not yet translated into prioritisation of physical activity initiatives, nor the development and implementation of national physical activity action plans and polices. This discrepancy between the evidence and the commitment points to a need to prioritise and resource strategic approaches to physical activity advocacy (Shilton, 2006).

If our ultimate measure of our effectiveness is increased population levels of physical activity, then clearly we have a long way to go. However, there is much from which we can take encouragement. A challenge is to identify why some programs have been able to demonstrate effectiveness, and how they have demonstrated effectiveness. The most significant challenge is one of advocacy, to ensure that global and national commitments are made to advancing physical activity action plans, mobilizing resources and affording priority to implementation of those plans.

References

ACSM (1978), American College of Sports Medicine position statement on the recommended quantity and quality of exercise for developing and maintaining fitness in healthy adults. *Medicine and Science in Sports*, 10(3), vii–x.

Bauman AE & Craig CL. (2005). The place of physical activity in the WHO Global Strategy on Diet and Physical Activity. *International Journal of Behavioural Nutrition and Physical Activity*, 2, 10.

Bauman AE & Miller Y. (2004). The public health potential of health enhancing physical activity (HEPA), in *Health enhancing physical activity, Vol 6, Multidisciplnary Perspectives of Physical Education and Sport Science*, Eds: Oja P, Borms J Meyer and Meyer Sport publishers, Oxford UK, 2004, pp 125–149.

Bauman AE, Nelson DE, Pratt M, Matsudo V & Schoeppe S. (2006a). Dissemination of physical activity evidence, programs, policies, and surveillance in the international public health arena. *American Journal of Preventive Medicine*, 31(4 Suppl), 57–65.

Bauman AE, Phongsavan P, Schoeppe S & Owen N. (2006b). Physical activity measurement – a primer for health promotion. *Promotion & Education*, 13, 92–103.

Bell AC, Ge K & Popkin BM. (2002). The road to obesity or the path to prevention: Motorized transportation and obesity in China. *Obesity Research*, 10(4), 277–283.

Bouchard C, Blair SN, Haskell WL. (eds) (2006). *Physical activity and Health*, Human Kinetics Publishers, Illinois.

Bull FC, Bellew B, Schöppe S & Bauman AE. (2004). Developments in National Physical Activity Policy: An international review and recommendations towards better practice. *Journal of Science and Medicine in Sport*, 7,1(Suppl), 93–104.

Ciclovías Unidas d las Américas. http://www.ciudadhumana.org/cicloviasunidas/red.htm. Accessed on October 2006.

Gebel K, King L, Bauman A, Vita P, Gill T, Rigby A, Capon A. *Creating healthy environments – a review of links between the physical environment, physical activity and obesity*. Sydney. NSW Health Department and NSW Centre for Overweight and Obesity. 2005. [monograph, http://www.coo.health.usyd.edu.au/publications/reports.shtml#CH].

Gomez LF, Mateus JC & Cabrera G. (2004). Leisure-time physical activity among women in a neighborhood in Bogotá, Colombia: Prevalence and socio-demographic correlates. *Cad Saude Publica*, 20(4), 1103–1109.

Gomez LF, Sarmiento OL, Lucumí D, Espinosa G & Forero R. (2005). Prevalence and factors associated with walking and bicycling for transport among young adults in two low-income localities of Bogotá, Colombia. *Journal of Physical Activity and Health*, 2, 445–459.

Gomez LF, Sarmiento OL, Mosquera J, Jacoby E. (2006). Influence of the built environment on physical activity and quality of life in Bogotá Colombia. *International*

Congress on Physical Activity and Public Health, 17–20, April 2006. Atlanta, Georgia USA.

Hallal PC, Victora CG, Wells JC & Lima RC. (2003). Physical inactivity: Prevalence and associated variables in Brazilian adults. *Medicine and Science in Sport and Exercise*, 35(11), 1894–1900.

Heath G, Brownson R, Kruger J, Miles R, Powell K, Ramsey L. and the Task Force on Community Preventive Services (2006). The effectiveness of urban design and land use and transport policies and practices to increase physical activity: A systematic review. *Journal of Physical Activity and Health*, 1, S55–S71.

Kahan B & Goodstadt M. (March, 2002). *IDM Manual for using the Interactive Domain Model approach to best practices in health promotion*, Centre for Health Promotion, University of Toronto, Toronto.

Kahn EB et al. (2002). The effectiveness of interventions to increase physical activity – A systematic review. *American Journal of Preventive Medicine*, 22(4S), 73–107.

Katzmarzyk PT, Janssen I. (2004). The economic costs associated with physical inactivity and obesity in Canada: An update. *Canadian Journal of Applied Physiology*, 29, 90–115.

Matsudo SM et al. (2006b). Evaluation of a physical activity promotion program: The example of Agita Sao Paulo. *Evaluation and Program Planning*, 29, 301–311.

Montezuma R, Neiman AB, Jacoby ER. (2006). Ciclovías de Las Americas. *International Congress on Physical Activity and Public Health*. 17–20, April 2006, Atlanta, Georgia USA.

Nutbeam D & Bauman A. (2006). *Evaluation in a Nutshell: A practical guide to the evaluation of health promotion programs*, McGraw-Hill, Sydney.

RAFA (2006), Physical Activity Network of the Americas. Available at http://www.rafapana.org/ Accessed on October 2006.

REDCOLAF (2006), Red Colombiana de Actividad Física REDCOLAF. Available at http://www.redcolaf.org/ Accessed on October 2006.

Parra D, Gómez LF, Pratt M, Sarmiento OL & Triche E. (2006). Urban changes in Bogotá and their possible influence with physical activity levels. *Active Living Research Meeting*, San Diego February 16–18, 2006.

Pratt M, Macera CA, Sallis JF, O'Donnell M, Frank LD. (2004). Economic interventions to promote physical activity: Application of the SLOTH model. *American Journal of Preventive Medicine*, 27,3(Suppl), 136–145.

Shilton TR. (2006). Advocacy for physical activity – from evidence to influence. *Promotion & Education*, 13(2), 118–126.

Sturm R. (2005). Economics and physical activity: A research agenda. *American Journal of Preventive Medicine*, 28,2(Suppl 2), 141–149.

U.S. Department of Health and Human Services. (1996). *Physical Activity and Health: A Report of the US Surgeon General*, National Centers for Disease Control, Atlanta, Georgia.

U.S. Department of Health and Human Services. (Accessed October 2006). www.thecommunityguide.org/pa/ U.S. Taskforce on Community Preventive Services, US Centers for Disease Control (CDC).

World Health Organization. (1986). *Ottawa Charter for Health Promotion*, World Health Organization, Geneva.

World Health Organization. (1997). *The Jakarta Declaration on Health Promotion in the 21st Century*, World Health Organization, Geneva.

World Health Organization. (2004). *The WHO Global Strategy on Diet Physical Activity and Health*, World Health Organization, Geneva.

World Health Organization. (2005). *Review of best practice in interventions to promote physical activity in developing countries. A report prepared by Bauman A, Schoeppe S, Lewicka M with technical assistance by Armstrong T, commissioned by WHO Headquarters/Geneva and funded by the WHO Centre for Health Development Kobe/Japan*, World Health Organization, Geneva.

World Health Organization. (2006). *Implementation framework for the global strategy on diet, physical activity and health*, World Health Organization, Geneva.

8
School Health Promotion
Achievements, Challenges and Priorities

LAWRENCE ST. LEGER, LLOYD KOLBE, ALBERT LEE,
DOUGLAS S. MCCALL AND IAN M. YOUNG

Health Promotion in Schools – The Context for a Consideration of Evidence

Are schools effective in building the health and well-being of their students? What evidence do we have to explore this question and what are the gaps? What do we need to do in the next decade to improve the quality of the evidence and the ways we collect, interpret and disseminate it?

This chapter addresses these questions. However, before they are examined, it is important to provide a brief explanation about school health and what actually happens in schools to promote the health and well-being of the school, its students and employees.

Schools have long been viewed as important settings for promoting the health and social development of children. In many countries, the first schools were often established by churches, charities and other Non Government Organisations (NGOs), to socialize and take care of the children whose parents had moved into cities during industrialization. Later, health education was introduced in schools, driven primarily by the medical fraternity with exhortations about the dangers of various diseases. The school was, and still is, seen by many as a site for health messages, materials, and prevention programs. Consequently, we have seen a wide variety of issue-specific and narrowly framed approaches to school health promotion come, stay or go across the educational landscape. Active schools (designed to increase physical activity), drug-free schools (designed to prevent drug use in, near, and beyond school), and safe schools (designed to prevent intentional and unintentional physical and psychological harm) are just three examples of approaches developed in response to specific societal health issues. Interestingly, these health driven models developed separately from models derived from the human services sector such as community schools (which utilize the school building, during and after school hours, and community agencies collectively to benefit principally students, but also the broader community) or full-service schools (which provide a wide range of medical, dental, psychological, social, and other services within or very near the school). The education sector also developed their own holistic models, including effective schools (with: a safe and orderly environment; climate of high expectations for success; effective instructional leadership; clear and focused mission, opportunity to learn and student time on task; frequent monitoring of student progress; and home-school relations) and learning communities which encourage teachers and local community groups collectively to design and adapt their teaching methods and goals to address the unique needs of students and stakeholders in their own communities).

Interestingly, the health driven models developed separately from models derived in the education sector such as community schools and full service schools. These were terms applied to a whole of school approach in addressing educational actions to build stronger links with the community, extend the services (e.g. psychological and health) available to students and staff, create supportive social and physical environments and extend the curriculum beyond the classroom. It is not surprising that those working within schools feel pressured by the expectations placed on them by of these congruent but sometimes competing frameworks, particularly where they see similarities or differences in the different models.

Another approach, which combined teaching and learning with the delivery of preventive health services and measures to maintain a healthy physical and social environment in the school, emerged in Europe and North America in the 1980s and 1990s (Allensworth & Kolbe, 1987; Young & Williams, 1989). This multi-faceted approach gained impetus from the emerging, concepts and principles about health promotion that were reflected in the Ottawa Charter (WHO, 1984; WHO, 1986).

The concept of school-based and school-linked health promotion evolved along similar, yet slightly different paths on five continents. In Europe it was called the Health Promoting School (Young & Williams, 1989). With the support of the European Commission and the Council of Europe, the European Network for Health Promotion Schools (ENHPS) was established and is now present in over 43 countries in the region. In North America, the concept of Comprehensive School Health Education was used widely in the 1980s denoting a curriculum-focused approach. This was broadened in the 1990s to "Coordinated" and "Comprehensive" programs and approaches to depict the use of multiple interventions from multiple agencies. (Kolbe, 1993; WHO, 1991). The Western Pacific Region of the WHO developed "Guidelines for Health Promoting Schools" for its 32 member states in 1995 (WHO, 1996). Developments similar to these have fostered Health Promoting Schools (HPS) and Coordinated School Health (CSH) in Latin America, North America, South America, the Middle East, Asia, and Africa.

However, there is still confusion about what school health is, which has major implications for assessing its effectiveness. The WHO Expert Committee (1997) noted some confusion with the concept. Is it an **outcome** (a "healthy" school), an **approach** (emphasis on different agencies working together), a set of **values** (based on a holistic view of health and well-being), an issue **specific program** (coordinated interventions to prevent one problem) or a **coordinated set of programs and services** (to address several health problems or to promote health in general)? Clearly, each of these perspectives led to different measures of success.

Schools are primarily focused on maximizing educational opportunities and outcomes for their students. How does the HPS/CSH approach contribute to enhancing learning processes and educational outcomes? If we truly recognize this as the main priority of the education sector, what does this mean for measuring effectiveness? Measurements of the effectiveness and quality of health promotion in schools need to take account of the mainstream methods used in the education system if they are to be valued by schools (Young, 2005).

There is a consolidated body of evidence which indicates that healthy students learn better and that improving the knowledge, competencies and health status of the young people will improve learning outcomes (WHO, 1997; Sinnott, 2005; National Foundation for Education Research, 2004; Scottish Council for Research in Education, 2002; Taras, 2005a; Taras, 2005b; Taras & Potts-Datema, 2005a; Taras & Potts-Datema, 2005b). In addition, in most countries, the health and education systems share similar values about what underpins educational experiences at school. Some of these common values include respect for self and others; respect for lifelong learning; respect for the environment; and upholding principles of social justice and equity.

We need to view schools as a means or setting through which several sectors can promote health, academic achievement and social development (Tones, 2005). This will mean that the measures for success and the evidence of effectiveness will include a mixture of health indicators and educational measures. What we choose to assess, and what values we place on the data, will affect how different sectors perceive the effectiveness of health-related initiatives in schools.

Evidence of Effectiveness of School Health

What Types of Evidence are Reported and Valued?

The answer to this question depends on the sector undertaking the evaluation. In schools, teachers usually wish to see if students have attained the knowledge and competencies of the health curriculum. Procedures are put in place to check knowledge, understanding, ability to analyze health data, skills in synthesizing and evaluating information and in creating or designing an action or strategy, e.g. a balanced diet for a week. Many believe the education sector should not measure personal health behavior changes as a result of the school-based health promotion program, nor attempt to assess an education program on health in terms of biological measures (e.g., reduce excessive BMI, cholesterol levels, etc.). Schools simply should assess if the educational components of their program have been achieved. Many school health programs are written in educational language focused on achieving educational outcomes relating to knowledge and understanding, skill development and to demonstrate an ability to explore attitudinal issues in the affective domain, e.g. gain an appreciation of . . .; list the factors which . . .; assess the issues . . .; evaluate alternatives to . . .; demonstrate the procedures to . . .

The health sector usually seeks evidence to ascertain if the "intervention" has resulted in a reduction in health risk behaviours and/or an increase in protective health behaviours, and sometimes changes in health status. The word "intervention" is often used as it indicates a special program or project over a finite amount of time, which focuses on a health issue, e.g. nutrition, sexuality, oral health. Evaluation of such studies regularly involves control groups and the application of evaluation methods designed to check if the intervention design produced the desired behavioral outcome(s) or health status changes. For example, in a physical activity program, the measures could include increased physical activity (behavior) and/or changes in aerobic capacity (health status).

The evidence suggests it is possible to have changes in student's health behaviors through school health initiatives. However, it appears that in order to achieve these outcomes the "intervention" (educational initiative or whole school program) needs to be of substantial intensity, exist over a number of years and connect with student's families, their peer group, relevant agencies, professionals, and the community. There is evidence to support the view that multiple approaches have stronger effects than, for example, a classroom-only approach if behavior changes or changes in health status are the goals. The resources to support these interventions are substantial and often rely on the health sector or donor organizations to fund them. This level of support is often beyond the expectations, priorities, and resources of schools.

Teachers adapt and modify programs and learning experiences according to needs, knowledge and interests of students. The classroom and school is a flexible place with lessons and activities being shaped, modified and contextualized by the issues of the day and certain school-based policies, practices and priorities (e.g., theme days, excursions, illnesses, and time limitations). The complexity of school communities can also make it difficult to find control groups that take account of all the important variables that could influence the outcomes in a comparative experimental study. In addition there are potential ethical issues in depriving control schools of particular innovative approaches which could be beneficial to improving education and/or health outcomes.

There is clearly a tension between what constitutes evidence for the education and health sectors and what benchmarks should be applied to the methodologies to ascertain if the evidence is admissible (Kemm, 2006). This tension occurs because both sectors often have different expectations of a school health program. Schools see learning as cumulative over the time a student is in school (up to 12 years and usually at least 6). Literacy, numeracy, and other core school programs build knowledge and competencies over many years, taking into account a student's cognitive and physical development. They don't expect major behavioral outcomes in less than one year, or even after two or three. The evidence shows that it is unrealistic to expect health "interventions" which are supported with limited and short-term funding, to make much difference in behavior change.

Recently, there has been an increased focus on looking at the evidence of quality practice in schools to assess if schools are undertaking their health promotion and education work in ways that reflect the evidence of effectiveness.

The frameworks of HPS/CSH are based solidly on the evidence of effective schooling, integrated approaches to health improvement and recognition of those components in school communities which influence health (e.g., policies, environment, partnerships, and skill acquisition). Evidence has been gathered extensively about what schools actually do in health promotion using the HPS/CSH framework (Lee, St.Leger & Moon, 2005; Marshall et al., 2000). This "audit" type evidence has provided schools and health and education authorities with comprehensive maps about what is happening and how comprehensive it is. It is proving very useful in assisting schools and authorities to concentrate on the gaps and to provide opportunities to affirm quality work in schools through award systems (Moon et al., 1999; Lee, Cheng & St. Leger, 2005).

Science has already demonstrated the benefits for young people of a healthy diet, appropriate physical activity, correct hygiene practices, social connectedness, etc. More effective and useful evaluations for school health initiatives need to unpack the circumstances that enable or inhibit the achievement of these goals, rather than only seek to prove that the program changes health status or certain behaviors.

Achievements of School Health Promotion

There have been many published evaluations of school health initiatives in the last twenty years. In the last decade researchers have interrogated this body of evidence in meta-analyses to synthesize the findings of the studies. These findings have subsequently generated evidence-based guidelines for school health promotion that also draw on evidence from the educational literature about innovation and change in schools, leadership and educational outcomes.

It is not the purpose of this chapter to summarise these studies in detail. Table 8.1 provides some of the examples of the meta-analyses and the evidence-based guidelines for whole school health.

Recent evidence suggests that the way the school is lead and managed, the experiences students have to participate and take responsibility for shaping policies, practices and procedures, how teachers relate to and treat students and how the school engages with its local community (including parents) in partnership work, actually builds many health protective factors and reduces risk taking behavior (Stewart-Brown, 2006; Blum et al., 2002, Patton, Bond, Carlin, Thomas, Butler, Glover, Catalano & Bowes, 2006). Many of these gains have occurred without a specific health "intervention." It appears that a whole school approach which encourages and recognizes student participation and which overtly addresses the building and maintenance of a caring school social environment may be the most effective way in achieving both health and educational outcomes.

The school health promotion programmes that were effective in changing young people's health or health-related behaviour were more likely to be complex, multifactorial and involve activity in more than one domain (curriculum, school environment and community). These are features of the health promoting schools approach, and to this extent these findings endorse such approaches. The findings of the synthesis also support intensive interventions of long duration. These were shown to be more likely to be effective than

TABLE 8.1. Major studies of effectiveness

Issue	Evaluations, Analyses and Reviews
• Nutrition	Gortmaker et al. (1999) Campbell et al. (2001) Sahota et al. (2001)
• Physical Activity	Dobbins et al. (2001) Timperio et al. (2004)
• Sexuality	Silva (2002) Kirby (2002)
• Drugs	Tobler & Stratton (1997) Lloyd et al. (2000) Midford et al. (2000) National Drug Research Institute (2002)
• Mental Health	Browne et al. (2004) Wells et al. (2003) Green et al. (2005) American Counselling Association (2006)
• Whole School Approach Health Promoting School (HPS) Coordinated School Health (CSH)	Lister-Sharp et al. (1999) Blum et al. (2002) West, Sweeting & Leyland (2004) Patton et al. (2006) Stewart-Brown (2006)
• Quality Practice Guidelines	European Network of Health Promoting Schools (1997) United States' Centers for Disease Control and Prevention (2003) Clift & Jensen (2005) Lee et al. (2006) St.Leger (2005) Task Force on Community Prevention Services (2006)

interventions of short duration and low intensity. This again reflects the Health Promoting Schools approach, which is intensive and needs to be implemented over a long period of time. (Stewart-Brown, 2006, p17)

A Framework for Research and Evaluation in School Health Promotion

School health initiatives have been or can be conceptualised with a focus, alternatively or in combination as:

A. Specific Outcomes
B. Essential School Health Promotion Processes
C. Evaluation Approaches (from both health and education perspectives)

As shown in Table 8.2, the *School Health Promotion Outcomes* component identifies all those outcomes where there is evidence to support the particular achievement. Part B, *School Health Promotion Processes*, identifies the diversity

TABLE 8.2. A framework for research and evaluation in school health promotion

A. School Health Promotion Outcomes
  - Health knowledge, attitudes, skills, intents
  - Health behaviours
  - Health outcomes
  - Education participation
  - Cognitive performance
  - Education achievement
  - Social outcomes
  - Economic outcomes

B. School Health Promotion Processes
  - Developing a nurturing and supportive psychosocial environment
  - Creating a safe and healthy physical environment
  - Delivering education that informs, motivates and empowers students and employees to assure individual, family, community, national and global health
  - Providing necessary health services
  - Developing healthy food and eating policies and practices
  - Creating opportunities and skills for enjoyable physical activity
  - Providing counselling, psychological and social services
  - Improving the health, productivity and quality of life of school employees
  - Integrating efforts of students, families, school employees and public, not-for-profit and private-sector community agencies – during both school hours and non-school hours
  - Implementing a Health Promoting School (HPS), or whole setting approach, integrating all of the above processes as an integral part of the school, instead of implementing a discrete process to attain a discrete outcome

C. Evaluation Approaches

Health Sector	Education Sector
• Research syntheses (including meta analyses)	• Case studies / action research / histories / biographies
• Randomised Control Trials (RCTs)	• Surveys / correlational studies / cohort analysis
• Cohort studies	• Group comparisons / controlled experimental design
• Outcome Research (case-control studies)	• Longitudinal studies / follow-up studies
• Case studies	• Research syntheses (including meta analyses)
• Expert opinion	

of successful processes (usually in complex combinations) which enable the outcomes to be achieved. Part C identifies the *Evaluation Approaches* mainly used by the health and education sections to collect the evidence. Traditionally, the health sector values Randomised Controlled Trials (RCTs) higher than case studies and expert opinion in terms of the significance of using such an approach. In educational evaluation the focus is on students, classrooms, schools and systems either separately or in combination. Whilst RCTs are occasionally used, it is impossible to ensure that which is implemented is uncontaminated by the teaching-learning dynamic that occurs in schools between teachers and students. Educational initiatives often change the conditions that made them work in the first place and are often difficult to replicate (Pawson, 2006).

Education research seeks to discover the factors that enable a program/intervention to have a reasonable chance of achieving the successful outcomes elsewhere. For the education sector to understand the causal connections in school health promotion it needs to " . . . understand outcome patterns rather than seek outcome regularities" (Pawson, 2006, p22).

The challenge is for both the health and education sectors to appreciate and understand what constitutes evidence in each sector and to recognize that there is a history of accepted approaches in each sector in gathering that evidence. Areas of overlap are present and need to be used as a starting point to ensure research and evaluation in school health promotion is more cognizant of the setting from which it is gathered and more in tune with how the findings will generate policy improvements and be more useful to practitioners, particularly teachers, in improving their practices.

Gaps in the Evidence

Whilst there is considerable evidence available about the outcomes of school health promotion on which to make some reasonable assumptions about policies, resource allocations, and priorities, there are still a number of gaps that need to be addressed.

Uncertainty about the Outcomes of School Health

What is the most valuable evidence concerning school health promotion? Is it the achievement or not of the goals of the program which may be evaluated in terms of, for example, knowledge, competencies, behaviors, biomedical changes, cognitive processes (e.g., analytical skills), and/or educational attributes? Or is it perhaps the unintended outcomes of the health promotion initiatives (e.g., new partnerships, increased parental involvement, and students being more questioning of policies and practices)? We risk missing out on the richness of school health activities by evaluating a narrow set of pre-determined outcomes. The importance of one's health (and education) are not levels of attainment that are only to be valued by certain designated standards (e.g., being within a certain body mass index (BMI) range, not smoking, high grades, such as an A in Mathematics). They are more than that. They are resources for living and have many components that have different degrees of importance to people as they go through life. There is the need, in addition to assessing standard outcomes for school health promotion interventions, to look more creatively at what constitutes successful outcomes and with an increased input from students, teachers and parents in determining them. This should give us a more holistic appreciation and understanding of all the effects of school based health promotion. Analyzing this data will enhance the quality of our models and programs.

Shared and Participatory Evaluation

Education systems, and many schools, often spell out in detail what expectations they have of students at certain ages, in terms of knowledge and competencies in the different aspects of the curriculum. This invariably includes health. Has the health sector done this? Should it do this? And should it be done in collaboration with the education sector and parents? What is the place of students in such negotiations? It is useful to explore these questions further.

Children's physical, mental, intellectual, emotional, and spiritual development proceeds at varying rates according to biological, social, cultural, environmental, and behavioral determinants. What "health assets" should a child have at the end of primary school, the end of secondary school, or at a certain age (e.g., 14 years of age)? Are there gender and cultural variations?

A case can be made for key stakeholders in each country and/or community to identify these age-related assets. This will enable groups to be more insightful about the relative importance of the assets, to be more strategic in collaboratively developing ways to facilitate the achievement of these assets and to be more empowered to own the local issues and collectively think of ways of addressing them. Most HPS/CSH frameworks and plans express explicitly the importance of school-family-community-health sector links. Yet, there is a major gap in the evidence about a shared set of student expectations regarding these health assets. It may be more effective for students and pivotal members of the local community to be involved more explicitly in identifying these, rather than as secondary and passive partners in a pre-determined program developed away from the school. This should ensure increased collaboration in evaluating initiatives designed to improve the health assets of school students. It will also mean methods of collecting the evidence are better aligned to the strategies used to achieve the outcomes.

The Paucity of Evidence from Low-Income Countries

The vast majority of evidence about the effectiveness of health promotion in schools is from developed countries. Many of the published reports of school health from low-income nations tend to describe what happened, and assess changes in knowledge before and after the intervention. Yet, the authors of this chapter have all seen examples of exciting and excellent approaches to school health in low-income regions of the world. There is much to learn from these approaches, but until priorities are set to better evaluate these approaches and initiatives, and allocate adequate resources, we will continue to have this as a major gap in the evidence.

Limited Recognition of Evidence from the Education Sector

There is a wealth of evidence from education research about the nature of what constitutes effective teaching and learning approaches; change and innovation in schools; leadership in schools; and effective schools. This is accessible through many peer reviewed journals, books and reports from governments, NGOs, research institutes, and universities. The findings have shaped the development of schools and their educational practices to varying degrees for many years. But, this evidence has too frequently been overlooked by the health sector as it has developed its own approaches to address those societal health issues which impact on school students now and in the future.

In some countries there is evidence of practical collaboration between the health and education sector in relation to measuring the effectiveness of Health Promoting Schools. In Scotland, for example, indicators of health promotion effectiveness have been built into the existing quality indicators which were used in the education sector to help embed health promotion actions within the education mainstream. Similar initiatives have occurred in Hong Kong, in many European countries, and in regions in North America. Such partnerships have demonstrated that whilst there are still substantial gaps in knowing about the full evidence picture, specialist groups and individuals are beginning to seek to understand what makes for effective schooling and health promotion actions, to utilize each others tools of measurement, to acknowledge the evidence from different disciplines and sectors, and to ask questions about it.

Evidence about Costs and Benefits

There have been very few cost-benefit and cost-effective studies about a whole school approach in the literature. Rothman and colleagues made a number of claims about whole school health in their detailed study in 1994. They argued an integrated whole school approach using the HPS/CSH framework was very cost-effective (Rothman, Ehreth, Palmer, Reblando & Luce, 1994). But Stewart-Brown and colleagues found no evidence of cost-effective studies examining whole school approaches in their two meta-analyses in 1999 or 2006 (Lister-Sharp, Chapman, Stewart-Brown & Sowden, 1999; Stewart-Brown, 2006).

There have been some topic-specific cost studies published. For example, school health promotion can be cost-effective and cost-saving in improving health, illustratively by preventing tobacco use (Wang, Crossett, Lowry, Sussman & Dent, 2001); obesity (Wang, Yang, Lowry & Wechsler, 2003); human immunodeficiency virus and other sexually transmitted diseases (Wang, Davis & Robin, 2000); and screening for Chlamydia (Wang, Burstein & Cohen, 2002).

What do these cost benefit/effective studies tell us about school health promotion? They suggest that certain topical approaches can be effective in terms of their costs. But what about a whole school approach? Are there cost-benefit/cost-effectiveness studies about the mainstream of schooling (e.g., school-based numeracy and literacy, and civic education)? The education sector rarely looks at cost-benefit/cost-effective approaches to the core areas of schooling because it is very difficult to identify valid indicators. The diversity of practices in the dynamics of the teacher-student, student-student engagements makes it methodologically complex to even design such studies.

The education sector views the processes and outcomes of school education as an important value and essential part of a society's obligations. School health promotion needs to be viewed in the same light.

Challenges in Evaluating School Health Promotion

Dissemination of the Evidence of Effectiveness

There has been considerable evidence published in the last decade about the effectiveness of interventions in schools to address health issues of young people, now and into their future. However, both the health and education sectors have not adequately summarized this evidence and made it accessible and understandable to specific groups and practitioners involved in school health. It is essential that teachers know what constitutes quality practice in classroom health programs and that they and principals, school nurses and counselors know about and understand the potential of whole school approaches to health which improve both educational and health outcomes for their students.

The educational research literature indicates school administrators play a major role in leading innovation and change. If more schools are to embrace a HPS/CSH framework to school health, then it is vital that they are informed about the benefits of HPS/CSH, particularly those related to educational outcomes. School administrators and teachers rarely, if ever, read the research and evaluation literature on school health. A challenge for both the health and education sectors is to interpret evidence-based information to school administrators and teachers specifically to enable them to facilitate better planning and implementation of school health initiatives without compromising the integrity of the research and evaluation findings.

Other key stakeholders who need ongoing and unambiguous access to research and evaluation data include public health administrators who connect with the education sector; curriculum designers who develop courses of study, classroom content, and practice guidelines; policy makers whose policies impact on schools – particularly those from the health, education, and community services sectors; and professionals who participate in school health programs (e.g., nurses, youth workers, and counselors).

Convincing the Health Sector about Realistic Expectations in Schools

A school's core business is to maximize learning outcomes, not solve health problems. A significant challenge for the health sector is to describe health issues more in educational terms and in ways that the education sector and schools in particular can embrace to enrich their educational mandate. This means expanding the evidence of effectiveness of school health to incorporate educational outcomes.

The time spent at school by students is finite. There are many priorities of schooling, including building numeracy and literacy skills; scientific and artistic competencies; societal, historical, and cultural dimensions; to name a few. Also, schools are expected to develop generic values (e.g., respect, honesty, trust, and tolerance). Too frequently, the "health program" is presented as an addition, rather than being integrated into the fundamental work of schools. It is often predicated on the assumption, that after the provision of some knowledge about the health issue and certain associated skills, healthy behaviors will follow. A challenge is to convince the health sector about the evidence of the major factors influencing young people's health viz. media, peer group, family, community, and to encourage health and education to work together to incorporate these influential factors in their school focused health promoting initiatives and associated evaluations.

Effective Ways of Persuading the Education Sector about the Values of School Health Promotion

Schools are busy places. The number of hours in the day, and number of weeks in the year that children attend school is finite. Teachers and school administrators are usually obligated to teach a prescribed curriculum program. They and their students are engaged in an interactive learning program which has certain milestones of accountability (e.g., regular tests of the students learning outcomes and teacher appraisal). School health, whilst integral to many school educational programs, is often raised to higher levels of importance by the health sector and governments to address certain community health issues (e.g., poor hygiene, drug misuse, including tobacco and alcohol, and obesity). This places pressure on schools and teachers. The argument from the health sector, for schools to embrace these extra funded programs, is often based on using the school as a site of access to be able to inform and skill students in healthy practices. Rarely have schools been informed and persuaded that "healthy students learn better."

More evidence needs to be established about the most effective ways of integrating school health programs into the regular routines of schools, school boards and education ministries. We need examples about how schools can integrate health into their school improvement planning and accountability procedures. How can education and health ministries do their planning and budgeting together as it relates to school health? What surveillance and monitoring activities can be jointly implemented effectively by both systems? How can local school boards and health authorities work together most effectively?

What evidence will convince schools and educational administrators that school health promotion will enhance student learning? For many years the health sector has assumed that because there is some data to suggest this may be the case, the schools will enthusiastically embrace health promoting initiatives. We need to interrogate this evidence more thoroughly and where studies are lacking, carry out research to see what health gains are most influential in improving learning outcomes.

Before we can persuade the education sector to embrace school health promotion and its organization frameworks of HPS/CSH more widely, we need to build a stronger and more specific evidence base to underpin our beliefs about the value of school health promotion to educational outcomes.

Equity and Social Justice Issues

School health promotion should be a fundamental component of education provision throughout the world. Sadly, in many low-income countries, poor sanitation and impure drinking water are the main health issues for young people. In many countries, it is a challenge to make clean water and sanitation available and to provide knowledge and skills for students on hygiene. The school as a setting where students can be accessed for immunization and student health checks is vital in building the health and well-being in most low income countries. The same also applies to many developed countries.

Evidence shows that if girls attend school, then not only their own health, but the health of their families will improve considerably (Blum et al., 2002; WHO, 1995). Girls, in some countries, are excluded from educational opportunities and also boys are sometimes forced to leave school early to assist with chores and generating the family income. Both these factors have substantial health impacts on these young people, now and into the future.

In many developed countries students feel alienated from school. There is a close correlation between their school attendance and participation and their health risk behaviors – the less attendance and involvement in school, the higher the risk behavior (Symons et al., 1997; Blum et al., 2002; Patton et al., 2006). This evidence from these and other researchers needs to be acknowledged more by the health sector in designing school based interventions. It appears some of these longer-term evaluations are strongly suggesting that it may be more important and effective to address the way the school is conducted and how participatory and democratic its processes are, than to take a health issue and seek to change specific student behaviors.

A challenge for schools is to make it a place where students want to be. The more students participate in and have some control over their learning, the more empowered they are. Higher educational achievements and increased health protective behaviors will follow. The HPS/CSH model is predicated on students being part of the planning and action scenarios. Supporting teachers to develop the skills and equipping them with resources to practice these principles is a challenging priority and there is little evidence about effective approaches. The increasing problems of obesity/overweight in developed countries provide schools with opportunities for staff to work collaboratively with students and the community to shape policies and engaging practices which facilitate students being more involved with food and eating, and physical activities in both the school and local community. School health promotion initiatives, such as this, will provide us with an excellent opportunity to be more rigorous and comprehensive in our research and evaluation studies as we seek evidence across all the components of the HPS/CSH approach to assess what works and why, and under what circumstances.

Empowerment and its Evaluation

The HPS/CSH framework places significant emphasis on empowering students and building their capacities in health behaviors, policies, and knowledge. This is where students can have a key role in running their schools' food services; deciding on policies and procedures around bullying; acting as mentors and friends to young students; and linking with community groups, to collectively address health impacting issues (e.g., environmental degradation and community safety). A challenge is to build students' "action competencies" (Jensen & Jensen, 2005) where it is appropriate and taking into account the students cognitive, physical, cultural and social developmental stages. As a consequence of this focus, teachers need to rethink school health away from focusing most efforts in the classroom. Challenges exist to have schools embrace whole school approaches to health promotion and to build the capacity of teachers to use teaching methods and techniques that facilitate student empowerment. This has implications for evaluations of such approaches. The evidence needed to make judgements about the effectiveness of health promotion initiatives directed at empowering students is more complex than simple measures testing students' knowledge or understanding. It places extra burdens on teachers to collect this data. Both the health and education sectors, and researchers in the field need to address this issue, and develop clear, practical and accessible techniques to collect information about student empowerment.

In the last decade many countries have begun to address staff health and well-being in addition to health promotion for students. But it raises questions. Where resources are finite, should the focus be both on students and staff health promotion, or on one group only? What is the evidence that suggests that interventions to promote staff health result in better teaching and enhanced student outcomes? Should the school as a Health Promoting Worksite be treated separately from the Health Promoting School? Who is more important when resources are limited? Where is the balance, if any, between empowering students and teachers?

Assessing School Health Outcomes

What should be evaluated in school health promotion? Who makes these decisions and is there a program logic in place that means the expected outcomes are related to the strategies used and the intensity of the intervention (e.g., resources and time)? The World Health Organisation's Expert Committee on School Health identified five types of indicators for school health interventions (WHO, 1995). They are:

1. Children's health status (e.g., height for age, total caloric intake);
2. Learning ability, attendance and learning achievement (e.g., literacy and numeracy skills, basic learning competencies);

3. Behaviors affecting health (e.g., tobacco use, physical activity);
4. Quality of the physical and psychosocial environment (e.g. water and sanitation quality, policies and practices in schools); and
5. School health program implementation (e.g. curriculum, access to health services, links with local community).

However most of the evaluations in the last decade appear to be focused on health behavior change. There has been a paucity of evaluations addressing educational outcomes on students (2) and not many which look at the changes in schools' policies and practices that enhance health (4). All five evaluation areas are necessary to gain an understanding of school health.

We need more studies which seek to inform the education sector, in particular, about the influence of school health activities on educational indicators for students, and school policies and practices. A challenge is to involve both the education and health sectors negotiating evaluation measures about any school health initiative or program at the beginning of the planning process.

School Health Promotion Effectiveness – Priorities for the Next 10 Years

There is now a considerable body of evidence to enable reasonable judgements about the effectiveness of school health promotion to be made. However there are a number of issues to be addressed in the next decade to enable a more complete and comprehensive picture to emerge. Consequently, administrators, practitioners, and policy makers can have a stronger evidence base on which to make decisions and enhance practice. The main priorities are:

- Increase collaboration between the health and education sectors in planning, implementing, and evaluating School Health Promotion.
- Improve the dissemination of the evidence of effectiveness to schools.
- Establish more realistic expectations for school health promotion.
- Build a stronger evidence base on effective School Health Promotion approaches in low-income countries.

Acknowledgments. The authors wish to acknowledge and thank Martha Perry from IUHPE for all her assistance, and also the many students, teachers, education and health administrators, community members and researchers, who plan, implement and evaluate the exciting initiatives in school health across so many countries.

References

Allensworth, D. & Kolbe, L. (1987). The comprehensive school health program: Exploring an expanded concept. *Journal of School Health, 57*, 10, 409–412.

American Counselling Association (2006). *Effectiveness of school counselling.* http://www.counseling.org/Files/FD.ashx?guid=4757e7f7-85ad-456b-88c3-5fb6a60 b9eba (accessed on October 11, 2006).

Blum, R., McNeely, C. & Rinehart, P. (2002). *Improving the odds: The untapped power of schools to improve the health of teens.* Center for Adolescent Health and Development, University of Minnesota.

Browne, G., Gafni, A., Roberts, J., Byrne, C. & Majumdar, B. (2004). Effective/efficient mental health programs for school age children: A synthesis of reviews. *Social Science and Medicine, 58*, 1367–1384.

Campbell, C., Waters, E., O'Meara, S. & Summerbell, C. (2001). Interventions for preventing obesity in childhood. A systematic review. *Obesity Reviews, 2*, 149–157.

Centers for Disease Control and Prevention (2003). *Stories from the field: Lessons learned about building coordinated school health programmes.* Washington: US Department of Health and Human Services.

Clift, S. & Jensen, B.B. (2005). *The health promoting school: International advances in theory, evaluation and practice.* Copenhagen: Danish University of Education Press.

Dobbins, M., Lockett, D., Michel, I., Beyers, J., Feldman, L., Vohra, J. & Micucci, S. (2001). *The effectiveness of school-based interventions in promoting physical activity and fitness among children and youth: A systematic review.* Ontario: McMaster University.

Gortmaker, S., Peterson, K., Weicha, J., Sobol, A., Dixit, S., Fox, M. & Laird, N.(1999). Reducing obesity via a school-based interdisciplinary intervention among youth: Planet Health. *Archives of Pediatric & Adolescent Medicine, 153*, 409–418.

Green, J., Howes, F., Waters, E., Maher, E. & Oberklaid, F. (2005). Promoting the social and emotional health of primary school aged children: Reviewing the evidence base for school-based interventions. *International Journal of Mental Health Promotion, 7*, 2, 30–36.

Jensen, B.B. & Jensen, B. (2005). Inequality, health and action for health-do children and young people in Denmark have an opinion? In: Clift, S. & Jensen, B.B. (eds) *The health promoting school: International advances in theory, evaluation and practice.* Copenhagen: Danish University of Education Press.

Kemm, L. (2006). The limitations of evidenced public health. *Journal of Evaluation in Clinical Practice, 12*, 3, 319.

Kirby, D. (2002). The impact of schools and school programs upon adolescent sexual behaviour *Journal of Sex Research, 39*, 1, 27–33.

Kolbe, L. (1993). An essential strategy to improve the health and education of Americans. *Preventative medicine, 22*, 4, 544–560.

Lee, A., Cheng, F. & St.Leger, L. (2005). Evaluating health promoting schools in Hong Kong: Development of a model. *Health Promotion International, 20*, 2, 177–186.

Lee, A., St.Leger, L. & Moon, A. (2005). Evaluating health promotion in schools: A case study of design, implementation and results from the Hong Kong Healthy School Award Scheme. *Promotion & Education, 12*, 3–4, 123–130.

Lee, A., Cheng, F., Fung, Y., St Leger, L. (2006). Can health promoting schools contribute to the better health and well being of young people: Hong Kong experience? *Journal of Epidemiology and Community Health, 60*, 530–536.

Lister-Sharp, D., Chapman, S., Stewart-Brown, S. & Sowden, A. (1999). Health promoting schools and health promotion in schools: Two systematic reviews. *Health Technology Assessment, 3*, 1–207.

Lloyd, C., Joyce, R., Hurry, J. & Ashton, M. (2000). The effectiveness of primary school drug education. *Drugs: Education, prevention and policy. 7*, 2, 109–126.

Marshall, B., Sheehan, M., Northfield, J., Carlisle, R. & St.Leger, L. (2000). School-based health promotion Across Australia. *Journal of School Health, 70*, 6, 251–252.

Midford, R., Lenton, S. & Hancock, L. (2000). *A critical review and analysis: Cannabis education in schools.* Sydney: New South Wales Department of Education and Training.

Moon, A., Mullee, M., Rogers, L., Thompson, R., Speller, V. & Roderick, P. (1999). Helping schools become health promoting: An evaluation of the Wessex Healthy Schools Award. *Health Promotion International, 14*, 111–122.

National Drug Research Institute (2002). *The prevention of substance use, risk and harm in Australia: A review of the evidence.* Canberra: Commonwealth Department of Health and Ageing.

National Foundation for Educational Research (2004).

Patton, G., Bond, L., Carlin, J., Thomas, L., Butler, H., Glover, S., Catalano, R. & Bowes, G. (2006). Promoting social inclusion in schools: A group-randomized trial on student health risk behaviour and well-being. *American Journal of Public Health, 96*, 9.

Pawson, R. (2006). *Evidence-based policy: A realistic perspective.* London: Sage.

Rothman, M., Ehreth, J., Palmer, C., Reblando, J. & Luce, B. (1994). *The potential benefits and costs of a comprehensive school health education program. Draft report.* Geneva: World Health Organization.

Sahota, P., Rudolf, M., Dixey, R., Hill, A., Barth, J. & Cade, J. (2001). Randomised control trial of a primary school based intervention to reduce risk factors for obesity. *British Medical Journal, 323*, 1–5.

Scottish Council for Research in Education (2002).

Silva, M. (2002). The effectiveness of school-based sex education programs in the promotion of abstinent behavior: A meta-analysis. *Health Education Research,17*, 4, 471–481.

Sinnott, J. (2005). *Healthy schools and improvements in standards, National Healthy Schools Program, England.* [Cited June 6, 2006]Available from: www.wiredforhealth.gov.uk/Word/improved_standards_05.doc.

St.Leger, L. (2005). Protocols and guidelines for health promoting schools. *Promotion & Education, 12*, 3–4, 145–147.

Stewart-Brown, S. (2006). *What is the evidence on school health promotion in improving school health or preventing disease and specifically what is the effectiveness of the health promoting schools approach?* Copenhagen: World Health Organization.

Symons, C., Cincelli, C., James, T. & Groff, P. (1997). Bridging student health risks and academic achievement through comprehensive school health programs. *Journal of School Health, 67*, 6, 220–227.

Taras, H. (2005a). Nutrition and student performance at school. *Journal of School Health, 75*, 6, 199–213.

Taras, H. (2005b). Physical activity and student performance at school. *Journal of School Health, 75*, 6, 214–218.

Taras, H. & Potts-Datema, W. (2005a). Obesity and student performance at school. *Journal of School Health, 75*, 8, 291–295.

Taras, H. & Potts-Datema, W. (2005b). Sleep and student performance at school. *Journal of School Health, 75*, 7, 248–254.

Task Force on Community Preventive Services (2006). Guide to Community Preventive Services: Systematic Reviews and Evidence Based Recommendations. Available at http://www.thecommunityguide.org/about/default.htm (accessed October 11, 2006).

Timperio, A., Salmon, J. & Ball, K. (2004). Evidence-based strategies to promote physical activity among children, adolescents and young adults: Review and update. *Journal of Science and Medicine in Sport, 7*, 1, 20–29.

Tobler, N. & Stratton, H. (1997). Effectiveness of school-based drug education programs: A meta analysis of the research. *Journal of Primary Prevention, 18*, 1, 71–128.

Tones, K. (2005). Health promotion in schools: The radical imperative. In: Clift, S. & Jensen, B.B. (eds) *The health promoting school: International advances in theory, evaluation and practice.* Copenhagen: Danish University of Education Press.

Wang, L., Burstein, G. & Cohen, D. (2002). An economic evaluation of a school-based sexually transmitted disease screening program. *Sexually TransmittedDiseases. 29*, 737–745.

Wang, L., Crossett, L., Lowry, R., Sussman, S. & Dent, C. (2001). Cost-effectiveness of a school-based tobacco-use prevention program. *Archives of Pediatric & Adolescent Medicine, 155*, 1043–1050.

Wang, L., Davis, M., Robin, L., Collins, J., Coyle, K. & Baumler, E. (2000). Economic evaluation of safer choices: A school-based human immunodeficiency virus, other sexually transmitted diseases, and pregnancy prevention program. *Archives of Pediatric & Adolescent Medicine, 154*, 1017–1024.

Wang, L., Yang, Q., Lowry, R. & Wechsler, H. (2003). Economic analysis of a school-based obesity prevention program. *Obesity Research, 11*, 1313–1324.

Wells, J., Barlow, J. & Stewart-Brown, S. (2003). A systematic review of universal approaches to mental health promotion in schools. *Health Education Journal, 103*,4, 197–220.

West, P., Sweeting, H. & Leyland, L. (2004). School effects on pupils' health behaviours: Evidence in support of the health promoting school. *Research Papers in Education, 19*, 31, 261–291.

World Health Organization (1984). *Health promotion: A discussion document on the concept and principles.* Copenhagen: World Health Organization.

World Health Organization (1986). The Ottawa charter for health promotion. *Health Promotion International, 1*, 4, 3–5.

World Health Organization (1991). *Comprehensive school health education suggested guidelines for action.* Geneva: World Health Organization.

World Health Organization (1995). *W.H.O. Expert committee on comprehensive school health education and promotion.* Geneva: World Health Organization.

World Health Organization (1996). *School health promotion – series 5: Regional guidelines: Development of health promoting schools: A framework for action.* Manila: World Health Organization.

World Health Organization (1997). *The health promoting school – an investment in education health and democracy.* Copenhagen: World Health Organization.

Young, I. & Williams, T. (1989). *The healthy school.* Edinburgh: Scottish Health Education Group.

Young, I. (2005). Health promotion in schools – a historical perspective. *Promotion & Education, 12*, 3–5, 112–117.

9
Health Promotion to Prevent Obesity
Evidence and Policy Needs

TIM LOBSTEIN AND BOYD SWINBURN

This chapter uses the International Obesity Taskforce framework on evidence-based obesity prevention and highlights key areas of evidence debate in this very important global epidemic. The existing evidence on the burden of obesity is sufficient to warrant action and the evidence on the determinants of obesity is also informative on *what* to do. The priority target groups (*who*) are mainly children and adolescents and high risk adults and schools are the favoured setting (*where*) although multiple settings are preferable. The strategies (*how*) also need to be multi-pronged with communications, programs, and policies being the main approaches. The evidence on effective interventions is quite limited although it is growing rapidly and a summary of recent literature reviews is included.

Primary school interventions dominate although the evidence suggests that multiple strategies across multiple settings are more likely to have a sustainable beneficial impact than single actions alone. While program interventions are more readily measured for effectiveness, environmental approaches are usually more sustainable and often have a greater effect on behaviour. An environment-centred approach often needs policy basis to initiate change.

Access to the target group and ability to introduce and measure the impact of specific interventions is paramount and this has created a strong "settings bias" (especially for schools) in the scientific evidence. This has limited the information available to policy-makers which means that the traditional definitions of "evidence-based policy or practice" are too narrow to be of use in areas of public health like obesity prevention where the need for action is high but the evidence base is limited.

Lastly, we suggest that in the absence of strong scientific evidence for *proven* strategies, action on obesity prevention can progress using an investment paradigm of *promising* strategies. In the absence of "safe" (evidence-based), "high-return" (very effective) "investments" (interventions), a portfolio of strategies could include a mixture of safe, low-return investments and "higher risk" (more uncertain), potentially high-return initiatives. Choosing the right portfolio of investments is the art and science of priority-setting and this ideally uses the best technical information available (including modelled estimates of effectiveness), but must also must include an appropriate process with stakeholders and incorporate informed, expert opinion.

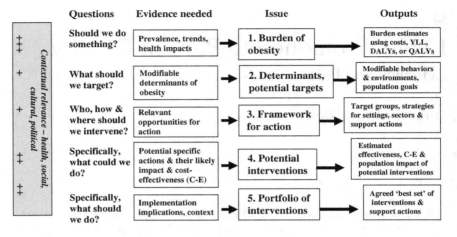

FIGURE 9.1. The international obesity taskforce framework for evidence-based obesity prevention.

Introduction

Obesity prevention is caught between the demands for action because obesity is a rapidly rising epidemic with serious health consequences and the demands that the programs, policies and practices implemented to counter the epidemic are evidence-based. The paradigm of evidence-based public health which grew from evidence-based medicine has brought with it both an awareness of the need to apply rigorous evidence more systematically to public health and an awareness that public health interventions are usually more complex than clinical interventions and less susceptible to randomised, controlled trials.

In an effort to clarify the role of evidence in obesity prevention, the International Obesity Taskforce (IOTF) published a framework (Swinburn, Gill & Kumanyika, 2005) which identified the key questions to be answered, the types of evidence needed and outputs produced, and the role of contextual factors (Figure 9.1). In the process of building this framework, there were a number of general concepts and specific issues to emerge about evidence as it applies to obesity prevention. These will be covered below along with a summary of the evidence from the literature for interventions in specific settings.

Definitions and Hierarchies of Evidence

Evidence, in its widest sense, is information that can provide a level of certainty about the truth of a proposition (Rychetnik, Hawe, Waters, Barratt & Frommer, 2004). This is a very broad definition, more along the lines of the legal, rather than the medical, concept of evidence and implies that this breadth of information is important and valid for decision-making. For the purposes of addressing the questions on obesity prevention, the IOTF framework grouped evidence into observational, experimental, extrapolated, and experience-based sources of evidence and information (Swinburn et al., 2005). Examples of these are outlined in Table 9.1.

Each type of evidence has its own strengths and weaknesses. Each can be judged on its ability to contribute to answering the question at hand. In practice, there is wide variation in the quantity and quality of information available in

TABLE 9.1. Examples of 'admissible evidence' for obesity prevention (adapted from Swinburn, Gill & Kumanyika, 2005)

Evidence	Examples
Observational	
Epidemiological studies that may involve comparisons of exposed and non-exposed individuals	Cross-sectional, case-control, or cohort studies of sweet drink consumption and obesity
Population monitoring data that can provide time series information	Trends in obesity prevalence, food supply data, car and TV ownership
Experimental	
Intervention studies where the investigator has control over the allocations and/or timings of interventions	Controlled trials of exercise programs among individuals, groups or whole communities
Program evaluation – assessing processes, impacts and outcomes	Health promotion programs to change behaviours, attitudes, environments, or policies
Extrapolated	
Modelling causative pathways to identify assign causality, size of effect, or intervention options	Structural modelling of influences that determine, mediate or moderate the relationship between TV viewing and obesity
Modelling effectiveness of interventions	Estimates of an education program's efficacy, uptake and population reach or the impact of
Modelling costs, cost-effectiveness, or cost-utility	farm policies on agricultural production, pricing, purchasing and consumption
Information allowing an inference ('indirect evidence')	patterns
	Costs and cost-effectiveness of an ongoing program across a population
	Continued, high investment in food marketing to children infers that such marketing increases children's consumption of those foods
Experience	
Evidence of intervention effectiveness from comparable fields ('parallel evidence')	The impact of taxes, social marketing, environmental changes in changing smoking prevalence
Expert and informed opinion from practitioners and stakeholders with practical experience	Input from paediatricians, marketing agencies, parents, school principals about the feasibility and sustainability of interventions
Theory and program logic	Regulations that ban vending machines from schools or TV advertising to children or health claims on products will result in those outcomes

respect of different settings, approaches and target groups for interventions to prevent obesity. There is virtually no evidence concerning the potential effects on obesity of altering social and economic policies, such as agricultural production policies or food pricing policies, while much more evidence is available on localised attempts to influence the consumer through educational and program-based approaches.

Traditional hierarchies of evidence are based on rankings of internal validity (certainty of study conclusions). These tended to be less valuable in the IOTF framework because of the tension between internal validity and the need for external validity (applicability of study findings). The importance of context on evidence and the need for external validity is greater in some areas than others (left-hand bar in Figure 9.1). It is especially important at the priority setting stage (issue 5), and this is where the informed opinions of stakeholders is paramount.

Modelled estimates of effectiveness and informed stakeholder opinion also become important sources of information where the empirical evidence is complex, patchy, and needs to be applied to different contexts. This means that assumptions and decisions must be made explicit and transparent. The acceptance of modelled estimates of effectiveness and informed opinion in the absence of empirical evidence means an acceptance of the best evidence *available* not just the best evidence *possible* (as occurred in systematic reviews with strict inclusion criteria).

Evidence on the Burden and Determinants of Obesity

These are the first two issues in the IOTF framework (Figure 9.1). In general, the size and nature of the obesity epidemic has been well enough characterised to have created the case for action. Of course many gaps and debates still remain such as the prevalence and trends in poorer countries, the psycho-social impacts of obesity in children, and the effect of the epidemic on life expectancy. Research will continue to build better pictures of the burdens of obesity.

Evidence on the determinants of obesity is very strong in most areas, although to date, most is focused on the more proximal biological and behavioural determinants rather than the more distal, but very powerful, social and environmental determinants. One poorly researched but very obvious set of determinants are the socio-cultural attitudes, beliefs, values and perceptions that may explain the very large differences in obesity prevalence rates seen across different cultures (1–2% in China and Japan to 25–50% in North America and the Pacific).

The strength of the evidence for various determinants of obesity has been used to justify and prioritise action on those factors with the highest levels of evidence. This was the evidence approach used by the World Cancer Research Fund (1997) and World Health Organization (2003) in their reports on the priorities for prevention of cancer and chronic diseases respectively. If the evidence for a particular determinant was rated as "convincing" or "probable" according to a hierarchy (based on internal validity), then it was considered a target for intervention. For example, it was considered that there was convincing evidence that a high fibre diet was protective and physical inactivity was causative of obesity but only "possible" evidence that low glycemic index diets were protective and "insufficient" evidence that alcohol was causative (Swinburn, Caterson, Seiddell & James, 2004).

Many issues arise in taking the leap from a list of determinants prioritised by strength of evidence to a list of priorities for action. Environmental determinants inevitably have a lower strength of evidence. For example, how strong is the evidence in the reported literature that supportive family environments are protective of obesity? This can never achieve a high level of evidence (randomised controlled trials) and there is no category for the "bleeding obvious" or "jump from a plane with no parachute" type of determinant. The evidence that high protein diets are protective against weight gain is very strong (high internal validity) supported by several randomised controlled trials, (Astrup, 2005) but the generalisability (external validity) is extremely low. The World Health Organization should not be recommending that the global population take up high protein diets, a policy which would be neither achievable nor environmentally sustainable.

The WCRF evidence review (World Cancer Research Fund, 1997) concluded (as will the updated review in progress) that obesity is an important determinant of the cancer burden. This is the equivalent of issue 2 on the IOTF framework (Figure 9.1). Another, totally different view of the evidence is then needed to work out what to do about it. As Robinson and Sirard (2005) eloquently point out, "problem-oriented" evidence (what is to blame?) is often quite different to "solution-oriented" evidence (what to do?). An obverse example is that the absence of dance may never be identified as part of the cause of obesity but dance could readily be part of the solution for teenage girls. Equally, occupational physical inactivity may be an important cause of obesity but it will not be an important solution because society will not revert to life without computers and labour-saving devices.

Opportunities for Action – Who, Where, How?

This is the third issue on the IOTF framework (Figure 9.1). Many countries have now created strategic plans for action on obesity either as an issue by itself or as part of promoting physical activity or health eating or reducing chronic diseases. Classic frameworks for health promotion specify "who" in terms of **target groups** (e.g. children, adolescents, pregnant women, minority ethnic groups, those on low incomes), "where" in terms of **settings or sectors** (e.g. workplace, schools, the commercial sector, the health sector), and "how" **approaches or strategies** (e.g. school education, community development, the use of mass media, environmental change, policy and infrastructure change) and the key issues on each of these will be considered.

Target Groups

Following the model given in the WHO Global Strategy on Diet, Physical Activity and Health (World Health Organization, 2004), target groups can be specified through reference to the life-course: this starts with maternal health and pre-natal nutrition and proceeds through pregnancy outcomes, infant nutrition, pre-school and school-age children, adolescents, adults and elderly people. Cross-cuttings of this sequence are groupings by gender, socio-economic status, ethnicity, and migrant status. The choice of target group will influence the nature of the approach used and the setting where the intervention takes place.

However, a potential limitation of identifying target groups is that they become too much the focus of the action (e.g. by encouraging them to make the healthy choices) rather than the players that influence the environments that determine those behaviours (those who can make the healthy choices easier for the target group). In this respect, the definition of target groups may need to be widened to include the providers of the determinants of health, such as the providers of health information – the health services, schools, the media, commercial producers – and widened still further to include those that set the policies which shape access to healthy lifestyles through, for example, pricing, distribution and marketing. In this sense, target groups may include shareholders in companies, professional groups, policy makers and public opinion leaders, including politicians and celebrities (Box 9.1).

Prevention strategies targeting adults make economic sense because it is the consequences of obesity occurring in middle aged and older adults that generate the economic costs of obesity – especially through type 2 diabetes and cardio-vascular diseases (Seidell, Nooyens & Visscher, 2005). Adults, especially those with other existing risk factors, are at high absolute risk of these diseases; there-fore they have the potential for high absolute gains. In addition, there is now very strong efficacy evidence that individual lifestyle interventions in high risk adults prevent diabetes and heart disease (Knowler, Barrett-Connor, Fowler, Hamman, Lachin, Walker, Nathan & The Diabetes Prevention Program Research Group, 2002; Ornish, Brown, Scherwitz, Billings, Armstrong, Ports, McLanahan, Kirkeeide, Brand & Gould, 1990).

BOX 9.1. Target groups versus beneficiaries

Jamie Oliver, a celebrity chef, provided an example of the need to widen the definition of target groups for health interventions. His TV series exposed the poor quality of food in English schools and led to a government pledge of money and a programme of raised school food standards. Jamie's intervention (which lacked a control group and was not systematically evaluated) targeted government policy-makers through public opinion, even though the ultimate beneficiaries were school children.

However, children have risen as the priority target group for most action on obesity and this has occurred for a number of reasons – some based on evidence, some based on societal principles, and some based on practicalities. Obesity prevalence among school-age children is rising in virtually all countries for which data are available (Wang & Lobstein, 2006). This is a relatively recent phenomenon, with little evidence of any change in the prevalence of childhood obesity before the 1970s, and signs of an accelerating increase in prevalence since the 1990s. An obese child faces a life-time of increased risk of various diseases, including cardiovascular disease, diabetes, liver disease and certain forms of cancer (World Health Organization, 2000). Even during childhood, obesity increases the risk of these diseases, and is a significant cause of psychological distress.

At present, paediatric services have few treatment options available. Once a child is substantially overweight, successful weight loss is difficult to achieve, as it is for adults, and requires intensive health care resources. However, younger children who are overweight do have a chance to "grow into" their weight. Prevention of obesity is, of course, preferred and as a general principle, it is better to start prevention early (childhood) rather than late (adulthood).

Known environmental risk factors for child obesity have been reviewed by several authors, (Lobstein, Baur, Uauy & The IASO International Obesity TaskForce, 2004; Parsons, Power, Logan & Summerbell, 1999; World Health Organization, 2000) and include parental body size, maternal smoking and diabetes status, infant feeding patterns, dietary energy density and meal patterns, and sedentary behaviour patterns such as TV watching. Children's behaviours are much more environmentally dependent than adults' behaviours and most of the evidence on obesity prevention has been in children (see below). However, far more powerful than the sum of the evidence are two other factors make children a priority target group: societal protection of children and access for interventions – especially through schools. Policy-makers have been especially sensitive to children because society has an obligation to protect them from ill-health. For adults, the societal obligation shifts towards protecting free choice – even if that choice is for unhealthy foods and physical inactivity.

Settings and Sectors

There are many potential settings for interventions (French, 2005; Swinburn & Egger, 2002), although the most powerful setting for influencing children, the home, has received little attention in relation to obesity prevention interventions because of the difficulty in access for interventions. The major options for influencing parents and homes are via mass media (usually very expensive) or via other settings (see below and Box 9.2).

Health care settings are in a key position to influence both their patients and the wider communities. Mother and baby clinics, health promotion programmes and outreach through community health workers (including school and workplace nurses and family health visitors) provide opportunities to monitor the practices of families and individuals, and to provide advice and information. There is a strong

Box 9.2. Policy driving environment and behaviour change

A national parliament may not seem a natural setting for health interventions, but in the broadest sense it is exactly that. In order to reduce the quantity of dairy fats being marketed and consumed, and to increase the amounts of fruits and vegetables available, the government of Finland proposed a new agricultural support policies which assisted farmers in converting from dairy to horticultural production. The parliamentary debate was an opportunity for health promotion through investment which was not entirely welcomed: moves to reduce butter consumption were resisted by commercial interests in the dairy farming sector and the cost of providing farm assistance for horticulture was not politically popular among some parliamentarians. However, the arguments for health eventually prevailed and the proposed polices were enacted, and have come to be recognised as the early drivers of change in the environments and behaviours which led to the reduction of cardiovascular disease in the country.

rationale for major health care organisations such as hospitals to take the lead as health promoting settings in promoting healthy eating.

Schools and other childhood settings such as kindergartens and day nurseries, provide a valuable opportunity to influence the dietary habits of people in a collective setting. Most of the trials of obesity prevention initiatives have been undertaken in schools. Nursery and pre-school settings are valuable opportunities for intervention at an early stage in the child's development, and have the potential to influence both the child and the family by setting an example of good practice.

The workplace has considerable potential to improve the health of the adult population because people spend a large proportion of their time at work and often eat there. It also has a role in supporting breast-feeding women and providing nursery facilities. In the US, workplace interventions are seen as a key strategy for obesity prevention (and weight reduction) and this is made feasible by the high health insurance costs borne by companies and thus the major financial benefits of a healthy workforce. Other countries without these levers will find it more difficult to get effective, sustainable workplace interventions implemented.

Other community settings include supermarkets, community and sports clubs and groups, churches and other religious settings, parks and recreational facilities. Several whole-of-community programs are underway which coordinate action across multiple settings and include local media.

The commercial sector, especially the food industry, has a huge influence on individual behaviours, although researching interventions in this sector is difficult. Proof of principle studies, such as the short-term effects of changes to food services, vending machine contents, labelling, and pricing of foods have shown significant effects on food selection (French, 2005). However, evidence on the wider application of such strategies is limited. Reducing portion sizes and altering food composition in order to reduce energy density are promising strategies which could have important impacts (Drewnowski & Rolls, 2005; Ledikwe, Ello-Martin & Rolls, 2005).

The built environment holds much promise for interventions, although most of the research to date has been limited to cross-sectional associations between aspects of the built environment and physical activity and obesity (Frank, Andresen & Schmid, 2004). Assessing the impact of cycle routes, walkways, sports and leisure facilities on population's body weight, fitness and cardiovascular health is difficult because these associations are prone to confounding and controlled interventions are difficult to design and implement. The retro-fitting of built environments to make them more conducive to health is likely to be a very long process which relies more on logic and these lower levels of evidence than high level evidence.

Approaches or Strategies

Approaches or strategies address *how* to bring about behavioural change in target groups, directly or indirectly. They can be broadly grouped into communication strategies (e.g. social marketing, education, information), programs (e.g. providing activities, increasing skills), and environmental change. The first two generally promote the healthy choices and the last one makes healthy choices easier – the so-called "upstream" approaches.

The environment, which is external to the individual, can be considered as physical, economic, policy and socio-cultural and these are all are very powerful influences on behaviours (Swinburn & Egger, 2004). For interventions, many environmental changes start at the policy level. For example: making the urban physical environment more walkable has to start with changes to urban planning regulations; exempting fruit and vegetables from a goods and services tax has to start with a policy; even changing the attitudes and perceptions about what is a "normal" school lunch can be accelerated through school food policies. Despite its central role in effecting change, the amount of research on the impact of policies is very limited.

For those who do not have the power to make the policy and environmental changes, advocacy for those changes becomes an important strategy (Box 9.3). Advocacy directed towards politicians on behalf of commercial interests (often referred to as lobbying) is sophisticated and well resourced with money and people. Advocates for public health are less well resourced but are often supported by professional, patient, and consumer groups and other non-governmental organisations. Advocacy organisations acting on behalf of public interests (such as consumer and environmental groups) tend to be trusted by the public at large to a greater extent than are commercial lobbying organisations or political parties (Eurobarometer, 2003). Advocacy no doubt has a major impact on public health but measuring the impact is difficult because it usually happens over long periods of time and in the context of many other changes (Chapman, 2001).

Box 9.3. Advocacy as an effective approach to policy

The protection of traditional, nourishing food sources against competition from less nourishing commercially produced foods can be of significant health benefit, but is likely to be undermined by a lack of market regulation to protect small producers and by economic policies which encourage modernization and a cash-based economy. In this context, advocacy can be one of the few defences of traditional products, and an example of this is given in the protection of breastfeeding undertaken by voluntary groups (involving professionals, parents and concerned individuals). Their advocacy to governments led to the WHO/UNICEF Code of Marketing of Breastmilk Substitutes and the development of some 20,000 Baby Friendly Hospitals in 150 countries, saving countless lives.

Further Caveats

We have described the traditional Targets-Settings-Approaches model for health promotion, but some extensions of this need to be considered.

Inequalities and the Locus of Responsibility

The traditional communications and program strategies (above) are dependent on the uptake of the messages or activities by the individual. Being individual-dependent, they are at risk of increasing health inequalities, because poorer people may not have the financial resources (e.g. to purchase healthier foods or use sports facilities) or the education and skills (e.g. in comprehending food labels and creating healthy recipes) or the "luxury" (e.g. their energy is taken up with coping with rent, jobs, and other problems) to hear the messages and convert them into behaviour changes (Cockerham, Rötten & Abel, 1997). An individual locus of responsibility (e.g. it is up to the parents to control what children eat and to get them involved in sports and other active programs) may pass the responsibility for disease prevention onto those at the most risk with the least capacity to achieve changes. Individualised or family-based health promotion, combined with the emphasis on personal responsibility or "making healthy choices" (Department of Health, 2004) may widen the health divide unless the strategy is supported by public interventions to ensure that healthier choices are fairly and widely available and their selection likely to be made by default.

"Settings Bias" in the Evidence

Although some interventions to prevent weight gain are undertaken within clinical settings (usually targeted at children already overweight or obese) the majority of primary prevention programmes aimed at children use schools. The reason for this is clear enough: that is where children are most accessible and where interventions can be implemented; controlled studies are feasible, usually using classes or schools as the unit of allocation; measurements are readily done within a school environment.

Care has to be taken with school-based interventions (e.g. contamination between intervention and control groups, effects of clustering, negative reactions to imposed notions of "health", stereotyping of body shapes, resource requirements and sustainability) although these problems are surmountable. However, there is a clear "settings bias" towards schools in the literature on child obesity prevention, leading to concerns that a traditional "evidence-based policy and practice approach" (demonstrated efficacy or effectiveness) will narrow the settings for obesity prevention to schools only and make a comprehensive approach impossible to justify (Swinburn et al., 2005; Lobstein, 2006). A wider view of converting broad evidence into agreed plans of action is outlined in the section on creating a portfolio of interventions.

Community Capacity Building

Community interventions will differ markedly depending on the targeted age group, ethnic mix, socio-economic status, urban/rural status, available settings, champions, existing activities and so on. To account for these contextual differences, one could look at "the intervention" broadly as building community capacity rather specifically as on-the-ground programs (e.g. after school activity program), communications (e.g. messages to parents about TV viewing), or environmental change (e.g. implementing school food policies). The science of measuring community capacity (leadership, resources, skills and knowledge, organisational relationships) is at in its early stages (Laverack, 2006) but since capacity building is an important part of the recipe for sustainability, much more research and better tools are needed in this area.

Effectiveness of Potential Interventions – An Evidence Review

This is the 4th issue in the IOTF framework (Figure 9.1) and asks "what are the potential, specific interventions and what is the evidence for their effectiveness?" In this section we summarise some of the evidence reviews of interventions to prevent overweight and obesity and to promote healthy body weights. We are not considering here the various measures available for obesity treatment or for weight loss in clinical patients.

It should be noted that, for most interventions, long-term follow-up was not undertaken, making it difficult to evaluate the efficacy of these interventions for population wide effects on obesity prevalence. Most of the studies were able to show improvements in eating and/or exercise habits and the large trials used for school-based interventions indicate the feasibility of implementing these sorts of programmes for children on a population basis. We are aware of no systematic reviews of interventions to prevent obesity in commercial settings, although various researchers have looked at the effects of price, labelling and marketing on food choices (French, 2005; Hastings, Stead, McDermott, Forsyth, MacKintosh, Rayner, Godfrey, Caraher & Angus, 2003).

The summary of the conclusions of systematic reviews given here is based on the Cochrane Library review (Summerbell, Waters, Edmunds, Kelly, Brown & Campbell, 2006) and 21 other published reviews (Carrel & Bernhardt, 2004; Casey & Crumley, 2004; Clemmens & Hayman, 2004; Dietz & Gortmaker, 2001; Doak, Visscher, Renders & Seidell, 2006; Flynn, McNeil, Maloff, Mutasingwa, Wu, Ford & Tough, 2006; Goran, Reynolds & Lindquist, 1999; Hardeman, Griffin, Johnston, Kinmonth & Wareham, 2000; Katz, O'Connell, Yeh, Nawaz, Njike, Anderson, Cory & Dietz, 2005; Micucci, Thomas & Vohra, 2002; Muller, Mast, Asbeck, Langnase & Grund, 2003; Mulvihill & Quigley, 2003; NHS Centre for Reviews and Dissemination, 1997; NHS Centre for Reviews and Dissemination, 2002; Reilly & McDowell, 2003; Schmitz & Jeffrey, 2002; Steinbeck, 2001; Story, 1999; Swedish Council on Technology Assessment in Health Care, 2002; Wareham, van Sluijs & Ekelund, 2005).

Breastfeeding Promotion

Four types of interventions have been shown to be useful in promoting breast-feeding:

- Peer-support programmes delivered in the ante- and post-natal periods increase initiation and duration rates among women on low incomes. Peer-support programmes should be targeted at women on low incomes who have expressed a wish to breastfeed.
- Informal, small-group health education sessions delivered during the ante-natal period have been shown to be effective in increasing initiation and duration among women of all income groups and women from minority ethnic groups.
- One-to-one health education can be effective at increasing initiation rates among women on low incomes. It may be more effective than group sessions in increasing initiation among women who have made a decision to bottle-feed.
- Changes in maternity ward practices to promote mother – infant contact and autonomy, such as "rooming in" (keeping the baby beside the mother) and breastfeeding support have been shown to be effective in increasing the initiation and duration of breastfeeding.

A more pronounced effect on both initiation and duration of breastfeeding has been found in studies of the Baby Friendly Hospital initiative promoted by UNICEF, including evidence of significant effects in European settings. In addition, initiation and duration of breastfeeding may be undermined by the physical hospital environment and by hospital routines e.g. feeding at set times, separation of mother and baby, use of infant formula, and by the attitudes and expectations of the health professionals who are involved.

Family-Based and Pre-School Settings

We are aware of no published systematic reviews of family-based interventions to prevent the development of overweight and obesity in pre-school children. A review in preparation suggests that the effectiveness of interventions targeted at

2–5 year olds and their families and carers, in terms of helping children maintain a healthy weight or prevent overweight or obesity, is equivocal (Summerbell, Brown & Ray, 2005). Three studies showed positive significant intervention effects, a further two studies failed to show significant improvements. The review suggests that small changes may be possible, and interventions are more likely to be effective if they are specifically focused on preventing obesity (rather than changing diet and physical activity behaviours), are intensive, costly (primarily a function of the intensity), targeted, and tailored to individual needs.

A review of the effectiveness of interventions to promote healthy eating in pre-school settings for children aged 1 to 5 years found that, while most studies demonstrated some positive effect on nutrition knowledge, the effect on eating behaviour was less frequently assessed and the results were inconsistent (Tedstone, Aviles, Shetty & Daniels, 1998). There were no data to evaluate long term effectiveness on knowledge or behaviour.

In the USA, a focus group involving 19 health care professionals in the Women, Infants and Child programme provided some insight into the barriers health professionals may face when counselling parents of overweight children (St Jeor, Perumean-Chaney, Sigman-Grant, Williams & Foreyt, 2002). They perceive that mothers: (1) were focused on surviving their daily life stresses, (2) used food to cope with these stresses and as a tool in parenting, (3) had difficulty setting limits with their children around food, (4) lacked knowledge about normal child development and eating behaviour, (5) were not committed to sustained behavioural change, and (6) did not believe their overweight children were overweight.

Effectiveness of family interventions targeted at older children, in terms of helping children maintain a healthy weight or prevent overweight or obesity, is also equivocal. Family based interventions may be less effective when trying to prevent obesity in adolescents. Studies of family-based treatment for overweight have indicated the need to consider the role of parents in the treatment process: one study indicated that treating the mother and child separately appeared to be significantly more effective than treating them together, or treating the child alone. In another study (10–11 year old children) there was no significant difference in effect on weight outcomes between treating the parent and child together or separately (McLean, Griffin, Toney & Hardeman, 2003). Interventions that link school and home activities appear to influence knowledge but not necessarily behaviour (Hopper, Gruber, Munoz & MacConnie, 1996). It is noteworthy to point out that family based interventions tend to be more expensive than child-based interventions conducted in schools.

School-Based Settings

Whilst school-based interventions appear able to show gains in children's nutrition understanding, increases in physical activity or improvements in diet, hardly any interventions appear able to demonstrate a significant effect on indicators of adiposity. Very few studies last longer than a year, and in those that follow children over a longer period find the initial advantages gained by the intervention may be reduced over time (Kafatos, Manios & Moschandreas, 2005).

Nearly all the reviews identify the combination of multiple approaches to obesity prevention – including education, food services and physical activity – as being more successful than single approaches. Increases in school physical activity opportunities and reduced television viewing time appear to be at least as important as classroom health education. Effectiveness may be increased by linking the school-based programme to out-of-school action, through the family and community.

Additional points raised are:

- Different age groups, ethnic groups and genders needed different approaches.
- For increasing physical activity, the most effective initiatives involved children through the whole school day, including lunch and recesses as well as class time and physical education lessons.
- Adults who had participated in school-based physical activities as children were more likely to be active in adulthood than those that had not.
- Breakfast clubs (food provided when children arrive early at school) can have a beneficial effect on behaviour, dietary intake, health, social interaction, concentration and learning, attendance and punctuality. They can reach lower income families and so address inequalities.
- School-based physical activity interventions that appear interesting and innovative to children (such as dance clubs), and interventions that aim to reduce television, videotape and video game use, are most effective.
- The most successful dietary interventions focus on promoting one aspect of a healthy diet, such as fruit and vegetables. Nutrition standards for food served in schools needs to be supported by measures to ensure that healthy options are selected. Restricting the choices of food available to children is associated with healthier eating.
- A comprehensive school food service policy should include snacks brought to school, vending machines, snack bars and access to local shops during breaks.
- Children will choose healthier options from vending machines, such as mineral water, pure fruit juice and skimmed milk: the key to success is pupil involvement, appropriate location of the vending machine close to the dining area, and ensuring continuity of provision (that the machine is full and in working order).
- Walking to school and cycling to school schemes may be effective, and may bring benefits besides preventing weight gain, but there is no good evidence available on which to base a recommendation.

A commentary by Lytle et al (Lytle, Jacobs, Perry & Klepp, 2002) noted the limited effects found in studies, and suggested several factors that may improve success rates, notably ensuring an adequate length of intervention and ensuring the involvement of all participants to prevent drop-out. The authors also note that heterogeneity, i.e. the involvement of participants from diverse cultural backgrounds, is rarely catered for in the experimental designs where "one size fits all", and this may compromise the ability to show significant effects. The authors recommend programmes which are more flexible and responsive to the social and cultural environments in which they occur, perhaps inviting the active participation of community members during the design of the intervention. They also note Richter et al's evidence that school and community interventions are more likely to be successful if they occur in the context of health-promoting environments (Richter, Harris, Paine-Andrews, Fawcett, Schmid, Lankenau & Johnston, 2000).

Workplace Settings

Strategies that target adults at their place of work include a number of different approaches: nutrition education, aerobic or strength training exercise prescription, training in behavioural techniques, changing workplace food (canteens, vending machines, catered food), and the provision of self-help materials. Evidence of effectiveness of workplace efforts to control overweight and obesity is not strong, but might encourage employers to provide such programmes. The literature supports an emphasis on interventions combining instruction in healthier eating with a structured approach to increasing physical activity in the worksite setting (Katz et al., 2005).

Further observations on the workplace setting include:

- Choose definable and modifiable risk factors which are a priority for the specific worker group.
- Strategies should not isolate health-related knowledge, values and behaviours from the social and material context in which the targeted employees live.
- Program cost-effectiveness data might increase employer interest.
- Given the frequency of weight rebound after short-term weight loss, additional research is needed regarding the most effective means of maintaining initial success.
- Visible and enthusiastic support and involvement from top management.
- Involvement by employees in the planning and implementation stages.

Community Settings

A summary of the evidence found inconclusive evidence regarding the effectiveness of community-based interventions (for example seminars, mailed educational packaged and mass media participation) for the prevention of obesity and overweight in adults (Mulvihill & Quigley, 2003). The review recommended that the effectiveness of community-based education programmes linked with financial incentives should be investigated further.

Examples of more imaginative approaches used in community settings include improved information and access to healthier food choices (for example, improving access to major stores and better provision at local shops, establishment of food co-ops, community cafes, growing clubs); health promotion activities for improving knowledge and skills (for example, through shopping tours, cook and eat classes); improved provision and safety of walking and cycling routes; and local voucher schemes (e.g. for local swimming pools).

Supermarket promotions appear to be effective in improving dietary intakes over the short term, particularly if accompanied by supporting information. Promotions in restaurants and cafes may have a greater impact than those in supermarkets. Using churches as a setting for health education may also have a positive impact on dietary intake (Weightman, Fry, Sander, Kitcher & Jenkins, 2005).

While the general promotion of active transport does not appear to be effective, targeted programmes with tailored advice do appear to change travel behaviour of motivated subgroups. Associated action, such as subsidies for commuters, may also be effective. Promotions which aim to motivate the use of stairs using posters and banners appear to have a positive effect (Kerr, Eves & Carroll, 2001; Marshall, Bauman, Patch, Wilson & Chen, 2002).

Cost Effectiveness

For policy-makers considering strategy options, the distinction between effectiveness and cost-effectiveness is critical. If a policy objective is to be pursued with no limitation on spending, then effectiveness (the beneficial effect of a strategy in practice) is the primary consideration. But when cost limitations apply (as they inevitably do), an evaluation of cost-effectiveness is essential if rational decisions are to be made (Brunner, Cohen & Toon, 2001).

A remarkable feature of the evaluations and systematic reviews of interventions described above is that they rarely mention the costs of the various programmes they examine, and make no estimates of cost-effectiveness. A recent review of workplace and community interventions noted that only two studies which met the criteria for inclusion provided cost-effectiveness analyses of worksite interventions to prevent and control overweight and obesity (Katz et al., 2005).

For child obesity prevention we have identified only one study which explicitly examined the costs of an intervention programme, the US Planet Health Program (Wang, Yang, Lowry & Wechsler, 2003). Planet Health's estimated cost-effectiveness ratio gives a value of $4305 per quality-adjusted life year gained, which compares favourably with interventions such as the treatment of hypertension, low-cholesterol-diet therapies, some diabetes screening programs and treatments, and adult exercise programs (Ganz, 2003).

Creating a Portfolio of Interventions

The evidence for obesity prevention covered thus far has shown: a substantial burden to warrant action; sufficient understanding of the determinants to know *what* to target; a determination of the priority target populations (*who*), the best settings to access (*where*), and the most appropriate strategies to use (*how*), and; a review of the literature about what has been shown to work or not work. The final challenge in the IOTF framework (prior to actually implementing and evaluating the work) is to create the "portfolio" of interventions to be implemented. This is a considerable challenge in priority setting of, because the aim of intervention selection is:

To agree upon a *balanced portfolio* of *specific, promising* interventions to reduce the *burden of obesity* and *improve health and quality of life* within the *available capacity* to do so

"Agreement" infers a process with decision-makers coming to a joint understanding. "Balanced portfolio" means a balance of content (both nutrition and physical activity), settings (not all school-based), strategies (policies, programs, communications), and target groups (whole population, high risk). Interventions need to be "specific" (not just "promote healthy eating") and can be "promising" rather than proven. The analogy of choosing a balance of products (shares, property, bonds) to create portfolio of financial investments has been used by Hawe and Shiell (1995) to conceptualise appropriate investment in health. The best investments are the safe, high return ones (i.e. high level of evidence, high population impact) but inevitably the choices come down to including some safe, lower return investments and some higher risk (i.e. less certainty), potentially higher return investments while excluding the high risk, low return ones. The IOTF framework (Swinburn et al., 2005) applies this investment concept to obesity prevention and presents a "promise table" which is a grid of certainty (strength of evidence) versus return (population impact) into which interventions can be placed according to their credentials.

The other key concepts in the priority setting aim are that the interventions reduce the "burden of obesity" and "improve health and quality of life". These issues are particularly important for obesity prevention because many of the interventions (healthier eating and physical activity) have their own independent effects on health and some interventions have the potential to do harm (such as increase stigmatisation and teasing) or increase health inequalities. Fitting the plan of action to the available capacity to achieve it is especially a challenge at the community level where the level of health promotion funding is usually very low and the enthusiasm for doing something is usually very high.

Given the challenging aim of intervention selection, how can this be achieved and what role does (or should) evidence play in the process? Certainly, the evidence of effectiveness is not sufficient by itself to guide appropriate decision-making, and, indeed, true evidence-based policy-making is probably quite rare. (Marmot, 2004) Some major policy decisions are made on the basis of extremely little evidence despite high costs (such as military interventions). A helpful concept to apply is that of "practice/policy-based evidence" (Marmot, 2004). Whereas evidence-based practice/policy starts in the library, assesses what has been published and then takes that intelligence to the policy-maker or practitioner to consider for implementation, practice/policy-based evidence starts at the table with the practitioner or policy-maker and assesses what could be implemented with the ideas coming from many sources: what is already happening here, what is happening elsewhere, what the literature shows, what the politicians want to implement and so on. Then some technical estimates are made using the best evidence available and these are brought back to the table to inform the priority setting. Two examples of this are given below.

Evidence and Priority Setting – National/State Level

The ACE-Obesity project (Assessing Cost-Effectiveness of Obesity Interventions) was funded by the Victorian Government in Australia to inform it on the best investments for reducing childhood obesity (Haby, Vos, Carter, Moodie, Markwick, Magnus, Tay-Teo & Swinburn, 2006). The ACE approach included extensive economic analyses around agreed, specified interventions to reduce childhood obesity at a state or national level, plus a process that engaged key stakeholders in first selecting the interventions for analysis and then secondly providing judgments on the modelling assumptions and a number of "second stage filters" (strength of evidence, feasibility, sustainability, acceptability, effects on equity, other positive or negative effects). The definition of evidence was wide and all assumptions in the modelling had to be explicit and have in-built uncertainty estimates. In this way, policies (such as banning food advertisements to children), programs (such as active transport to school) and services (such as gastric banding for very obese teenagers) which lacked trial evidence could still be modelled.

The outputs were estimates of total cost, population health gains (body mass index [BMI] units saved or disability-adjusted life years [DALY] saved), cost-effectiveness ($/BMI saved, $/DALY saved), and the second stage filter judgements. Table 9.2 shows some of these outputs for the 13 interventions modelled (Department of Human Services, 2006; Haby et al., 2006).

From this set of data, there are clear pointers for decision-makers such as the low cost of policies compared to programs and the importance of the reach of an intervention (another advantage of policies over programs). It poses problems

TABLE 9.2. Modelled estimates of costs and impacts of obesity prevention interventions for children and adolescents (ranked by population impact – total DALYs saved)

Intervention	Total DALYs saved	Total BMI units saved	Gross cost (AUD $m)	Net cost (AUD $m)
Bans on TV food advertising to children	37 000	400 000	0.13	−300
Laparoscopic adjustable gastric banding for obese teenagers	12 000	55 000	130	55
School-based programs to reduce TV viewing	8 600	122 000	54.6	−2.1
Multi-faceted school-based including active PE	8 000	124 000	40.4	−28.7
School-based programs to reduce sweet drinks	5 300	69 000	3.3	−5.2
Family-based program for overweight children	2 700	3 400	11	−4.1
Multi-faceted school-based without active PE	1 600	23 000	24.3	11.2
GP delivered program for overweight children	510	2 300	6.3	3.0
Active After School Communities program	450	4 200	40.3	36.6
Orlistat therapy for obese teenagers	450	600	6.4	4.0
Multi-faceted school-based program for overweight children	360	2 000	0.56	−0.1
'TravelSMART' active transport program	50	470	13.1	12.5
Walking School Bus program	30	270	22.8	22.6

DALY = Disability-adjusted life year, BMI = body mass index, AUD = Australian dollars
Adapted from Haby et al (2006) and Department of Human Services (2006).

however when some effective interventions are not very acceptable to stake-holders like governments (such as bans on television advertising to children and gastric banding for teenagers), or when popular programs (such as walking school bus and active after school programs) are not very effective or cost-effective. These and other second stage filters are essentially stakeholder judgements which are either not included or are on the bottom rung of evidence hierarchies as expert opinion, yet they carry such weight in real life policy decisions. The aim here is to make them transparent. It may be perfectly appro-priate to fund a Walking School Bus program even though it is costly and ineffective for obesity prevention. It could be justified for other benefits (e.g. reducing congestion and pollution) or as an "icon" program (e.g. as a visible, leader program for active transport in general) but high expectations cannot be placed on the program for contributing to reducing obesity.

Evidence and Priority Setting – Community Level

Well-evaluated community demonstration projects are an excellent strategy to build the evidence for obesity prevention at the community level. However, the same challenges of defining what *could* be done and then undertaking a priority setting process to determine what *should* be done apply at the community level as much as they apply at a state or national level. Similar principles to ACE-Obesity, but a simplified process, were applied in the formative stages of six demonstration projects in Australia, New Zealand and the Pacific (Schultz, Utter, Mathews, Cama, Mavoa & Swinburn, 2007). The central feature is the ANGELO workshop (so-called because it uses an Analysis Grid for Elements Linked to Obesity – see Swinburn, Egger & Raza, 1999) which brings together the literature-based evidence and the local context expertise so that stakeholders can prioritise a number of specified behavioural targets, knowledge and skills gaps and environmental barriers for action. At the end of a 2-day workshop, they have a draft action plan that they own and is truly "practice-based evidence" because the three critical features have been brought together: the evidence (all parts of the IOTF framework), the context (stakeholder judgements) and a transparent process.

Effects of Globalisation

Food supply, food prices, food policies and food marketing at a community and national level are heavily influenced by global forces. It is clear from the recent economically-based analyses for the UK Treasury (Wanless, 2002) that interven-tions to reduce smoking, obesity and physical inactivity require economic modelling including analyses of the effects of product prices and marketing practices on consumers' purchasing patterns. These approaches have been used by the EU in its agricultural policies for manipulating the production of cereals, meat, milk, butter, sugar, wine, fruit and vegetables by altering subsidy and tariff levels, controlling minimum prices and shaping markets (e.g. by destroy-ing fish catches and fruit and vegetable crops). Routine economic planning approaches have not often been applied sufficiently to analyses of options for social policy change. The evidence required to show how policy changes in these areas might affect consumption patterns and subsequent chronic disease rates has received too little attention.

In a review of the determinants of dietary trends, Haddad (2003) notes the need to consider several macro-economic factors, including income growth, urbanisation, and the relative prices of foods and their availability which are affected by mass production technology and commodity costs, along with retail distribution chains and catering outlets. One study of US food supply price elasticities showed that an increase in the price of oils would lead to a decrease in fat consumption and total energy intake, and an increase in the consumption of most other nutrients (Huang, 1996).

Prices of foods are in turn affected by the cost of commodities, which are in turn affected by agricultural support policies and trade regulations. Food prices must also absorb marketing and promotion budgets.

Marketing itself interacts with consumer awareness and cultural practices. There is remarkably little publicly available data on the impact of commercial marketing strategies on children's behaviour, including the effects on diet and physical activity and consequential weight gain. It is highly likely that some valuable data is held by the commercial interests themselves. A government initiative to acquire this data on behalf of consumers would be a valuable research resource, on a par with the commercial papers that were released during litigation against the tobacco companies. In respect of marketing, the evidence needed should include not only direct marketing strategies, such as television advertising and promotional internet sites, but also product placement on film and television programmes, cross branding of recognisable elements of food brands on non-food items, the use of colouring and flavour-boosting food additives to promote sales, the use of sponsorship and celebrity endorsement of products, the licensing of children's cartoons for use on food labels and other techniques aimed to influence children's food and leisure choices. Evidence is needed to show how these various promotional methods affect dietary choices and subsequent health.

Similarly, more evidence is needed on the impact of investment strategies, such as foreign direct investment in sectors affecting food supplies – agriculture, food manufacturing, retailing and catering (e.g. fast food catering) – for their potential effects on diet and health, mediated through food prices and availability.

In all the above suggestions, similar analyses could be undertaken relating to the "products" (including buildings, vehicles, parks and streets, television entertainment etc) which affect the physical environment and influence physical activity, or which encourage sedentary behaviour. The marketing of products affecting physical activity are all in need of better research understanding in order to demonstrate to policy-makers that interventions can be a worthwhile investment opportunity.

Evidence Needs

In this chapter we have reflected on the shortcomings of the current evidence base for obesity prevention and the difficulties in obtaining relevant evidence for policy-making. These problems were also considered at the WHO Kobe expert meeting on childhood obesity (World Health Organization, 2005) which made several recommendations, including:

- All interventions should include process evaluation measures, and provide resource and cost estimates. Evaluation can include impact on other parties, such as parents and siblings.
- Interventions using control groups should be explicit about what the control group experiences. Phrases like "normal care" or "normal curriculum" or "standard school PE classes" are not helpful, especially if normal practices have been changing over the years.
- There is a need for more interventions looking into the needs of specific sub-populations, including immigrant groups, low income groups, and specific ethnic and cultural groups.
- There is a shortage of long-term programmes monitoring interventions. Long-term outcomes could include changes in knowledge and attitudes, behaviours (diet and physical activity) and adiposity outcomes.
- New approaches to interventions, including prospective meta-analyses, should be considered.
- Community-based demonstration programmes can be used to generate evidence, gain experience, develop capacity and maintain momentum.
- There is a need for an international agency to encourage networking of community-based interventions, support methods of evaluation and assist in the analysis of the cost-effectiveness of initiatives.

The Kobe meeting also expressed concern at the role of interested parties in the funding and evaluation of research and recommended that research reviews should not be funded by commercial interests. The meeting identified a need to evaluate the impact of programs funded by industry and other sources of potential bias, in order to examine their contribution to the evidence base.

Conclusions

The traditional approach to evidence is based on a medical model but this needs to be adapted to suit obesity prevention, retaining the rigour of evidence assessments and uses while incorporating the flexibility and complexity needed for public health intervention research. The IOTF framework attempts to achieve this by articulating the various questions that the evidence needs to address, by expanding the definitions of evidence, by highlighting the need for modelling where there are gaps in the empirical data, by lifting the value of informed stakeholder input for those research questions where contextual factors are important, by taking a "solution-oriented" approach to determining interventions, and by defining how a "policy/practice-based evidence" paradigm can better align evidence with the realities of decision-making.

Acknowledgements. We would like to acknowledge the input of Tim Gill and Shiriki Kumanyika in the IOTF evidence framework, the work of Rob Carter, Theo Vos, Michelle Haby, Anne Magnus, Alison Markwick, Marj Moodie, and Mike Ackland on the ACE-Obesity project, and Colin Bell, Andrea Sanigorski, and Anne Simmons on the community-based intervention approaches.

References

Astrup, A. (2005). The satiating power of protein – a key to obesity prevention? *Am J Clin Nutr, 82*, 1–2.

Brunner, E., Cohen, D. & Toon, L. (2001). Cost effectiveness of cardiovascular disease prevention strategies: A perspective on EU food based dietary guidelines. *Public Health Nutr, 4*, 711–715.

Carrel, A.L. & Bernhardt, D.T. (2004). Exercise prescription for the prevention of obesity in adolescents. *Curr Sports Med Rep, 3*, 330–336.

Casey, L. & Crumley, E. (2004). *Addressing Childhood Obesity: The Evidence for Action.* Canadian Association of Paediatric Health Centres: Ottawa.
See http://www.caphc.org/childhood_obesity/obesity_report.pdf.

Chapman, S. (2001). Advocacy in public health: Roles and challenges. *Int J Epidemiol, 30*, 1226–1232.

Clemmens, D. & Hayman, L.L. (2004). Increasing activity to reduce obesity in adolescent girls: A research review. *J Obstet Gynecol Neonatal Nurs, 33*, 801–808.

Cockerham, W.C., Rütten, A. & Abel, T. (1997). Conceptualizing contemporary health lifestyles. Moving beyond Weber. *Sociol Q, 38*, 321–342.

Department of Health. (2004). *Choosing Health: Making Healthier Choices Easier.* Public Health White Paper. The Stationery Office: London.

Department of Human Services. (2006). *ACE Obesity. Assessing Cost-Effectiveness of obesity interventions in children and adolescents. Summary of results.* Department of Human Services, Victorian Government: Melbourne.
See http://www.dhs.vic.gov.au/health/healthpromotion/downloads/ace_obesity.pdf.

Dietz, W. & Gortmaker, S. (2001). Preventing obesity in children and adolescents. *Annual Review of Public Health, 22*, 337–353.

Doak, C.M., Visscher, T.L.S., Renders, C.M. & Seidell, J.C. (2006). The prevention of overweight and obesity in children and adolescents: A review of interventions and programmes. *Obes Rev, 7*, 111–136.

Drewnowski, A. & Rolls, B.J. (2005). How to modify the food environment. *J Nutr, 135*, 898–899.

Eurobarometer. (2003). European Union citizens and sources of information about health. *Eurobarometer special report 58.0.* European Opinion Research group, for the European Commission: Brussels, March 2003.

Flynn, M.A., McNeil, D.A., Maloff, B., Mutasingwa, D., Wu, M., Ford, C. & Tough, S.C. (2006). Reducing obesity and related chronic disease risk in children and youth: A synthesis of evidence with "best practice" recommendations. *Obes Rev, 7 Suppl 1*, 7–66.

Frank, L.D., Andresen, M.A. & Schmid, T.L. (2004). Obesity relationships with community design, physical activity, and time spent in cars. *Am J Prev Med, 27*, 87–96.

French, S.A. (2005). Public health strategies for dietary change: Schools and workplaces. *J Nutr, 135*, 910–912.

Ganz, M.L. (2003). Commentary: The economic evaluation of obesity interventions: Its time has come. *Obes Res, 11*, 1275–1277.

Goran, M., Reynolds, K.D. & Lindquist, C.H. (1999). Role of physical activity in the prevention of obesity in children. *Int J Obes, 23 Suppl 3*, 18–33.

Haby, M.M., Vos, T., Carter, R., Moodie, M., Markwick, A., Magnus, A., Tay-Teo, K.S. & Swinburn, B. (2006). A new approach to assessing the health benefit from obesity interventions in children and adolescents: The assessing cost-effectiveness in obesity project. *Int J Obes, 30*, 1463–1475.

Haddad, L. (2003). Redirecting the diet transition: What can food policy do? *Development Policy Review, 21*, 599–614.

Hardeman, W., Griffin, S., Johnston, M., Kinmonth, A.L. & Wareham, N.J. (2000). Interventions to prevent weight gain, a systematic review of psychological models and behaviour change methods. *Int J Obes, 24*, 131–143.

Hastings, G., Stead, M., McDermott, L., Forsyth, A., MacKintosh, A.M., Rayner, M., Godfrey, C., Caraher, M. & Angus, K. (2003). *Review of research on the effects of food promotion to children. Final report*. Prepared for the Food Standards Agency, London. See http://www.ism.stir.ac.uk/projects_food.htm.

Hawe, P. & Shiell, A. (1995). Preserving innovation under increasing accountability pressures: The health promotion investment portfolio approach. *Health Prom Aust, 5*, 4–9.

Hopper, C.A., Gruber, M.B., Munoz, K.D. & MacConnie, S.E. (1996). School-based cardiovascular exercise and nutrition programs with parent participation. *Journal of Health Education, 27*, 32–39.

Huang, K.S. (1996). Nutrient elasticities in a complete food demand system. *Am J Agric Econ, 78*, 21–29, cited in Haddad, L. (2003) *op cit*.

Kafatos, A., Manios, Y. & Moschandreas, J. (2005). Preventive medicine & nutrition clinic university of crete research team. Health and nutrition education in primary schools of Crete: Follow-up changes in body mass index and overweight status. *Eur J Clin Nutr, 59*, 1090–1092.

Katz, D. L., O'Connell, M., Yeh, M.C., Nawaz, H., Njike, V., Anderson, L.M., Cory, S. & Dietz, W. (2005). Task force on community preventive services. Public health strategies for preventing and controlling overweight and obesity in school and worksite settings: A report on recommendations of the task force on community preventive services. *MMWR Recomm Rep, 7*, 1–12.

Kerr, J., Eves, F. & Carroll, D. (2001). Six-month observational study of prompted stair climbing. *Prev Med, 33*, 422–427.

Knowler, W.C., Barrett-Connor, E., Fowler, S.E., Hamman, R.F., Lachin, J.M., Walker, E.A., Nathan, D.M. & The Diabetes Prevention Program Research Group. (2002). Reduction in the incidence of type 2 diabetes with lifestyle intervention or metformin. *N Engl J Med, 346*, 393–403.

Laverack, G. (2006). Evaluating community capacity: Visual representation and interpretation. *Community Development Journal, 41*, 266–276.

Ledikwe, J.H., Ello-Martin, J.A. & Rolls, B.J. (2005). Portion sizes and the obesity epidemic. *J Nutr, 135*, 905–909.

Lobstein, T. (2006). Comment: Preventing child obesity – an art and a science. *Obes Rev, 7 Suppl 1*, 1–5.

Lobstein, T., Baur, L., Uauy, R. & The IASO International Obesity TaskForce. (2004). Obesity in children and young people: A crisis in public health. *Obes Rev, 5*, 4–104.

Lytle, L.A., Jacobs, D.R., Perry, C.L. & Klepp, K-I. (2002). Achieving physiological change in school-based intervention trials: What makes a preventive intervention successful? *Brit J Nutr, 88*, 219–221.

Marmot, M.G. (2004). Evidence based policy or policy based evidence? *BMJ, 328*, 906–907.

Marshall, A.L., Bauman, A.E., Patch, C., Wilson, J. & Chen, J. (2002). Can motivational signs prompt increases in incidental physical activity in an Australian health-care facility? *Health Educ Res, 17*, 743–749.

McLean, N., Griffin, S., Toney, K. & Hardeman, W. (2003). Family involvement in weight control, weight maintenance and weight-loss interventions: A systematic review of randomised trials. *Int J Obes Relat Metab Disord, 27*, 987–1005.

Micucci, S., Thomas, H. & Vohra, J. (2002). *The Effectiveness of School-Based Strategies for the Primary Prevention of Obesity and for Promoting Physical Activity and Nutrition, the Major Modifiable Risk Factors for Type 2 Diabetes: Review of Reviews.* Public Health Research, Education and Development Program, Hamilton: Canada.

Muller, M.J., Mast, M., Asbeck, I., Langnase, K. & Grund, A. (2003). Prevention of obesity – is it possible? *Obes Rev, 2*, 15–28.

Mulvihill, C. & Quigley, R. (2003). The management of obesity and overweight An analysis of reviews of diet, physical activity and behavioural approaches *Evidence briefing 1st Edition.*Health Development Agency: London.

NHS Centre for Reviews and Dissemination. (1997). The prevention and treatment of obesity. *Effective Health Care No 3, 2*, 1–12.

NHS Centre for Reviews and Dissemination. (2002). The prevention and treatment of childhood obesity. *Effective Health Care Bulletin No 7, 6*, 1–12.

Ornish, D., Brown, S.E., Scherwitz, L.W., Billings, J.H., Armstrong, W.T., Ports, T.A., McLanahan, S.M., Kirkeeide, R.L., Brand, R.J. & Gould, K.L. (1990). Lifestyle changes and heart disease. *Lancet, 336*, 741–742.

Parsons, T.J., Power, C., Logan, S. & Summerbell, C.D. (1999). Childhood predictors of adult obesity: A systematic review. *Int J Obes Relat Metab Disord, 23 Suppl 8*, S1–107.

Reilly, J.J. & McDowell, Z.C. (2003). Physical activity interventions in the prevention and treatment of paediatric obesity: Systematic review and critical appraisal. *Proc Nutr Soc, 62*, 611–619.

Richter, K.P., Harris, K.J., Paine-Andrews, A., Fawcett, S.B., Schmid, T.L., Lankenau, B.H. & Johnston, J. (2000). Measuring the health environment for physical activity and nutrition among youth: A review of the literature and applications for community initiatives. *Preventive Medicine, 31*, 98–111.

Robinson, T.N. & Sirard, J.R. (2005). Preventing childhood obesity: A solution-oriented research paradigm. *Am J Prev Med, 28*, 194–201.

Rychetnik, L., Hawe, P., Waters, E., Barratt, A. & Frommer, M. (2004). A glossary for evidence based public health. *J Epidemiol Community Health, 58*, 538–545.

Schmitz, K.H. & Jeffrey, R.W. (2002). Prevention of obesity. In: Wadden, T.A. & Stunkard, A.J. (eds) *Handbook of Obesity Treatment.*Guilford Press: New York. pp. 556–593.

Schultz, T., Utter, J., Mathews, L., Cama, T., Mavoa, H. & Swinburn, B. (2007). The Pacific OPIC Project (Obesity Prevention in Communities) – Action plans and interventions. *Pac Health Dialogue* (in press).

Seidell, J. C., Nooyens, A.J. & Visscher, T.L. (2005). Cost-effective measures to prevent obesity: Epidemiological basis and appropriate target groups. *Proc Nutr Soc, 64,* 1–5.

St Jeor, S.T., Perumean-Chaney, S., Sigman-Grant, M., Williams, C. & Foreyt, J. (2002). Family-based interventions for the treatment of childhood obesity. *Journal of the American Dietetic Association, 102,* 640–644.

Steinbeck, K. (2001). The importance of physical activity in the prevention of overweight and obesity in childhood: A review and an opinion. *Obes Rev, 2,* 117–130.

Story, M. (1999). School-based approaches for preventing and treating obesity. *Int J Obes, 23 Suppl 2,* 43–51.

Summerbell, C., Brown, T. & Ray, P. (2005). A systematic review of the effectiveness of interventions, including family interventions (in children aged 5–12), to prevent excess weight gain or maintain a healthy weight in children aged between two and five years. *Obesity Guideline Development Group: Public Health Sub-Group.* CPHE Collaborating Centre: University of Teesside.

Summerbell, C.D., Waters, E., Edmunds, L.D., Kelly, S., Brown, T. & Campbell, K.J. (2006). Interventions for preventing obesity in children. *The Cochrane Database of Systematic Reviews, 2006 (1).*

Swedish Council on Technology Assessment in Health Care. (2002). Obesity – problems and interventions. *Report No 160.* The Swedish Council on Technology Assessment in Health Care. Stockholm, Sweden. See http://www.sbu.se/Filer/Content0/publikationer/1/obesity_2002/obsesityslut.pdf.

Swinburn, B. & Egger, G. (2002). Preventive strategies against weight gain and obesity. *Obes Rev, 3,* 289–301.

Swinburn, B. & Egger, G. (2004). Influence of obesity-producing environments. In: Bray, G.A. & Bouchard, C. (eds) *Handbook of Obesity – Clinical Applications.*Marcel Dekker, Inc.: New York. pp. 97–114.

Swinburn, B.A., Caterson, I., Seiddell, J.C. & James, W.P.T. (2004). Diet, nutrition and the prevention of excess weight gain and obesity. *Public Health Nutr, 7,* 123–146.

Swinburn, B.A., Egger, G.J. & Raza, F. (1999). Dissecting obesogenic environments: The development and application of a framework for identifying and prioritising environmental interventions for obesity. *Prev Med, 29,* 563–570.

Swinburn, B., Gill, T. & Kumanyika, S. (2005). Obesity prevention: A proposed framework for translating evidence into action. *Obes Rev, 6,* 23–33.

Tedstone, A., Aviles, M., Shetty, P. & Daniels, L. (1998). *Effectiveness of interventions to promote healthy eating in preschool children aged 1 to 5 years: A review.* Health Education Authority: London.

Wang, L.Y., Yang, Q., Lowry, R. & Wechsler, H. (2003). Economic analysis of a school-based obesity prevention program. *Obes Res, 11,* 1313–1324.

Wang, Y. & Lobstein, T. (2006). Worldwide trends in childhood overweight and obesity. *Int J Ped Obesity, 1,* 11–25.

Wanless, D. (2002). *Securing Our Future Health: Taking a Long-Term View. Final report.* HM Treasury: London.

Wareham, N.J., van Sluijs, E.M. & Ekelund, U. (2005). Physical activity and obesity prevention: A review of the current evidence. *Proc Nutr Soc, 64,* 229–247.

Weightman, A., Fry, S., Sander, L., Kitcher, H. & Jenkins, E. (2005). *A rapid review of broader community-based interventions to prevent obesity.* Obesity Guideline

Development Group: Public Health Sub-Group.CPHE Collaborating Centre: Cardiff University.

World Cancer Research Fund. (1997). Food, nutrition, and the prevention of cancer: A global perspective. American Institute for Cancer Research. American Institute for Cancer Research: Washington.

World Health Organization. (2000). *Obesity, preventing and managing the global epidemic – Report of a WHO consultation.* WHO Technical Report Series, 894. World Health Organization: Geneva.

World Health Organization. (2003). WHO Technical Report Series 916. Diet, nutrition and the prevention of chronic diseases. Joint FAO/WHO expert consultation: Geneva.

World Health Organization. (2004). Global Strategy on Diet, Physical Activity and Health. Endorsed at the 57th World Health Assembly, May 2004. World Health Organization: Geneva.

World Health Organization. (2005). *Obesity in childhood: Draft report of an expert committee held in Kobe, Japan, June 2005.* WHO: Geneva. (unpublished).

10
Effective Health Promotion Against Tobacco Use

KAREN SLAMA, CYNTHIA CALLARD, YUSSUF SALOOJEE AND BUNGON RITHIPHAKDEE

The development of tobacco control policies and programs has been shaped by two concurrent forces. The first is the public health tradition of evidence-based decision making, which compels the abandonment of ineffective strategies and the continuous improvement of effective ones. The second is the tobacco industry tradition of resisting public health initiatives in order to maintain tobacco sales. This on-going battle has slowed progress in reducing death and disease from tobacco. Nonetheless, after five decades of research on, and evaluation of public health strategies, a consensus on a set of effective measures to curb the tobacco epidemic has emerged (Jha & Chaloupka, 1999).

The lessons learnt in changing tobacco use behaviors have given impetus to the development of the science of health promotion. In the early stages health authorities relied on giving individuals "the facts," but soon recognized that that this was not sufficient and that additional measures were needed. These included not only making health education more persuasive and motivating, but changing the environment so as to make "healthy choices, easy choices."

Creating environments that allow people to choose not to use tobacco means enacting tobacco control legislation to limit tobacco industry marketing strategies, to regulate tobacco product contents and emissions, to regularly increase price through taxes, and to protect people from exposure to tobacco smoke in public places. It also means that tobacco control laws be enforced and that smuggling is kept under control.

Tobacco control seeks to change social norms and individual motivations related to tobacco use through media campaigns and other health education initiatives, easy access to cessation treatment, community involvement, and lobbying and advocacy. Governments also had to recognize their changed role from one of non-intervention in private lifestyle decisions to one of principled acceptance of their public health responsibilities.

Indicators of the Effectiveness of Tobacco Control Programs

Tobacco control interventions try to influence the social, economic and environmental factors that affect a population's use of tobacco. A fall in consumption should, in time, result in better health for populations as a result of both a reduction in premature death and disease from tobacco-related causes and the reallocation of resources used in the production of tobacco products. Evidence continues to build of the impact of government policy on tobacco use and of programs for cessation and prevention in a form that can be used for the Cochrane reviews (http://www.cochrane.org/reviews/en/topics/94.html).

A number of strategic performance indicators of the effectiveness of tobacco control interventions have been identified by the World Health Organization (WHO) (Chollat-Traquet, 1996). These are:

- Political outcomes – the number of policies and programs adopted and implemented by governments.
- Educational outcomes – public awareness of risks, attitudes on tobacco use and opinions towards policies.
- Environmental outcomes – increase in smoke-free environments, decreased availability and affordability of tobacco products.
- Behavioral outcomes – reductions in the prevalence of tobacco use, in consumption, increase in self-protective behavior (e.g., attempts to quit, use of smoke-free facilities) and personal involvement in tobacco control programs (e.g., advocacy or physician advice to patients to quit).
- Economic outcomes – impact on personal and public finance (e.g., lower household spending on tobacco, reductions in medical care costs, improved productivity) and on business sectors.
- Health outcomes – improved quality of life, decreased tobacco-related morbidity and mortality for smokers and nonsmokers.

There is, typically, a considerable gap between changes in behavior and measurable improvements in health. The political, economic, social and behavioral impacts of these policies are better short- and medium-term indicators of progress.

Reducing levels of tobacco use is a fundamental goal of tobacco control interventions. Adult per capita tobacco consumption and smoking prevalence are therefore the most frequently used measures of effectiveness. The utility of these measures as a link between behavioral changes and final health outcomes has been shown. In countries with long-standing tobacco control policies like the USA and UK, where large numbers of people have stopped smoking for decades, decreases in lung cancer and heart disease have been observed (Peto, Darby, Deo, Silcocks, Whitley & Doll, 2000; Jemal, Cokkinides, Shafey & Thun, 2003).

Countries where the tobacco epidemic has only recently spread can benefit from the current understanding of the tobacco industry to impede the industry's attempts to delay implementation of legislative measures and to adopt policies and programs that affect people's behaviors and counteract industry tactics. This means giving precedence to population measures over individual approaches. Examples of population-based approaches will be demonstrated in the section on tobacco control in different parts of the world.

After five decades of research on and evaluation of public health strategies, a set of population measures defined as effective by health authorities throughout the world has been agreed and codified in an international treaty for health protection by governments and sets global standards for the production, marketing and use of tobacco products (WHO, 2003). The WHO Framework Convention on Tobacco Control (FCTC) entered into force in February, 2005, and has been ratified by 138 nations, as of September 1, 2006.

There is great variability in the population measures that have been adopted and in the general acceptance of tobacco use in society, or by governments. The existence of the WHO FCTC and its ratification is an example of a new consensual end-point. Whether or not the measures included in the treaty are adopted and enforced will be the result of civil society demand and government readiness.

Effective Tobacco Control Programs in Different Regions

Tobacco Control in the Americas

The American Regional Office of the World Health Organization (the Pan American Health Organization, PAHO) defines effective tobacco control measures as those that prevent initiation, increase quitting, reduce consumption and exposure to toxins by smokers who continue to smoke and which protect non-smokers from exposure to second-hand smoke (PAHO, 2006). PAHO considers the most cost-effective tobacco control measures to be imposing higher tobacco taxes, ending tobacco advertising and promotion, ensuring smoke-free environments and requiring strong, graphic health warnings on tobacco packaging. PAHO recognizes that these measures have diverse and mutually strengthening impacts: smoke-free environments protect nonsmokers, assist quitting by smokers and reduce the social acceptability of smoking, which helps prevent smoking initiation. PAHO cautions governments that only implementing programs for specific groups to stop smoking or prevent starting can deplete resources but may have limited impact on the population in the absence of broader policy measures.

Countries and sub-national jurisdictions in the PAHO region have taken very different approaches to tobacco control, and have achieved varying levels of success. Canada has had most of the elements of the Framework Convention on Tobacco Control in place (with significant levels of funding) since 2001. Severe restrictions on tobacco promotions were phased into effect during this period; large graphic health warnings were required on all cigarette packages; most workplaces and public places became smoke-free; taxes on cigarettes were increased; community programs were expanded and public education enhanced. Support for quitters was provided through a network of quit-lines, community programs, and health services. Support for community change (such as smoke-free bylaws) was provided through federal funding to non governmental organizations and other levels of government. Some provinces implemented school-based programs, but attempted to address the poor evidence of their success by focusing on "engaging" youth to create smoke-free culture in their schools rather than "teaching" them about smoking. During this period, for the first time in modern Canadian history, the number of smokers fell (from 6 million to 5 million, and from a prevalence rate of 25% to 20% of the population over 15 years of age). Cigarette consumption has fallen almost as dramatically. The appropriate attribution of this success to the varying elements of this comprehensive campaign has not yet been determined (Health Canada, 2005).

Other jurisdictions have taken very different approaches and achieved significant successes. California, for example, which does not have the power to impose graphic cigarette warnings or to ban advertising, has developed a different mix of comprehensive strategies. California has focused on ensuring a high volume of activities and programs, on smoke-free public and private spaces, on denormalizing tobacco companies, on establishing appropriate programs for minority populations, and on the provision of cessation services. California has seen significant reductions in smoking following the implementation of tax increases, smoke-free policies, mass media and community programming. The California government reports that Californians now smoke approximately half as many cigarettes as smokers in the rest of the United States (California Department of Health Services, 2006), and that the chief challenge in achieving this has been the opposition and tactics of the "relentless" tobacco industry.

Some South American jurisdictions have launched or implemented tobacco control programs, which include advertising bans, e.g., Brazil, and smoke-free measures (Da Costa e Silva Goldfarb, 2003); Uruguay, and graphic warning labels; e.g., Brazil, Uruguay, Venezuela.

Tobacco Control in Europe

In Europe, as in other areas in the world, there is great diversity in tobacco control progress. The European Union has not adopted a full tobacco control agenda as recommended in the EU commissioned report on tobacco control (Aspect Consortium, 2004), but various directives have pushed the agenda forward for legislation on stricter product regulation, tobacco advertising bans and eliminating duty-free sales within the European community. The WHO Regional Office for Europe has developed a database of indicators of national tobacco control programs available on their website (WHO EURO). Most countries in Europe have introduced tobacco control legislation, 20 countries have total tobacco taxes over 70% of retail price, and 48 have bans on advertising in at least some of the following: media, press, point of sale, sports. The first country-wide comprehensive clean air policies were instigated in Ireland, with Norway and Scotland following the lead. Malta, Sweden, and Italy have enacted comprehensive bans with designated smoking rooms in bars and restaurants. England and other parts of the UK will have comprehensive bans in 2007. While the prevalence of smoking has been dropping for many years among men and women in Scandinavia and Northern Europe, women's smoking rates in some Southern and Eastern European countries are still rising (Slama, 2004). The differences in progress are still emerging in mortality rates, as Eastern Europe overtook Western Europe in tobacco mortality among men (Heartstats, 2000). European Union Directives against tobacco advertising and sponsorship, misleading descriptors, more pertinent and visible health warnings, etc., have influenced the countries of Eastern Europe into developing tobacco control measures at a much faster rate than might otherwise be expected. The most pertinent international factor in progress is the Framework Convention on Tobacco Control, of which 38 out of 54 countries in Europe are Parties, as of June, 2006. Parties include Germany, the country that has been a major barrier to developing policy measures for tobacco control within the European Union (23 Parties out of 25 countries) and in influencing similar policies among neighbors to the East. So the window is open for progress. Countries around Europe vary greatly in their appreciation of the role of tobacco industry in the growth of tobacco use across the continent; many European governments use tobacco company school prevention campaigns; within all countries of course, there are pro-tobacco forces in government and in civil society.

Tobacco Control in Africa

Tobacco is, at present, not a major cause of death in Africa. Tobacco consumption rates are still comparatively low on the continent, so primary prevention of the epidemic is possible. However, African governments have traditionally given low priority to prevention just as most nations do.

By 1999, about half the governments in sub-Saharan Africa had taken some steps to regulate tobacco. Some 20 countries have enacted laws regulating smoking in public places, 16 require health warnings on tobacco products and 10 have total or strong partial bans on tobacco advertising and promotion. However, apart from South Africa, Botswana, Mauritius, and Mali most countries have not passed comprehensive tobacco control laws and the legislation is weak.

South Africa has made the most progress in regulating tobacco, with consumption falling by 33% between 1990 and 2000. The South African Parliament prohibited all tobacco advertising, sponsorship, and promotions in 1999. No advertisement may contain trademarks, logos, brand names, or company names of tobacco products. The law also bans smoking in all enclosed places, including workplaces, and the free distribution of tobacco products, and awards or prizes to induce the purchase of tobacco. The government has also increased tobacco excise taxes for "health reasons," so as to discourage consumption (Saloojee, 2000).

In 1996 Mali prohibited the advertising of tobacco products in most media, and smoking in public places requires health warnings and ingredient disclosure on cigarette packs. Mauritius enacted similar legislation in 1995.

Tobacco Taxes and Smuggling

The most cost-effective way to control tobacco, especially in low-income countries, is to raise the price of cigarettes through increasing tobacco taxes. The World Bank estimates that an increase of 10 per cent in the price of a pack of cigarettes across all sub-Saharan African countries would persuade 3 million smokers in the region to quit smoking and prevent 0.7 million premature deaths from diseases caused by smoking (Jha & Chaloupka, 1999).

Every tobacco tax decision is therefore a health decision, and maintaining the price of tobacco above the rate of increase in real (inflation-adjusted) incomes is an important public health goal. Between 1990 and 2000 the real price of cigarettes in eight African countries increased by an average of 2.14 per cent annually (Table 10.1), which is well below the rate of increase in countries with progressive tobacco control policies like France (9.25%), Hong Kong (8.63%), or Australia (6.54%) (Guindon, Tobin & Yach, 2002). The rate of tobacco taxes in African countries is also low compared to say the European Union (EU). The EU adopted a directive in 1992 that fixed a minimum tax level of at least 70% of the retail price of a pack of cigarettes. In ten African countries, for which data was available, in 1999 the average tax was 46% of the retail price. The rate was lowest in Nigeria (32%) and highest in Ghana (66%) (Jha & Chaloupka, 1999).

Recognizing the implications that higher taxes and prices have on their sales volumes, the tobacco manufacturers have strongly opposed these through various strategies, including smuggling.

The once-secret internal tobacco industry documents reveal the industry's practices. These show that the tobacco companies not only colluded with smugglers by knowingly supplying them with cigarettes, but also centrally organized the process and collected hundreds of millions of pounds worth of black market proceeds (Campbell & Maguire, 2001). The tobacco companies monitored and watched over the smuggling of their brands in about 30 African countries including Benin, Cameroon, Central African Republic, Nigeria, Niger, and Sudan.

TABLE 10.1. Cigarette price in selected African countries

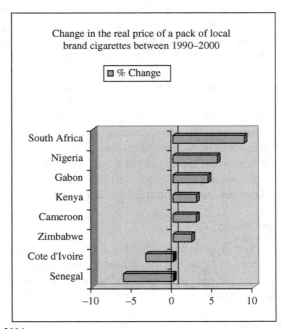

Source: Saloojee, 2004.

During the negotiations on the Framework Convention of Tobacco Control, the African region was a staunch proponent of evidence-based regulations. African governments formed a common front, pressing both for progressive regulatory measures (advertising bans, tax increases, restrictions on smoking in public places, anti-smuggling measures, etc.,) and for provisions to assist in providing alternative livelihoods for tobacco workers. The common front included both tobacco growing and non-tobacco growing countries. By June, 2006, 27 of 46 countries in the WHO-AFRO region had ratified the FCTC.

Tobacco Control in Southeast Asia

Tobacco use has increased considerably in the Southeast Asia region, disproportionately affecting the poor. With one of the highest smoking prevalence rates in the developing world, especially amongst men, it is estimated that over half of Cambodian and Laos men smoke and around more than one third of adult men in Vietnam, Thailand and Malaysia. With the region's population base of almost 500 million, and a total trade of US$ 720 billion (ASEAN website), it is a big market and prime target for the transnational tobacco companies as they seek to expand their markets and to compensate for a declining market in many developed western countries. But in recent years, governments of the region have shown interest in the need for strong and effective national tobacco control policies. Getting tobacco control policies put in place is a big step forward and getting effective enforcement and implementation is usually a next step.

Thailand, Singapore, and Malaysia are the countries in the region that have the most extensive population measures for tobacco control, including comprehensive tobacco control legislation, mass education campaigns, research to develop an evidence base, and tobacco cessation programs. These countries are regularly obliged to amend their tobacco control policies to counter new marketing and promotion strategies of tobacco companies which use loopholes in laws already in place. Countries which have not adopted comprehensive tobacco control policies such as Cambodia, Vietnam, Philippines, Laos, and Indonesia have nevertheless seen policy initiatives put forward.

Key measures to curb the increasing prevalence of tobacco use in this region are the same as in other parts of the world: tobacco taxation, total bans on tobacco advertising, sponsorship and promotions, prominent health warnings on tobacco packaging, smoke free workplaces and public places and public awareness campaigns. However success and progress vary from country to country.

One of the World Bank recommendations to all governments for controlling tobacco is to raise tobacco taxes, but it has not been easy to convince policy makers in Southeast Asia to increase taxes on cigarettes, due to opposition from the tobacco industry. When this was discussed in Thailand, studies were put forward which showed that cigarette price increases would decrease the number of Thai children starting to smoke as well as providing additional government revenue. These studies helped to convince the cabinet to approve increasing cigarette taxes from 55% to 60% in late 1993. The government has continued to raise cigarette taxes every other year since then, because as tobacco taxes have increased and government revenues have increased, tobacco consumption has decreased. The current excise tax on cigarettes in Thailand is 79% of the retail price.

Policy and action to ban smoking in public places and workplaces in Southeast Asia are expected to help to establish a non-smoking norm. In addition, although women for the most part do not smoke, as there is high smoking prevalence among men, smoke-free policy would protect women from passive smoking. The reduction in exposure to tobacco from banning smoking in public places and workplaces has been the object of reflection by the tobacco industry. According to a Philip Morris internal document from 1992, "if smoking were banned in all workplaces, the industry's average consumption would decline, and the quitting rate would increase . . ." (Hieronimus, 1992).

Thailand, for example, has extended its smoking ban to all air-conditioned dining premises and 18 other kinds of public places, such as hotel lobbies, Internet cafes, barbershops and beauty salons. Singapore first banned smoking in cinemas and theaters in 1970 and extended the ban to include air-conditioned restaurants in 1989 and air-conditioned shopping centers in 1995. Starting July of next year, the smoking ban will also cover entertainment outlets such as pubs, discos and karaoke lounges, but operators will be allowed to have a designated smoking room. In the Philippines, the Tobacco Regulation Act of 2003 includes an absolute smoking ban in all public places including bars and restaurants; phasing out of tobacco advertisements by January 2007, with a total ban on any form of tobacco advertising by July 2008. Indonesia is planning to prohibit smoking in public places such as public transit, and government and private buildings. Malaysia is currently launching a campaign drive in several cities in the country to ensure the strict enforcement of anti-smoking laws in the country. Vietnam has banned smoking in government buildings, schools, and hospitals and is considering extending this to all public places. Smoking was also banned at the Southeast Asian Games hosted by Vietnam in December, 2003. In the Lao People's Democratic Republic, the Lao school of Medicine declared the faculty to be smoke-free.

Cambodia has strengthened community action by engaging religious leaders to play an active role in creating smoke free temples and encouraging smoking cessation among monks. Utilizing Buddhist principles and the influence of Buddhist monks has not only raised awareness among Buddhists but also garnered support in advocacy for smoke free public places and FCTC ratification.

Asia exemplifies the variable end-points of tobacco control endeavors. Despite setbacks, progress is being made throughout the region – albeit at various speeds – to protect the public health through tobacco control efforts.

Tobacco Control in Other Regions

Similar variation and progress can be found in the other regions of the world not included in this report. All regions of the world include countries of very high tobacco consumption and rising tobacco-related mortality rates. In the Western

Pacific area, Australia, and New Zealand have created societies where many in the population are not drawn to tobacco use. In the Eastern Mediterranean Region, great increases in tobacco use have encouraged governments to enact legislation for tobacco control.

Issues in Measuring Effectiveness

The extent of national legislation and its enforcement is one of the best indicators of the strength of tobacco control forces in a country. Success in getting legislation enacted requires protracted media advocacy, winning community support, and strong lobbying of legislators. The advocacy "process", however, remains poorly documented. The lessons that have been learnt by countries that have successfully (or unsuccessfully) tackled tobacco are not easily generalized and passed on to others.

In assessing what works in tobacco control a number of factors that may ameliorate outcomes need to be taken into consideration. Firstly, evaluations may be time-sensitive, with results varying with time. Interventions need time to be implemented, time to exert their effects, and with time there may be an erosion of the effect. Outcomes may thus be very different if evaluated after a few weeks, a few months or a few years. Some policies too may reduce tobacco use more rapidly than others. For example, price increases produce results relatively quickly, while the effects of an advertising ban may take longer to become apparent. Policies often also have a major impact when first introduced, and then as populations either become sated or familiar with the measure the impact declines.

Secondly, competing influences, or societal influences unrelated to the intervention, may undermine the impact of a measure. For instance, the public may receive mixed messages as a result of industry disinformation campaigns, which may dilute the effect of an educational intervention. The industry also uses counter-strategies to make continuation of tobacco use easier for smokers (such as price-discounting and promotions, or advocating for smoking and non-smoking areas in public places). In the face of such challenges effective programs may only be able to stabilize smoking prevalence or may act to minimize an increase. The success of an intervention should therefore not just be measured in terms of declines in prevalence, but against the expected prevalence rates in the absence of the intervention. Few systematic attempts have been made to incorporate industry actions into evaluation methods for tobacco control programs.

Thirdly, tobacco control programs are often introduced as a comprehensive package and separating out the part played by the individual components is not always possible. For instance, if a ban on tobacco advertising and tax increases are introduced concurrently, the impact of the ban on declines in youth smoking may be difficult to measure. On the other hand, there may also be synergy between interventions. For example, a reduction in adult smoking may change the normative environment, so that there is less explicit modeling of smoking as an adult behavior and thus reduce smoking by youth. Determining the optimal policy mix for any given society remains a challenge.

Fourthly, the introduction of tobacco control laws is almost always preceded by public debate and the educational value of these debates may contribute significantly to reductions in tobacco usage.

Finally, there is a need for more and better data particularly from lower-income countries. Often there is no baseline data, insufficient information on the quality of the intervention or the extent of implementation, and little information on tobacco industry counter measures.

Conclusions

The Ottawa Charter for health promotion recommends healthy public policy, supportive environments, strengthened community action, development of personal skills and reorientation of health services as key elements of the health promotion movement to protect the public from the harms of tobacco use. Countries around the world are slowly enacting these measures. With the WHO FCTC, the nations of the world have been given the opportunity to join together to fight a pervasive and powerful industry and to counteract the progression in tobacco use that is still occurring. The treaty contains current standards of best practice, but the goals of tobacco control strategies and the application of agreed measures need frequent updating to respond to both the tobacco industry and the evolution of tobacco use in populations.

References

ASEAN Website. http://www.aseansec.org/ Aspect Consortium. (2004). *Tobacco or Health in the European Union. Past, present and future.* European Communities.

California Department of Health Services. *Confronting a Relentless Adversary: A Plan for Success. Toward a Tobacco-Free California 2006–2008.* (2006, March). Californian Department of Health Services, Accessed June 15, 2006.
http://www.dhs.ca.gov/tobacco/documents/pubs/MasterPlan05.pdf.

Campbell, D., Maguire, K. (2001, August 22). Clarke company faces new smuggling claims. *The Guardian*,
http://www.guardian.co.uk/guardianpolitics/story/0,540558,00.html.

Chollat-Traquet, C. (1996). *Evaluating Tobacco Control Activities: Experiences and Guiding Principles.* Geneva: World Health Organization.

Da Costa e Silva Goldfarb, L.M. (2003). Government leadership in tobacco control: Brazil's experience. In: J. De Beyer J, L. Waverley Brigden (eds) *Tobacco Control Policy: Strategies, Successes & Setbacks* (pp. 38–70). Washington DC: World Bank.

Guindon, G.E., Tobin, S., Yach, D. (2002). Trends and affordability of cigarette prices: Ample room for tax increases and related health gains. *Tobacco Control, 11*, 35–43.

Health Canada. (2005). *The National Strategy: Moving Forward – the 2005 Progress Report on Tobacco Control.* Cat. H128–1/05–442. ISBN 0–662–69369–8. Health Canada.

Heartstats website. (2000) Total numbers of deaths and numbers of deaths due to smoking by cause, adults aged 35 and over, by sex & country, 2000, Europe (Table) Source: Peto R et al (2003). Oxford University Press. http://www.heartstats.org.

Hieronimus, J. (1992, January 22). *Impact of Workplace Restrictions on Consumption and Incidence.* Philip Morris. Bates No. 2023914280.
http://tobaccodocuments.org/landman/2023914280–4284.html.

Jemal, A., Cokkinides, V.E., Shafey, O., Thun, M.J. (2003). Lung cancer trends in young adults: An early indicator of progress in tobacco control (United States). *Cancer Causes and Control, 14,* 579–585.

Jha, P., Chaloupka, F.J. (1999). *Curbing the Epidemic.* Washington DC: World Bank.

Pan American Health Organization. *Effective Tobacco Control Measures.* PAHO. http://www.paho.org/English/ad/sde/ra/Tobmeasures.htm Accessed June 15, 2006.

Peto, R., Darby, S., Deo, H., Silcocks, P., Whitley, E., Doll, R. (2000). Smoking, smoking cessation, and lung cancer in the UK since 1950: Combination of national statistics with two case-control studies. *British Medical Journal, 321,* 323–329.

Saloojee, Y. (2000). Tobacco Control in South Africa. *South African Health Review* (pp. 429–440). Durban: Health Systems Trust. http://www.hst.org.za/sahr.

Saloojee, Y. (2004). Tobacco in Africa: More than a health threat. In: P. Boyle, N. Gray, J. Henningfield, J. Seffrin,W. Zatonski (eds) *Tobacco and Public Health: Science and Policy* (pp. 267–287). Oxford: Oxford University Press.

Slama, K. (2004). Tobacco control. In: H. Sancho-Garnier, A. Anderson, A. Biedermann, E. Lynge, K. Slama (eds) *Evidence-Based Cancer Prevention: Strategies for NGOs. A UICC Handbook for Europe* (pp. 74–93). Geneva: UICC.

World Health Organization. (2003). *WHO Framework Convention on Tobacco Control.* Geneva: World Health Organization.

World Health Organization, European Regional Office. Database on tobacco control: http://data.euro.who.int/tobacco.

11
Effectiveness of Health Promotion in Preventing Alcohol Related Harm[*]

PETER HOWAT, DAVID SLEET, BRUCE MAYCOCK AND
RANDY ELDER

About 4% of the global burden of disease is attributed to alcohol, which contributes to 3.2% of deaths and 4.0% of the disability-adjusted life years lost. Of the 2 billion alcohol consumers worldwide, over 76 million have been diagnosed with alcohol use disorders (Room et al., 2005). As well as being the leading risk factor for disease burden in low mortality developing countries, alcohol consumption is the third largest risk factor for developed countries (Doran, 2003; WHO, 2004).

Despite the scope of alcohol related problems globally and the difficulty in preventing them, there is increasing evidence of effectiveness of some prevention strategies, especially those aimed at reducing alcohol-related traffic injuries. Over the past three decades, high-income countries have experienced a substantial reduction in mortality and morbidity from alcohol-related traffic crashes (Peden et al., 2004). The majority of this reduction is attributed to behavioral changes associated with public education, organizational policies, legislation, law enforcement, and economic actions, in multiple settings involving multiple sectors (Commonwealth Department of Health and Aging, 2003; Hingson & Sleet, 2006).

This chapter reviews evidence regarding the effectiveness of interventions aimed at reducing alcohol-related problems, considered within a health promotion framework (Howat et al., 2004). It illustrates these interventions, using examples primarily drawn from high income countries, and discusses the potential benefits of a synergistic application of these interventions. There is a paucity of literature on the effectiveness of interventions aimed at minimizing alcohol-related problems in low-income countries. While these countries can learn much from the high-income countries (Doran, 2003), caution is recommended in extrapolating the likely effectiveness of these interventions.

---

[*] The findings and conclusions in this chapter are those of the authors and do not necessarily represent the views of the Centers for Disease Control and Prevention of the Department of Health and Human Services or Curtin University.

The Health Promotion Framework

Although people must assume personal responsibility for maintaining their health, there is wide recognition that environmental cues and reinforcers exert an important influence on behavioral choices and outcomes (Geller et al., 1991). Drinking behavior is shaped by individual choices and motivation, and also strongly influenced by organizational, economic, environmental, and social factors (WHO, 2004; WMA, 2005). Therefore, approaches that attempt to bring about change in drinking behavior through education alone are likely to have limited or no success (Gielen & Sleet, 2003; Howat et al., 2004; Peden et al., 2004; Sleet et al., 1989), whereas those that combine educational with other behavioral, environmental, policy and organizational changes are likely to be the most effective (Shults et al., 2001; Waller 1998; WHO, 1986)

During the past two decades there has been a significant increase in evidence that various aspects of the environment influence alcohol use. These influences may include social cues, such as use by family members and peers, or images of alcohol use promulgated by advertising and media (USDHHS, 1997a). Environmental influences also include availability, cost and the nature of the alcoholic beverages offered for sale (Stockwell et al., 1997). Measham and Brain (2005) in their recent review on binge drinking and British alcohol policy identified that intoxication was encouraged by economic deregulation and constrained by legislative change, highlighting that poor policy can contribute to alcohol related harm.

A health promotion approach to the prevention of alcohol-related problems incorporates an appropriate balance of individually-focused behavior change strategies and those that produce environments that support healthy behaviors. One definition of health promotion is:

a combination of *educational, organizational, .economic* and *political* actions designed with consumer participation, to enable individuals, groups and whole communities to increase control over, and to improve health through changes in knowledge, attitudes, behavior, policy, and social and environmental conditions (Howat et al., 2003)

This definition builds on and incorporates aspects of earlier definitions of health promotion (Green & Kreuter 1999; WHO, 1986). An example of how this approach could be applied to alcohol-related problems is provided (Figure 11.1). Figure 11.1 presents a logic model and framework for how the components of health promotion (economic actions, policy actions, organizational actions, and health education) can cumulatively contribute to changes in knowledge, attitudes, behaviors, policies, and the social and physical environment that are necessary to reduce alcohol-related problems. These changes have the potential to reduce alcohol-related harm, ultimately improving health status of individuals and the community (Pinder, 1994; USDHHS, 1997b; WHO, 1984)

Within each component, there is a wide range of strategies employed to reduce alcohol related problems. For some strategies, there is While some

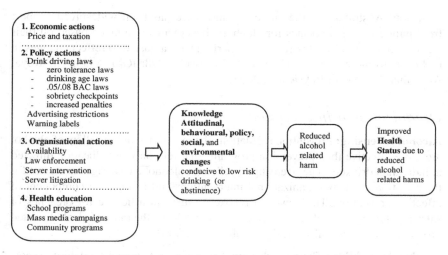

FIGURE 11.1. A health promotion framework for reducing alcohol related harm.

single interventions serve as strong supporting actions, they might not be proven to be effective on their own; therefore, although advocating for strategies with demonstrated effectiveness within a comprehensive framework is critical, practitioners should also continue to support research on interventions that currently have only moderate or insufficient evidence. This chapter reviews these strategies embedded within the components of the health promotion framework.

Economic Interventions

Price and taxation: Pricing policies are regarded as among the most effective measures to reduce total alcohol consumption and hence alcohol-related problems. Studies have indicated that a rise in price will lead to a drop in consumption (Babor et al., 2003; Waller, Naidoo & Thom, 2002; WHO, 2004) and a decrease in price will likely result in additional alcohol related deaths (Schancke, 2005). One estimate indicated that a 10% increase in the price of alcoholic beverages in the United States would reduce alcohol-impaired driving by about 8% for females and about 7% for males (Babor et al., 2003). Another estimate is that a 17% increase ($1) in the price of alcohol for a six pack of beer could lead to a 3.3% reduction of current alcohol-attributable mortality in the USA (Hollingworth et al., 2006). Pricing policies are likely to be particularly effective in reducing consumption by young people, as they are more likely to be sensitive to price changes due to their smaller disposable incomes. Moreover, an increase in the real price of alcohol has been shown to significantly reduce alcohol attributable harms among Indigenous peoples where high levels of overall alcohol consumption and related harms are of particular concern (Chikritzhs et al., 2005)

In both Australia and the United States, there has been widespread support from public health advocates for alcoholic beverages to be taxed based on their alcohol content, and for tax rates to be periodically adjusted to reflect changes in real costs to the consumer (Crosbie & Stockwell 1998; IOM, 2003; The Royal Australian College of Physicians, 2005).

Organizational Interventions

Alcohol Licensing: Prevention regulations that are aimed at the sellers of alcohol are more effective than prevention programs that rely only on education directed at individual drinkers. The licensing of sellers of alcoholic beverages is crucial for the adoption of many organizational interventions and is a central component of effective prevention. The power to revoke or suspend a license for breaches of sales regulations is an effective strategy for controlling the rates of alcohol related problems, including traffic crashes (Babor et al., 2003).

Alcohol Availability: There is substantial evidence that alcohol availability is correlated with levels of consumption and ultimate harm (Waller et al., 2002; WHO, 2004). Some studies have described a clear epidemiological link between alcohol consumption and suicide and violence (Rossow, 2000; Rossow, Grøholt & Wichstrom, 2005). Availability of alcohol can be controlled by restrictions on hours and days of sales, and by controlling the number, location, and type of liquor outlets. There is evidence of the benefits of bans on sales to specific groups such as minors (Shults et al., 2001), or in specific circumstances such as during sporting events (Douglas, 1998; Gray et al., 1995).

There is strong evidence that off-premise monopoly systems can limit both the levels of alcohol consumption and alcohol related problems (WHO, 2004). Examples from Finland and Sweden illustrate substantial rises in consumption, including by minors, associated with availability of alcohol in grocery stores (Babor et al., 2003). When Swedish grocery stores were no longer permitted to sell 4.5% beer, a significant drop in traffic crashes followed (Babor et al., 2003).

There is inconsistent evidence on the effectiveness of changing hours of sale of alcohol, but strategic restrictions on hours of alcohol sales and service appear to be beneficial. A number of studies indicate that changing the hours or days of alcohol sales can influence the incidence of alcohol related problems (Babor et al., 2003; Chikritzhs & Stockwell, 2002; Chikritzhs & Stockwell, 2006, McMillan & Lapham, 2006)

Server intervention and drinking environments: Server intervention programs involve training servers employed to serve alcohol beverages in alcohol retail establishments, often in conjunction with training for managers and door staff. Their main objective is to prevent intoxication and drunk driving by their clients. Recommended serving practices include providing food, slowing service to drinkers showing signs of intoxication, refusing service to intoxicated or underage drinkers, and taking steps to prevent intoxicated patrons from driving. Increasing attention is being paid to such issues of server training and the safety of drinking environments in the United States, Australia, Sweden and Canada (Babor et al., 2003; Daly et al., 2002; Loxley et al., 2004; Shults et al., 2001). A review of server interventions found evidence of effectiveness, under conditions of face-to-face instruction and strong management support (Shults et al., 2001) and mandatory regulations and meaningful enforcement (Stockwell, 2006).

The introduction of voluntary "Alcohol Accords" or codes of practice in Australia between local alcohol retailers, police, local government and community representatives is one method to promote responsible service policies. Despite a number of Alcohol Accords in place throughout Australia, the evidence of their effectiveness is equivocal (Daly et al., 2002), and they are likely to have only minimal impact on reducing alcohol-related harm

Server litigation: In Australia, alcohol-consuming patrons involved in subsequent traffic crashes have successfully sued bar and hotel proprietors following traffic crashes, claiming they were served dangerous levels of alcohol (Stockwell, 2001). These actions may have the potential to reduce the prevalence of driving while intoxicated (DWI), especially if they foster improved service practices (Stockwell, 2001). Studies from the United States have found that alcohol-related crashes decreased following high-profile server liability cases (Wagenaar & Holder, 1991), and that states with statutes or case law permitting server liability tend to have lower fatality rates from alcohol-related crashes (Chaloupka et al., 1993; Whetten-Goldstein et al., 2000).

Policy Interventions

McGinnis et al., (2002) argue for the central role of policy development in health promotion. The clearest evidence of the impact of policy interventions comes from the literature on alcohol related traffic crashes.

Drink driving legislation: The enactment of laws, along with enforcement and informational efforts, have resulted in substantial declines in the rate of alcohol related traffic crashes in countries such as the United States, Australia and New Zealand (Henstridge et al., 1997; Jones & Lacey, 2001; Dellinger et al., 2007). Some examples of laws where evidence supports such benefits include:

- A reduction of the legal BAC to .05% in Australia and .08% in the United States (Howat et al., 1992; Shults et al., 2001)
- Sobriety checkpoints and testing (Jones & Lacey, 2001; Shults et al., 2001)
- Stricter enforcement of drink driving legislation (Holder, 1998)
- An increase in the legal drinking age (Shults et al., 2001)

Reducing Blood Alcohol Concentration (BAC) limits: Many countries have laws, known as illegal "per se" laws that specify BAC limits at which it is illegal to operate motor vehicles. Recent literature reviews indicate that lowering the "per se" limit to 0.08 g/dL or lower has been effective for decreasing alcohol-related crashes in the United States (Shults et al., 2001) and other countries (Mann et al., 2001; Howat et al., 1991). In the United States, Congress required States to .08 g/dL BAC laws by October 2003 to avoid the withholding of federal highway construction funds (Shults et al., 2001). Lower BAC limits specifically for young or inexperienced drivers are also effective at decreasing alcohol-related crashes (Shults et al., 2001). All 50 U.S. states have such laws, as do Australia, New Zealand, Austria and parts of Canada (Homel, 1994; Hollingworth et al., 2006; Shults et al., 2001).

There is an interesting benefit of tougher DWI laws that set low legal blood alcohol limits for drivers under the age of 21 years. An estimated reduction of 7% to 10% in suicide for among young males between 15 and 20 years is attributed to such laws in the USA for the period 1981–1998 (Carpenter, 2004).

Sobriety checkpoints: Sobriety checkpoints allow law enforcement officers to assess drivers for alcohol impairment. In Australia and a number of European countries, drivers are systematically stopped and given a breath test to measure their blood alcohol concentrations (BACs). In the United States, police must suspect a driver has consumed alcohol before they can demand a breath test. Both of these breath test procedures are usually accompanied by extensive publicity in an attempt to alert drivers to the consequences of drink driving and to increase their perceived risk of arrest (Jones & Lacey, 2001; Shults et al., 2001). Evaluations of the effects of sobriety checkpoints on crashes in the United States and Canada indicate that they decrease alcohol-related crashes by approximately 20% (Elder et al., 2002; Jones & Lacey, 2001). In Australia, sobriety checkpoints are credited with about 30% of the reduction of fatal traffic injuries (Henstridge et al., 1997). The success of checkpoint programs is dependent on both the level of enforcement and on publicity campaigns (Elder et al., 2002; Henstridge et al., 1997; Jones & Lacey, 2001).

Increased penalties for drink driving: Australian data indicates that harsh penalties for drink-drivers has the highest level of public support (89%) among the many policy-oriented interventions (AIHW, 1999), yet there is little evidence of substantial benefits from increased fines or mandatory jail time (Homel, 1981; Villaveces et al., 2003).

Drinking age: A recent global review of alcohol policies (WHO, 2004) indicated a relationship between raising the drinking age and a reduction in alcohol consumption and alcohol related problems among young people. Conversely, there is new evidence of an increase in hospitalized injuries associated with alcohol-related traffic crashes when the legal drinking age was lowered from 20 to 18 years in New Zealand (Kypri et al., 2006). Studies in the United States have produced strong evidence that increasing the drinking age to 21 years resulted in substantially fewer alcohol-related crashes among young people (Shults et al., 2001; Wagenaar & Toomey, 2002). Similarly, alcohol related problems in the UK decreased after the minimum age for drinking in public places was raised (Waller et al., 2002).

Multiple policy interventions: The implementation of multiple policies to reduce alcohol-related harms is generally preferable to reliance on any single strategy due to the potential for synergistic effects (Howat et al., 2004; Green & Kreuter, 2005; Howat et al., 2003; Shults et al., 2002).

An analysis of alcohol control policies in 97 American cities showed a relationship between the number of regulations and alcohol related traffic fatalities. Cities with less than 10 of 20 listed alcohol control regulations had 1.46-times more deaths than cities with 15 or more of these regulations (Cohen et al., 2001). Economic research in Australia indicated substantial economic benefits from employing multiple interventions and the combination of strategies (such as sobriety checkpoints, lower legal BAC limits, mass media publicity, higher penalties and stricter enforcement of penalties) was considered particularly effective (Commonwealth Department of Health and Aging, 2003).

The key to the success of drink driving legislative interventions is a change in the public perception of the risk of being involved in an alcohol related crash, of being arrested for drink driving, or both (WHO, 2004). Public media campaigns can be effective in raising awareness, increasing knowledge, and improving the acceptance of traffic regulations, making legislation both possible and acceptable (Stockwell et al., 1998). Public information and education was a major factor for the success of sobriety checkpoints in Australian States in the 1980's (Henstridge et al., 1997; Homel, 1994; Howat et al., 1992), and was essential in a successful US community-based intervention (Holder, 1998).

Restrictions on advertising and promotion: The alcoholic beverage industry has vigorously promoted its products through direct and indirect advertising. Advertising and marketing strategies once used by the tobacco industry have been employed to increase the market share of alcoholic beverages (Jernigan et al., 2005; Mosher & Johnsson, 2005; USDHHS, 1997a) An aim of alcohol promotion is to "normalize" regular drinking, to encourage non-drinkers to try alcoholic products, and to encourage current drinkers to consume more (Donovan et al., 2007; WHO, 2004).

There is increasing evidence that advertising and promotion act as reinforcing factors for consumption (WHO, 2004; Wyllie et al., 1998) and there seems to be a link between advertising and increased consumption of alcohol by young people (Hastings et al., 2005; Wyllie et al., 1998). Hollingworth and colleagues (2006) estimated that a complete ban on alcohol advertising could result in a 16.4% decrease in alcohol-related life years lost in the USA. A partial ban could lead to a 4% reduction.

In Australia, the United States, and other countries, regulations governing the promotion of alcohol have been relatively ineffective at reducing alcohol-related harms (Donovan et al., 2007; Roberts, 2002). Voluntary codes of advertising have been adopted by the industry as part of a philosophy of self-regulation (ICAP, 2001). Mosher (1994) concluded that the codes adopted by the alcohol industry were "vague, too narrow and unenforceable." In a recent review, Casswell and Maxwell (2005) reiterated this view that attempts to restrict marketing globally, primarily by voluntary codes, are inadequate. This apparent failure of voluntary restrictions has led some researchers to conclude that restrictions on the advertising and promotion of alcohol should be only one part of the implementation of more comprehensive set of alcohol control policies (Donovan et al., 2007; Jones & Donovan, 2002;).

Mandatory health and safety warnings: Mandated alcoholic beverage container warning labels were introduced in the United States in 1989. The dangers of operating machinery or driving a vehicle when impaired by alcohol are prominent among these warnings (Babor et al., 2003). However, the long-term efficacy of warning labels on consumption and risk behaviors is unproven (The Royal Australian College of Physicians, 2005; WHO, 2004).

Health Education, School and Community Interventions

Direct health education aimed at altering alcohol related behaviors has met with limited success, although few interventions have been well designed or adequately evaluated, and many suffer from inadequate data reporting and analysis (Foxcroft et al., 2003; McBride, 2003). While the evidence is mixed on the relation between education alone and sustained behavior change, it is important to recognize that education underpins all of the other interventions discussed in this paper. Without a clear understanding by policy makers and community members of the harms associated with alcohol and the need for specific interventions to address these harms, there would be little support for such initiatives.

The evidence suggests that for behavior change to be effective, a supportive environment (via organizational, economic and political actions) is usually necessary (Hingson et al., 1996; Holder, 1998; Howat et al., 2004). It is important, therefore, that education programs encourage community members to seek changes in policies and practices that help reduce alcohol related problems. Specific education efforts also need to be directed at opinion leaders and policy makers, to support structural changes.

School programs: Evidence for the effectiveness of school-based alcohol interventions is unclear. Many designs and program evaluations are methodologically flawed (Black et al., 1998; Foxcroft et al., 2003; McBride, 2003; Waller et al., 2002; White & Pitts, 1998). Many school programs have been short term and have operated in isolation from other alcohol control initiatives in the broader community (Catford, 2001). Even for those programs with sound research designs, their effects on behavior are often small (Foxcroft et al., 2003; McBride et al., 2004; White & Pitts, 1998).

School programs resulting in positive outcomes have been generally grounded in educational and behavioral change theory and used life skills training to target drinking behaviors of young people (Marlatt & Witkiewitz, 2002; McBride et al., 2004). There is some evidence indicating that well designed and implemented peer led prevention programs are more effective than those led by a teacher (Black et al., 1998), as are those that use interactive approaches fostering interpersonal skills (Tobler et al., 2000; Elder et al., 2005)

School policies in Australia, the UK, and other European countries are increasingly adopting a harm reduction rather than abstinence focus (McBride, 2003). Empirical studies demonstrate that harm reduction approaches are at least as effective as abstinence oriented strategies in reducing alcohol consumption and alcohol related harm (Marlatt & Witkiewitz, 2002). In addition to providing opportunities to engage students, the school setting may also be appropriate as a venue to engage parents in programs, but such approaches have not undergone sufficient empirical research to measure effectiveness.

Tertiary institution programs: Research suggests that most prevention programs in the university setting have had limited success in preventing hazardous drinking (Mitic, 2003). Research in NZ and the USA has investigated the efficacy of brief interventions as a harm-reduction approach to alcohol consumption (Baer et al., 2001; Kypri & Langley, 2003; Marlatt et al., 1998). Findings from a study among high-risk students who were provided with a brief intervention based on principals of motivational interviewing showed significant reductions in drinking rates and harmful consequences, as well as a significantly greater deceleration of drinking rates and problems over time compared with a control group (Baer et al., 2001; Marlatt et al., 1998). A study reported by Newman et al., (2006) used a health promotion approach to develop and implement a combination of individual and environmental interventions. Reductions in binge drinking and self reported harms followed implementation of these interventions.

Mass media campaigns: Mass media strategies have been used extensively to promote health-enhancing behaviors and are the most common examples of counter advertising. There is evidence that well devised and adequately resourced programs incorporating mass media can improve health related behaviors (Donovan & Henley, 2003; Henley et al., 2007).

Mass media campaigns in isolation have had limited effectiveness in reducing or preventing alcohol-related problems (Donovan & Henley, 2003; Loxley et al., 2004). Furthermore, despite evidence of cost-effectiveness at the societal level (Elder et al., 2004), they can be costly and more difficult to sustain than policy or organizational interventions. Nonetheless, mass media campaigns can play an important role in:

- Raising awareness about alcohol issues, and generating public debate;
- Reinforcing health related messages;
- Changing perceived norms regarding alcohol use and drink driving; and
- Providing support for other health promotion initiatives, including policies and environmental and organizational changes.

A recent systematic review (Elder et al., 2004) found strong evidence that mass media campaigns that are carefully planned, well-executed, attain adequate audience exposure, and are implemented in conjunction with other ongoing prevention activities, such as law enforcement, are effective in reducing alcohol-impaired driving and alcohol related crashes. Such campaigns can be effective whether they are focused on publicizing laws and enforcement activities or on the health and social consequences of drinking and driving.

Community mobilization: There is some evidence that community mobilization or community action projects involving local groups have been effective in contributing to changes related to reducing alcohol-related harm (Hanson et al., 2000; Hingson et al., 2005; Howat et al., 1992). In New Zealand the use of community organization along with mass media were effective in influencing support for alcohol policy changes (Casswell & Gilmore, 1989). In the US, using a variety of community interventions resulted in a 42% reduction in fatal crashes involving alcohol (Hingson et al., 1996) and a five-community comprehensive intervention significantly reduced alcohol availability and fatal traffic crashes (Hingson et al., 2005)

Media advocacy and public communication efforts can shape policies that have significant benefits to the community. Local leaders are generally supportive of such an approach, which is consequently likely to be more sustainable than other approaches that depend on substantial funding, such as ongoing community education programs. For example, Mothers Against Drunk Driving in the United States has been very effective in organizing community action for change in drunk driving (El-Guebaly, 2005; Webb, 2001).

Discussion

Effective health promotion leads to changes in the determinants of alcohol-related problems, both those within the control of individuals (such as decision-making) and those outside their direct control in the social, economic and environmental arenas (such as pricing, promotion, sales, availability, peer pressure, and alternative transportation) (IUHPE, 2000). According to this perspective, the most effective means of changing drinking behavior is through a combination of educational, organizational, economic and political actions.

The evidence of effectiveness for various component strategies within the health promotion framework varies, from strong evidence for some policies to inadequate evidence for some education efforts directed at individuals. Effective component strategies include economic and retailer interventions, taxation tied to alcohol content, reducing alcohol availability, server litigation, sobriety checkpoints, random breath testing, lowering the legal BAC limit, minimum legal drinking age laws, supportive media promotions and other relevant laws/regulations. These interventions have had their greatest impact when administered in the context of other on-going interventions in the community (Foxcroft et al., 2003; Gielen & Sleet, 2003; Shults et al., 2001; Shults et al., 2002; Waller et al., 2002).

The effectiveness of other component approaches is moderate, with evidence for some isolated interventions either absent or inconclusive. Strategies such as those that restrict advertising and promote counter advertising may under some conditions be influential in addressing alcohol related harm. Although some authors have demonstrated that interventions specifically focusing on server responsibility, modifying physical drinking environments, conducting school drug and alcohol education programs, incorporating community mobilization initiatives, college and worksite programs, and enforcing compulsory health and safety warning labels can have some positive outcomes, the overall evidence supporting their individual efficacy is inconclusive (Hingson et al., 2007).

In this review of component strategies within the health promotion framework, one of the weaknesses is that many of the interventions reviewed were implemented and evaluated without benefit of understanding and controlling other potential synergistic effects. The ecologic effects of implementing numerous interventions simultaneously are difficult to evaluate, but important to consider in any multi-level effort to reduce alcohol-related problems.

A second limitation in this overview is that the impact of specific interventions was limited to research in high-income countries. Consequently, the generalizability of these data to other countries may be questionable. The transferability of these strategies from high-income to low or middle-income countries needs further examination (Peden et al., 2004; WHO, 2004). There is potential to fund some of these interventions from revenue gained from enforcement of policies and ultimately from reductions in health care costs.

Educating and informing the public and policy-makers regarding effective prevention strategies, and the need for them, is an important aspect of health promotion. This information can be helpful in modifying community attitudes and behaviors, and fostering a receptive climate for implementing effective policies and organizational change.

Approaches with limited evidence of effectiveness on their own may nevertheless prove useful in a multi-faceted program, as the stronger components in the framework will drive change, and the weaker ones may reinforce and support change. Consequently, while advocating for strategies with demonstrated effectiveness within a comprehensive framework, practitioners should not stop supporting research on interventions that currently have only moderate or insufficient evidence. Health promotion approaches require consideration of the many ways in which change in alcohol related harms can occur, and the many opportunities for leveraging a community's resources to reduce alcohol related problems and improve health. Use of the health promotion framework to plan and implement comprehensive community-based programs to reduce alcohol related problems offers our best hope for success.

Acknowledgments. We acknowledge the contributions of Dr. Ruth Shults at the US Centers for Disease Control and Prevention, Jenny Smith, Lynda Fielder, Dr Alexandra McManus and Leza Duplock at WACHPR, and Dr.Tanya Chikritzhs and Professor Steve Allsop of the National Drug Research Institute for their helpful input. This chapter is a condensed version of a complete report prepared by the authors for the IUHPE publication *Effectiveness of health promotion in preventing alcohol related harm (2006).*

References

AIHW. Australian Institute of Health and Welfare. 1999, *1998 National drug strategy household survey: First results*, AIHW, Canberra.

Babor, T, Caetano, R, Casswell, S, Edwards, G, Giesbrecht, N, Graham, K, Grube, J, Gruenewald, P, Hill, L, Holder, H, Homel, R, Osterberg, E, Rehm, J, Room, R & Rossow, I. 2003, *Alcohol: No ordinary commodity – research and public policy*, Oxford University Press, Oxford.

Baer, J, Kivlahan, D, Blume, A, McKnight, P & Marlatt, G. 2001, "Brief intervention for heavy-drinking college students: 4-year follow-up and natural history", *American Journal of Public Health*, vol. 91, no. 8, pp. 1310–1316.

Black, D, Tobler, N & Sciacca, J. 1998, "Peer helping/involvement: An efficacious way to meet the challenge of reducing alcohol, tobacco, and other drug use among youth?" *J. School Health*, vol. 68, no. 3, pp. 878–893.

Carpenter, C. 2004, "Heavy alcohol use and youth suicide: Evidence from tougher drunk driving laws", *Journal of Policy Analysis and Management*, vol. 23, no. 4, pp. 831–842.

Casswell, S, Maxwell, A. 2005, Regulation of alcohol marketing: A global view, *J Public Health Policy*. vol. 26, no. 3.

Casswell, S & Gilmore, L. 1989, "An evaluated community action project on alcohol", *J. Stud. Alc.*, vol. 50, pp. 339–346.

Catford, J. 2001, "Illicit drugs: Effective prevention requires a health promotion approach", *Health Promotion International*, vol. 16, no. 2, pp. 107–110.

Chaloupka, F, Saffer, H & Grossman, M. 1993, "Alcohol control policies and motor vehicle fatalities", *J. Legal Stud.*, vol. 22, pp. 161–186.

Chikritzhs, T, Stockwell, T & Pascal, R. 2005, "The impact of the Northern Territory's Living With Alcohol Program", 1992–2002: Revisiting the evaluation. *Addiction*, no.100, pp. 1625–1636.

Chikritzhs, T & Stockwell, T. 2002, "The impact of late trading hours for Australian public houses (hotels) on levels of violence", *To stud. Alc.,* vol. 63. pp. 591–599.

Chikritzhs, T & Stockwell, T. 2006, "The impact of later trading hours for hotels on levels of impaired driver road crashes and driver breath alcohol levels", *Addiction*, no. 101, pp. 1254–1264.

Cohen, D, Mason, K & Scriber, R. 2001, "The population consumption model, alcohol control practices, and alcohol-related traffic fatalities", *Prev. Med.*, vol. 34, pp. 187–197.

Commonwealth Department of Health and Ageing. 2003, *Returns in investment in public health*, Canberra, Australia.

Crosbie, D & Stockwell, T. 1998, *Alcohol, taxation reform and public health in Australia'*, National Centre for Research into the Prevention of Drug Abuse, Perth.

Daly, J, Campbell, E, Wiggers, J & Considine, R. 2002, "Prevalence of responsible hospitality policies in licensed premises that are associated with alcohol related harm", *Drug Alc. Rev.*, vol. 21, pp. 113–120.

Dellinger, A, Sleet, DA, Jones, BH. 2007, Drivers, Wheels, and Roads: Motor Vehicle Safety in the Twentieth Century. In: J. Ward & C. Warren (eds) *Silent victories: The history and practice of public health in twentieth-century America*. Oxford University Press, New York. pp. 343–362.

Donovan, K, Donovan, R, Howat, P & Weller, N. 2007, "The content and frequency of alcoholic beverage advertisements and sales promotions in popular magazines", *Drug Alc. Rev.*, vol. 26, no.1, pp. 73–81.

Donovan, R & Henley, N. 2003, *Social marketing: Principles and practice* IP Communications, Melbourne.

Doran, C. 2003, *Economic impact assessment of non-communicable diseases on hospital resources in Tonga, Vanuatu and Kiribati. A report for the Pacific Action for health project: Secretariat of the Pacific Community, AusAID*, National Drug and Alcohol Research Centre, Sydney.

Douglas, M. 1998, "Restriction of the hours of sale of alcohol in a small community: A beneficial impact", *Australian and New Zealand Journal of Public Health*, vol. 22, no. 6, pp. 714–719.

El-Guebaly, N. 2005, "Don't drink and drive; the successful Mothers Against Drunk Driving (MADD)", *World Psychiatry*, vol. 4, no. 1, pp. 35–36.

Elder, R, Shults, R, Sleet, D, Nichols, J, Thompson, R, Rajab, W & Services. 2004, "Effectiveness of mass media campaigns for reducing drinking and driving and alcohol-involved crashes: A systematic review", *Am. J. Prev. Med.*, vol. 27, no. 1, pp. 57–65.

Elder, R, Shults, R, Sleet, D, Nichols, J, Zaza, S & Thompson, R. 2002, "Effectiveness of sobriety checkpoints for reducing alcohol-involved crashes", *Traffic Inj. Prev.*, vol. 3, pp. 266–274.

Elder, RW, Nichols, JL, Shults, RA, Sleet, DA, Barrios, LC, Compton, R, and Task Force on Community Preventive Services. 2005, Effectiveness of school-based programs for reducing drinking and driving and riding with drinking drivers: A systematic review. *American Journal of Preventive Medicine* vol. 28, no. 5S, pp. 288–304.

Foxcroft, D, Ireland, D, Lister-Sharp, D, Lowe, G & Breen, R. 2003, *Primary prevention for alcohol misuse in young people*, The Cochrane Library, Oxford.

Gielen, A & Sleet, D. 2003, "Application of behavioral-change theories and methods to injury prevention", *Epidemiol. Rev*, vol. 25, pp. 65–76.

Geller, ES, Elder, J, Hovell, M, Sleet, D. 1991, Behavioral Approaches to Drinking-Driving Interventions. In: W. Ward, F.M. Lewis (eds) *Advances in health education & promotion*, Jessica Kingsley Press, UK. vol. III, pp. 45–68.

Gray, D, Drandich, M, Moore, L, Wilkes, T, Riley, R & Davies, S. 1995, "Aboriginal well-being and liquor licensing legislation in Western Australia", *Australian Journal of Public Health*, vol. 192, pp. 177–185.

Green, L & Kreuter, M. 1999, *Health promotion planning: An educational and ecological approach*, Mayfield, Mountain View.

Green, L & Kreuter, M. 2005, *health program planning: An educational and ecological approach (4th edition)*, McGraw Hill, New York.

Hanson, B, Larrson, S & Rastam, L. 2000, "Time trends in alcohol habits – results from the Kirseberg Project in Malmo, Sweden", *Subst. Use Misuse*, vol. 35, no. 1 & 2, pp. 171–187.

Hastings, G, Anderson, S, Cooke, E & Gordon, R. 2005, "Alcohol marketing and young people's drinking: A review of the Research", *J Public Health policy*, vol. 26, no. 3, pp. 296–311.

Henstridge, J, Homel, R & Mackay, P. 1997, *The long-term effects of random breath testing in four Australian states: A time series analysis, CR 162*, Federal Office of Road Safety, Canberra.

Henley, N, Donovan, R, Francas, M. 2007, Developing and implementing communication messages. In: L. Doll, S. Bonzo, J. Mercy, D. Sleet (eds) *Handbook of injury and violence prevention*. Springer, New York.

Hingson, R & Sleet, DA. 2007, Modifying alcohol use to reduce motor vehicle injury. Chapter 11 In: AC. Gielen, D.A. Sleet, R. DiClemente (eds) *Injury and violence prevention: Behavior Change theories, methods and applications*. Jossey-Bass, San Francisco, CA. pp. 234–256.

Hingson, R, Swahn, M, Sleet, DA. 2006, Interventions to prevent alcohol-related injuries. Chapter 16. In: L. Doll, S. Bonzo, J. Mercy, D. Sleet (eds) *Handbook of injury and violence prevention*. Springer, New York.

Hingson, R, McGovern, T, Howland, J et al. 1996, "Reducing alcohol-impaired driving in Massachusetts: The Saving Lives Program", *Am J Public health*, vol. 86, pp. 791–797.

Hingson, R, Zakocs, R, Heeren, T, Winter, M, Rosenbloom, D & DeJong, W. 2005, "Effects on alcohol related fatal crashes of a community based initiative to increase substance abuse treatment and reduce alcohol availability", *Injury Prevention*, vol. 11, pp. 84–90.

Holder, H. 1998, "Can local action on alcohol reduce harm? Results of the community trials project in the United States", In: T. Stockwell (ed) *Drug trials and tribulation: Lessons for Australian drug policy*, Curtin University, Perth.

Hollingworth, W, Ebel, B, McCarty, C, Garrison, M, Christakis, D & Rivara, F. 2006, "Prevention of deaths from harmful drinking in the United States: The potential effects of tax increases and advertising bans on young drinkers", *Journal of Studies on Alcohol*, vol. 67, no. 2, pp. 1–9.

Homel, R. 1981, "Penalties and the drink-driver: A study of one thousand offenders", *Aust. NZ J Criminol.*, vol. 14, pp. 225–241.

Homel, R. 1994, "Drink driving law enforcement and the legal blood limit in New South Wales", *Accid. Anal. Prev.*, vol. 26, pp. 147–155.

Howat, P, Maycock, B, Cross, D, Collins, J, Jackson, L, Burns, S & James, R. 2003, "Towards a more unified definition of health promotion", *Health promotion Journal of Australia*, vol. 14, no. 2, pp. 82–84.

Howat, P, Sleet, DA, Smith, DI. 1991, "Alcohol and driving: Is The 0.05% blood alcohol concentration limit justified?" *Drug and Alcohol Review* (Australia), vol. 10, no. 1, pp. 151–166.

Howat, P, O'Connor, J & Slinger, S. 1992, "Citizen action groups and health policy", *Health Promotion Journal of Australia*, vol. 2, no.3, pp. 16–22.

Howat, P, Sleet, D, Elder, R & Maycock, B. 2004, "Preventing alcohol related traffic injury: A health promotion approach", *Traffic Inj. Prev. (special issue)*, vol. 5, no. 3, pp. 208–219.

Institute of Medicine. National Research Council. 2003, *Reducing underage drinking: A collective responsibility. Committee on developing a strategy to reduce and prevent underage drinking*, The National Academies Press, Washington, DC.

International Centre for Alcohol Policies. 2001, *Self-regulation of beverage alcohol advertising*, ICAP, Washington DC.

International Union for Health promotion and Education. 2000, *The Evidence of Health Promotion Effectiveness: Shaping Public Health in a New Europe* (A report for the European Commission). 2nd edition. Paris: Jouve Composition & Impression.

Jernigan, D, Ostroff, J & Ross, C. 2005, "Alcohol advertising and youth: A measured approach", *J Public Health Policy*, vol. 26, no. 3, pp. 312–325.

Jones, R & Lacey, J. 2001, *Alcohol and highway safety*, National Highway Traffic Safety Administration, Washington DC.

Jones, S & Donovan, R. 2002, "Self-regulation of alcohol advertising: Is it working for Australia", *J Public Affairs*, vol. 2, no. 3, pp. 153–165.

Kypri, K & Langley, J. 2003, "Perceived social norms and their relation to university student drinking", *Journal of studies in Alcohol*, vol. 64, pp. 829–834.

Kypri, K, Voas, R, Langley, J, Stephenson, S, Begg, D, Tippetts, A & Davie, G. 2006, "Traffic crash injuries among 15–19 year olds and minimum purchasing age for alcohol in New Zealand", *American Journal of Public Health*, vol. 96, no.1, pp. 126–131.

Loxley, W, Toumbourou, J & Stockwell, T. 2004, *The prevention of substance use, risk and harm in Australia: A review of the evidence.*, The National Drug Research Institute and the Centre for Adolescent Health, Ministerial Council on Drug Strategy, Commonwealth of Australia, Canberra.

Mann, R, Stoduto, G, Macdonald, S, Sheikh, A, Bundy, S & Jonah, B. 2001, "The effects of introducing or lowering legal per se blood alcohol limits for driving: An international review", *Accid. Anal. Prev.*, vol. 33, pp. 61–75.

Marlatt, G, Baer, J, Kivlahan, D, Dimeff, L, Larimer, M, Quigley, L et al. 1998, "Screening and brief intervention for high-risk college student drinkers: Results from a 2-year follow-up assessment", *Journal of Consulting and Clinical psychology*, vol. 66, no. 4, pp. 604–615.

Marlatt, G & Witkiewitz, K. 2002, "Harm reduction approaches to alcohol use: Health promotion, prevention, and treatment", *Addictive Behaviors*, vol. 27, pp. 867–886.

McBride, N. 2003, "A systematic review of school drug education", *Health Educ. Res.*, vol. 18, no. 6, pp. 729–742.

McBride, N, Farrington, F, Midford, R, Meuleners, L & Phillips, M. 2004, "Harm minimization in school drug education: Results of the School Health and Alcohol Harm Reduction project (SHAHRP)", *Addiction*, vol. 99, pp. 278–291.

McGinnis, JM, Williams-Russo, P, Knickman, J. 2002, "The case for more active policy attention to health promotion", *Health Affairs*, vol. 21, no. 2, pp. 78–86.

McMillan, G & Lapham, S. 2006, "Effectiveness of bans and laws in reducing traffic deaths: legalized Sunday packaged alcohol sales and alcohol-related traffic crashes and crash fatalities in New Mexico", *American J Public Health*. vol. 96, no. 11, pp. 1944–1948.

Measham, F & Brain, K. 2005, " 'Binge' drinking, British alcohol policy and the new culture of intoxication", *Crime, Media, Culture*, vol. 1, no. 3, pp. 262–283.

Mitic, W. 2003, "Alcohol and university student drinking – not a class act", *Canadian Journal of Public Health*, vol. 94, pp. 13–15.

Mosher, J. 1994, "Alcohol advertising and public health: An urgent call for action", *American Journal of Public Health*, vol. 84, pp. 180–181.

Mosher, J & Johnsson, D. 2005, "Flavored alcohol beverages: An international marketing campaign that targets youth", *J Public Health Policy*, vol. 26, no. 3, pp. 326–342.

Newman, I, Shell, D, Major, L, Workman, T. 2006, "Use of policy, education, and enforcement to reduce binge drinking among university students: The NU Directions project", *The International J Drug Policy*, vol. 17, pp. 339–349.

Peden, M, Scurfield, R, Sleet, DA, Mohan, D, Hyder, AA, Jarawan, E, Mathers, C. (eds) 2004, World report on road traffic injury prevention. Geneva, Switzerland: World Health Organization.

Pinder, L. 1994, *The federal role in health promotion: Art of the possible*, WB Saunders, Toronto.

Roberts, G. 2002, *Analysis of alcohol promotion and advertising*, Centre for Youth Drug Studies, Australian Drug Foundation, Available: [www.adf.or.au/cyds/alcohol_advertising.pdf].

Room, R, Babor, T & Rehm, J. 2005, "Alcohol and Public Health", *www.thelancet.com*.

Rossow, I. 2000, "Suicide, violence and child abuse: A review of the impact of alcohol consumption on social problems", *Contemporary Drug Problems*, vol. 27, no. 3, pp. 397–433.

Rossow, I, Grøholt, B & Wichstrom, L. 2005, "Intoxicants and suicidal behaviour among adolescents: Changes in levels and associations from 1992 to 2002", *Addiction*, vol. 100, no. 1, pp. 79–88.

Schancke, VA. 2005, *Forebyggende og helsefremmende arbeid, forskning til praksis*, Nordnorsk kompetansesenter-Rus, ved Nordlandsklinikken, Narvik.

Shults, R, Elder, R, Sleet, D, Nichols, J, Alao, M, Carande-Kulis, V, Azaz, S, Sosin, D & Thompson, R. 2001, "Reviews of evidence regarding interventions to reduce alcohol-impaired driving", *Am J Prev. Med.*, vol. 21, no. 4S, pp. 66–88.

Shults, R, Sleet, D, Elder, R, Ryan, G & Sehgal, M. 2002, "Association between state level drinking and driving countermeasures and self reported alcohol impaired driving", *Injury Prevention*, vol. 8, pp. 106–110.

Sleet, D, Wagenaar, A & Waller, P. 1989, "Drinking, driving and health promotion", *Health Educ. Quartely*, vol. 16, no. 3, pp. 329–333.

Stockwell, T. 2001, "Responsible alcohol services: Lessons from evaluations of server training and policing initiatives", *Drug Alc. Rev.*, vol. 20, pp. 257–265.

Stockwell, T, Single, E, Hawks, D & Rehm, J. 1997, "Sharpening the focus of alcohol policy from aggregate consumption to harm and risk reduction", *Addiction Research,* vol. 5, pp. 1–19.

Stockwell, T, Masters, L, Philips, M, Daly, A, Gahegan, M, Midford, R & Philp, A. 1998, "Consumption of different alcoholic beverages as predictors of local rates of night-time assault and acute alcohol-related morbidity", *Australian & New Zealand Journal of Public Health,* vol. 22, no. 2, pp. 237–242.

Stockwell, T. 2006, "Alcohol supply, demand, and harm reduction: What is the strongest cocktail?" *International Journal of Drug Policy,* vol. 17, no. 4, pp. 269–277.

The Royal Australian College of Physicians. 2005, *Alcohol policy: Using evidence for better outcomes,* Sydney.

Tobler, N, Rooner, M, Ochshorn, P, Marshall, D, Streke, A & Stackpole, K. 2000, "School-based adolescent drug prevention programs: 1998 meta-analysis", *J. Prim. Prev.,* vol. 20, pp. 275–336.

US Department of Health and Human Services. 1997a, *Youth drinking: Risk factors and consequences. Alcohol Alert No. 37 July 1997,* National Institute on Alcohol Abuse and Alcoholism, Rockville.

US Department of Health and Human Services. 1997b, *Reducing tobacco use among youth: Community based-approaches,* Substance Abuse and Mental Health Services Administration. Centre for Substance Abuse Prevention, Rockville, DHHS Publication No. (SMA)97–3146.

Villaveces, A, Cummings, P, Koepsell, T, Rivara, F, Lumley, T & Moffat, J. 2003, "Association of alcohol-related laws with deaths due to motor vehicle and motorcycle crashes in the United States, 1980–1997", *Am J. Epidemiology,* vol. 157, pp. 131–140.

Wagenaar, A & Holder, H. 1991, "Effects of alcohol beverage server liability on traffic crash injuries", *Alcohol Clin. Exp. Res.,* vol. 15, pp. 942–947.

Wagenaar, A & Toomey, T. 2002, "Effects of minimum drinking age laws: Review and analyses of the literature from 1960–2000", *J. Stud. Alc.,* vol. Suppl. 14, pp. 206–225.

Waller, P. 1998, "Alcohol, aging and driving", In: E. Gomberg, A. Hegedus & R. Zucker (eds) *Alcohol problems and aging: NIAAA research monograph No. 33 NIH Pub No. 98–4163,* NIAAA, Bethesda.

Waller, S, Naidoo, B & Thom, B. 2002, *Prevention and reduction of alcohol misuse,* Health Development Agency, London.

Webb, M. 2001, "Research as an advocate's toolkit to reduce motor vehicle occupant deaths and injuries", *Am J Prev. Med.,* vol. 21, no. 4S, pp. 7–8.

Whetten-Goldstein, K, Sloan, F, Stout, E & Liang, L. 2000, "Civil liability, criminal law and other policies and alcohol-related motor vehicle fatalities in the United States: 1984–1995", *Accid. Anal. Prev.,* vol. 32, pp. 723–733.

White, D & Pitts, M. 1998, "Educating young people about drugs: A systematic review", *Addiction,* vol. 93, no. 10, pp. 1475–1487.

World Health Organisation. 1984, *Discussion document on the concept and principles of health promotion,* European Office of the World Health Organization, Copenhagen.

World Health Organisation. 1986, *Ottawa charter for health promotion,* WHO, Geneva.

World Health Organisation. 2004, *Global status report: Alcohol policy,* WHO, Geneva.

World Medical Association. 2005, *WMA Statement on reducing the global impact of alcohol on health and society,* World Medical Association, France.

Wyllie, A, Zhang, J & Caswell, S. 1998, "Responses to televised alcohol advertisements associated with drinking behaviour of 10–17 year olds", *Addiction,* vol. 93, pp. 361–371.

Section 3
Global Areas of Interest that Challenge the Assessment of Health Promotion Effectiveness

12
Globalization and Health Promotion
The Evidence Challenge

RONALD LABONTE

"We no longer inhabit, if we ever did, a world of discrete national communities. [T]he very nature of everyday living – of work and money and beliefs, as well as of trade, communications and finance . . .connects us all in multiple ways with increasing intensity" (Held, 2004).

The *Ottawa Charter for Health Promotion* (World Health Organization, 1986) identified in shorthand many of the strategies and tasks in an emerging field and literally wrote its practice into being. Each subsequent international health promotion conference probed a different area of the *Charter's* defining *raisons d'être*. Each subsequent conference also involved an increasing number of health promotion workers, policy-makers and scholars from developing countries, internationalizing what had been seen as an elite field concerned primarily with changing unhealthy rich world lifestyles. There were several plausible reasons for this:

- The end of the epidemiological transition: poorer countries were adding chronic diseases associated with Western consumption patterns without diminishing their burden of infectious ills, and richer countries were experiencing costly skirmishes with new or re-emerging pandemics as microbes became 24 hours from anywhere.
- The rising importance of Asian countries within a global economy: the West could no longer give short shrift to the Rest.
- A growing consciousness of one planet, one people: From the moonwalk to Greenpeace to climate change, new technologies and new social movements were thrusting a new awareness of the slender threads of planetary survival upon all of those within media reach.
- And beneath it all, the lurking late millennial behemoth of "globalization," a contested and already weary term that describes the accelerating global integration of trade in goods and services, and financial flows unimpeded by national borders.

Unsurprisingly, one of the foci of the 2005 Bangkok gathering was globalization itself. As the *Bangkok Charter for Health Promotion* expressed: "Health promotion must become an integral part of domestic and foreign policy and international relations" (World Health Organization, 2005).

Doing so raises two fundamental questions about the nature of evidence as it pertains to globalization: First, what is the evidence for globalization's impacts on health status, and how do we adjudicate it? Second, how do we measure the impacts of interventions aimed at a target as large as the planet and all its peoples?

It's About the Money

Before turning to these questions, let's consider the shibboleth itself: globalization. To some, it describes a function of technology, culture and economics leading to a compression of time (everything is faster), space (geographic boundaries begin to blur) and cognition (awareness of the world as a whole) (Lee, 2002). While undoubtedly true, these have been societal qualities for as long as there have been written records of societies. The recent and important qualitative shift lies in the intensity of these changes. Others have argued (convincingly) that "economic globalization has been the driving force behind the overall process" (Woodward et al., 2001), i.e., the source of globalization's recent intensification, bringing with it new challenges to health and its promotion. The major forms of economic globalization include:

1. The scale of cross-border private financial flows (most of it speculative) resulting from capital market liberalization. Daily currency trades dwarf the total foreign exchange reserves of all governments reducing their ability to stabilize their currencies when speculators decide to cash in their winnings. Each country experiencing a currency crisis (from Mexico and Thailand to Russia and Brazil) has seen increased poverty and inequality, and decreased health and social spending (O'Brien, 2002; Cobham, 2002), with women and children disproportionately bearing the burden (Gyebi et al., 2002).

2. The establishment of binding trade rules, primarily through the World Trade Organization (WTO). These trade rules limit the policy flexibilities of national governments in ways that could imperil public health (Labonte & Sanger, 2006b; Labonte & Sanger, 2006a). As the "Doha Development Round" of negotiations intended to benefit disproportionately developing countries continues to sputter to an inconclusive end due to rich world mercantilism, bilateral and regional agreements multiply in which the economic might of the wealthier countries invariably eclipses the nominal democracy that inheres in the WTO.

3. The reorganization of production across national borders. At least one third (and as much as two-thirds) of global trade is intra-firm between affiliated companies of transnational corporations (TNCs) (Gyebi et al., 2002; World Commission on the Social Dimensions of Globalization, 2004). The emergence of these global production or commodity chains allows TNCs to locate labour intensive operations in low-wage countries (often in exclusive export processing zones or EPZs, known for poor wages and working conditions), carry out research and development in countries with high levels of publicly funded education and public investment in research, and declare most of their profits in low-tax countries.

4. The crisis of climate change. For over 20 years health promotion has recognized the centrality, if not primacy, of the physical environment as a prerequisite

to health (Labonte, 1991a; Labonte, 1991b). Virtually all environmental markers show deterioration in our life support. Climate change is undoubtedly the most urgent global health issue and its linkage to global market integration is straightforward: Moving goods around the world consumes fossil fuel and exhausts greenhouse gases. In the UK, increases in trade-related shipping are now cited as the principle reason why that country will not meet its Kyoto commitment.

In crude summary, if we want to interrogate the evidence-base for how globalization is affecting health we need to follow the flows of finance capital, and how its creation and accumulation is affecting health risks.* In particular, we need to assess how the economic drivers of globalization are affecting equity in both health opportunities (the determinants of health, or what the *Ottawa Charter* called the "prerequisites to health") and health outcomes, and at different levels – from the household, to the community, the region, the nation. The evidence task is daunting.

First: Moving from International to Global

In apprising the evidence-base (essential with respect to knowing where and how to intervene) we first need to distinguish a *global* approach to health promotion from an *international* approach. Until recently, researchers, development agencies and non-governmental organizations (NGOs) mobilized around "international health:" the greater burden of disease faced by poorer groups in poorer countries. Actions on health remained, at best, a partnership between wealthier and poorer countries on diseases or health issues within the poorer partners' borders. International health as a practice paradigm is still important. If nothing else, there is a global obligation under various human rights treaties (e.g. Article 12 on the Right to Health in the International Covenant on Economic, Social and Cultural Rights) and development commitments (such as the Millennium Development Goals and their associated targets) for those countries with more financial and human capital to spend some of it on the problems of those with less. But a number of recent world events have changed the landscapes of what we once called "international relations" – and hence international health – irrevocably.

The first event was the 1970s recession in the industrialized world, compounded by the "oil crisis" and US monetary policies that dramatically increased interest rates. These events led many developing countries to default on international loans from rich world creditors that had been thrust upon them indiscriminately (perhaps even as a deliberate form of creating economic servitude) and as requisites to pay for the quadrupled price of oil imports. The "debt crisis," in turn, re-shaped the

---

* One small indication of this: In 2005, the net capital flow from developing to developed countries (based on [debt payments + profit repatriation] – [development assistance + foreign direct investment] came to over US$483 billion (UN DESA, 2006). This is a striking reversal of the early 1990s when developed countries managed to trickle a very small positive capital flow in the other direction. Today, world's poor are indirectly but no less perversely subsidizing the debt-fuelled excess consumption and lifestyle venality of the rich.

International Monetary Fund (IMF) and World Bank into watchdogs for developing countries to keep them on a policy track that would allow them to repay most of their debts and to open their markets for international investors. This policy track of "structural adjustment" embodied the neo-liberal economic orthodoxy and conservative politics of the wealthier countries that dominate decisions in both institutions: reductions in public spending, privatization of productive state assets, welfare minimalism, cost-recovery for remaining services and rapid liberalization of financial markets and lowering or elimination of tariffs (Schrecker & Labonte, 2006).

Other transformative events included:

- The fall of the Berlin Wall, which established the United States as the world's only superpower and created a normative vacuum for alternative models of development that could no longer experiment with "third way" blends of state centralism and market capitalism.
- The 1992 United Nations Conference on Environment and Development, which fostered a "global environmental consciousness" with special emphasis on the developing world's need for both economic growth and environmental protection.
- The diffusion of information and communications technologies (ICTs), which transformed the nature of global capitalism, while increasing the speed and scale with which civil society could analyze and mobilize responses to capitalism's more egregious abuses.

In this new landscape, a shift is needed in how health promotion is conceptualized, from an international concern with poorer countries' greater burden of disease to a more critical recognition that both the determinants and the consequences of this burden are inextricably linked to processes of globalization.

Second: Mapping the Linkages

How do we show these inextricable linkages? The pathways between globalization and health are neither short nor direct; as a health determinant, globalization represents perhaps the most distal causal element. In assembling the evidence base for its health impacts, a heuristic is needed against which the multiple arrays of research findings might be organized into defensible causal pathways.* Many such heuristics (or models) exist; I will use one that I developed not because it is best, but because it is the one I am most comfortable explicating.

This framework (Fig. 12.1) argues that globalization – simply defined as increased interdependence through accelerating global market integration – will have different

---

* It is important to note here that "causal" is not used here in the narrow sense of scientific certainty or statistical probability, but more in the legal sense of "burden of proof." As will be seen in the discussion of narrative syntheses that follows, conventional scientific notions of causality cannot apply when investigating such complex social phenomena as globalization.

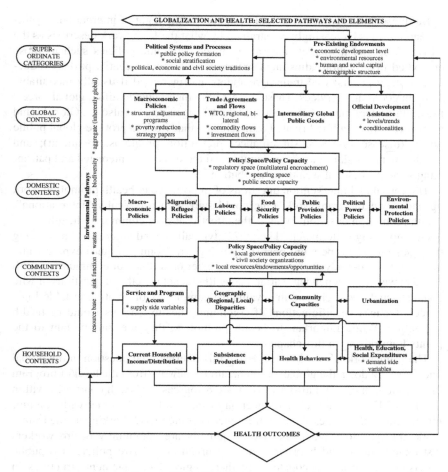

FIGURE 12.1. Globalization and health.

health effects depending on the political history and resource endowments of different countries or regions. The most obvious and important differences relate to existing stocks of capital – financial (wealth), human (educational and health levels), natural (resource base), social (an imprecise term that I will not try to shorthand). A small, landlocked African country facing critical health crises and with low population literacy rates and technologically unsophisticated industry will not adjust to the competitive pressures of open markets as well as a rich, economically advanced nation with well-developed social infrastructures. But even at similar development levels, political traditions play an important role. Post-tax/transfer child poverty is much less in the social democratic Nordic countries than in the market-liberal Anglo-American countries. HIV prevalence is much higher in Africa than other parts of the world and, within Africa, in some countries but not in others due at least partly to differing national policy choices.

But these policy choices (or "policy space" in the argot of international political economy) is increasingly constrained by what the framework describes as the "drivers" of global market integration: macroeconomic policies such as those embodied in structural adjustment programs and, more recently, poverty reduction strategy papers; free trade agreements and increased if usually inequitable flows in goods and services. These drivers have their countervailing global forces: those multilateral institutions – such as the UN agencies, but also the Global Fund and other Global Public Private Partnerships – that work to provide global public goods (disease research, surveillance, prevention programs, treatment); and development assistance as an inadequate and too often self-interested and patronizing system of global wealth redistribution.[*]

The causal and intervention questions of importance to health promotion work up and down the framework. One could start with a typically "international" health promotion question: What is the effectiveness of community health workers in improving maternal/child health? A typically sound approach to answering this question would be a pre-post study using a randomized, quasi-experimental or multiple case-study design where the number or skill-set of community health workers was the independent variable. (I will bracket the ethical questions of who conducts such research, and the evaluative complexity of creating testable logic models for *why* specific actions of community health workers would be health promoting. While important to health promoters, they are unimportant to the points I am raising in this chapter.)

The framework allows us to re-define this international question into a global one. Working down the globalization/health framework from the level of program intervention, one would also ask: How are resources for health controlled within the home? How do household education or income levels interact with community health workers in explaining differences in outcomes? Working up the framework, the questions would be: How equitably are community health workers distributed within and between rural and urban areas? Are policies for public provision of services adequate? Are there regional management structures in place to ensure service quality and continuity?

But working even further up – to the national and global levels – one would need to ask: What are the constraints on national government expenditures to ensure an adequate and equitable supply of community health workers? What role do international aid agencies or multilateral institutions play in worsening or lessening these constraints? How does the proliferation of "siloed" global health

---

[*] The Global Fund (to fight AIDS, Tuberculosis and Malaria) was established by the Group of 7 (G7) countries in 2001. Reliant on donations – almost all of which come from governments – the Fund has always struggled to secure enough resources to meet the competitive demand from developing countries. Regarding development assistance, only a few countries have ever reached the long-agreed target of 0.7% of their Gross National Income to aid; and much aid remains tied to the purchase of goods or services from the donor country. For a fuller discussion of these issues, see (Labonte et al., 2005; Labonte & Torgerson, 2005; Schrecker & Labonte, 2006).

programs affect the development of a more integrated and effective public provision system? What role do trade agreements play, particularly in employment conditions or income generation that might affect household resource levels? How does the "brain drain" of skilled health workers from poor to rich countries affect the supply of community health workers or, more importantly, the supply of nurses or physicians needed as more highly skilled back-ups? How does capital flight or the existence of offshore tax havens constrain expenditures, or promote corruption that, in turn, might ripple down the public and private systems of delivery? Each of these questions, in turn, begs an analysis that locates the answers within the historical and political contexts of a particular country, while incorporating findings from cross-country analyses that might determine whether elements of the key globalization "drivers" are primarily responsible, or more domestic factors afford the predominant explanation.[*]

Case Example: HIV in Zambia

Zambia is one of the southern African countries hard hit by the HIV/AIDS pandemic. Using the trope of a woman I will call Chileshe and key elements of the globalization/health framework, a different set of health promotion policy issues emerges than the more traditional (though still essential and often effective) interventions of prevention through education and treatment through antiretroviral treatment (ART) roll-out.

Chileshe, like tens of thousands other Zambian women, is waiting to die from AIDS. Prevention programs and expanded treatment campaigns are too little, too late. She acquired the disease from her now dead husband, who lost his job in a textile plant and moved to the capital, Lusaka, where he sold used clothing as a precarious street vendor. Alone and lonely, he traded money for sex with women desperate to support their own lives, and those of their children. And so the epidemic spread eventually reaching Chileshe.

What has Chileshe's plight to do with globalization? The answer lies principally with the macroeconomic policies imposed by the World Bank and the International Monetary Fund as conditions for new loans to help Zambia cope with its debt crisis. In 1992, Zambia was required to open its borders to textile imports, including cheap, second-hand clothing. Its domestic state-run clothing

---

[*] Much of the debate on globalization and health has been framed by cross-country regression analyses using various measures of economic globalization (e.g. inward and outward trade and financial flows, depth of liberalization), domestic performance (e.g. economic growth, "good governance") and health (e.g. average life expectancy). The problems with such studies are that the choice of variables and time frames can produce contradictory findings, the reliability of required data points for many countries is questionable and there is little attention paid to distributional equity within countries. The "stylized" findings of such studies may be useful as stimuli to discussion but are no substitute for detailed, country- or region-specific historical analyses.

manufacturers, inefficient in both technology and management by wealthier nation standards, could not compete, especially when the importers of second-hand clothing had the advantage of no production costs and no import duties. (Ironically, many of the second-hand clothes that flooded Zambia and other SSA countries began as donations to charities in Europe, the USA and Canada.) Within eight years, 132 of 140 clothing and textile mills closed operations and 30,000 jobs disappeared, which the World Bank later acknowledged as "unintended and regrettable consequences" of the adjustment process (Labonte et al., 2005).

For conventional economists, this is a textbook example of how and why trade liberalization works: Consumers get better and cheaper goods (at least for a while) and inefficient producers are driven out of business. However Chileshe's husband, and then Chileshe herself, paid a heavy price that cascaded throughout other sectors of Zambia's limited manufacturing base, with some 40 per cent of manufacturing jobs disappearing during the 1990s. Other facets of structural adjustment also played a role in Chileshe's HIV infection. Part of the standard adjustment package is privatization of state industries to raise short-term revenue to continue servicing overseas debts. This privatization robs a country of the ability for profitable state-run sectors to cross-subsidize social spending in such crucial areas as education and health. Liberalization of financial markets makes it easier, in turn, for foreign-owned firms to move their profit offshore and avoid having it taxed for public spending or re-invested for domestic growth within the country. This is precisely what happened in Zambia. As well, the assumption that growth would inevitably follow such shock treatment, leading to new forms of employment and taxation to replace the sources lost by unemployment and tariff revenues, proved theoretically sound but empirically false. The net result was a dramatic drop in the monies available to the state to invest in health or education. This was buttressed by other adjustment requirements – a decrease in public spending, a cut in public sector wages and the introduction of cost-recovery (user-fee) programs in health and other social services. All of this was imposed just at a time when the AIDS pandemic was starting to surge.

In varying degrees this story recurred throughout many southern Africa countries. While the economic outcomes of adjustment remain equivocal (some countries weathered the changes better than others), and the World Bank and IMF argue that things would likely have been worse without these changes, in Africa the economic outcomes were largely negative and, in the case of health impacts, singularly destructive (Breman & Shelton, 2001). In effect, African people not responsible for the debts that precipitated the adjustment process were required to sacrifice their health to ensure the debts would be repaid.

As evidence and global campaigning on the "death by debt" mounted, the Bank, IMF and their major shareholders – the wealthier industrialized countries – initiated the "Heavily Indebted Poor Countries" (HIPC) program of debt relief. This program did free up monies for investing in health and education, and requirements for cost-recovery were slowly dropped, but the discredited economic policies of structural adjustment still resided in the background of the newer and mandatory "poverty reduction strategy papers." One key element is the imposition of public spending ceilings, based on two neo-liberal economic principles: public debt is bad, so public spending must be constrained; and inflation is bad, so increases in public spending must be slow and small. To qualify for debt-relief, Zambia agreed to keep its public salary spending below 8% of its GDP. A few years ago, Zambia increased its salaries for health workers and teachers to help stem their exodus to wealthier countries, and provided incentives to those working in grossly underserved rural areas. Combined with a drop in the price of its primary export commodity (copper) and increases in other sector spending, Zambia crossed the 8% threshold and was summarily dropped from the debt relief program. It then had to pay over US$300 million in debt servicing costs, money that did *not* go into HIV prevention programs or to rebuild and sustain its fragile public health system. A subsequent rebound in global copper prices and an agreement by a major donor country to pay directly the salaries of some of its teachers (thereby taking the costs off the government's books) allowed Zambia to re-qualify for debt relief a year later.

HIV/AIDS prevention programs, using the "best practice" lessons of health promotion past, have worked in slowing or decreasing the pandemic in countries like Zambia, but their expansion has not kept pace with the disease (UNAIDS, 2006). One key reason – despite such new Global Public Private Partnerships as the Global Fund – is a lack of funds, a problem partly embedded in the fiscal, lending, debt-recovery, trade and intellectual property policies of wealthier nations, and the economic prescriptions the international financial institutions that they dominate continue to impose of poor countries. Another key reason is that such prevention programs continue to be disease-specific and fail to rise to the health promotion future challenge posed by the recent (2005–2008) World Health Organization's Commission on the Social Determinants of Health: What good does it do to treat a disease and then send people back to the conditions that made them sick?

Back to the Evidence

Chileshe's story is what is now referred to as *evidence-informed* rather than the more narrowly construed concept of *evidence-based*. In areas of health promotion intervention where the causes and policy implications are complex and contested, evidence alone will never be sufficient or persuasive in itself. As most health promoters have long known, "healthy public policy" usually arises from the entwined efforts of those who provide as much evidence as possible and those who then lobby its importance. While evidence matters, policy battles are won as much through influence networks and individual testimonies as by the reasoned arguments of narrative syntheses or systematic reviews.

Chileshe's story, and the claims I have just made about structural adjustment and HIV/AIDS in Zambia, derive from a form of research synthesis that is important in evidence-gathering in global health research: narrative syntheses – referred to in comparative historical sociology as process tracing – in which "hundreds of observations are marshaled to support deductive claims regarding linkages in a causal chain" (Goldstone, 2003, p. 49). Narrative syntheses incorporate several elements which, in Chileshe's case, include: (a) description of the national and international policy context; (b) country- or region-specific studies that describe changes in determinants of health, such as the level and composition of household income, labour market changes, access to education and health services; (c) evidence from clinical and epidemiological studies that relates to demonstrated or probable changes in health outcomes arising from those impacts; (d) ethnographic research, field observations, and other first-hand accounts of experience "on the ground." In assembling such evidence – aided by whatever globalization framework appears best suited to the need (health promotion research or evaluation) – it is necessary to recognize that rarely can conclusions be stated with the degree of confidence in findings that is possible in a laboratory situation or even in many epidemiological study designs, where almost all variables can be controlled. As Sir Michael Marmot, chair of the WHO's Commission on the Social Determinants of Health, expresses: "The further upstream we go in our search for causes," and globalization is the quintessential upstream variable, "the less applicable is the randomized controlled trial," and the greater the need to rely on "observational evidence and judgment in formulating policies to reduce inequalities in health" (Marmot, 2000).

An example that more formally applied the techniques of process tracing than my account of Chileshe is a recent study that identified the multi-step pathways that lead from globalization to increased vulnerability to HIV infection among women and children in sub-Saharan Africa (De Vogli & Birbeck, 2005). The researchers identified five manifestations of, or responses to, globalization at the national level: currency devaluations, privatization, financial and trade liberalization, implementation of user charges for health services and implementation of user charges for education. An array of existing research studies was assembled to interrogate each of these pathways. The first two pathways were found to operate by way of reducing women's access to basic needs, either because of rising prices or reduced opportunities for waged employment. The third operated by way of increasing migration to urban areas, which simultaneously may reduce women's access to basic needs and increase their exposure to risky consensual sex. The fourth pathway (health user fees) reduced both women's and youth's access to HIV-related services, and the fifth (education user fees) increased risk of exposure to risky consensual sex, commercial sex and sexual abuse by reducing access to education. The explanatory approach the researchers adopted complements recent systematic reviews of research on determinants of vulnerability not only to HIV/AIDS but also to tuberculosis and malaria. These reviews concluded that vulnerability to all three diseases is closely linked; that poverty, gender inequality, development policy and health sector reforms that involve user fees and reduced access to care are important determinants of vulnerability; and that "[c]omplicated interactions between these factors, many of which lie outside the health sector, make unravelling of their individual roles . . . difficult" (Bates et al., 2004, p. 268).

Health Promoting Globalization Interventions in Fact

To date, health promotion interventions into globalization as a health determinant have been limited. Any effort to establish the globalization/health promotion evidence and effectiveness link is premature and perhaps even misplaced. As with all complex phenomena, the ability to single out a particular intervention (or even sets of interventions) as probabilistically formative in changes to the economic practices of globalization is methodologically impossible. Within a normative frame of strategic assumptions, however, akin to economists' reasoned but no less idealized models for which they are annually awarded Nobel science prizes, it is possible to assess certain actions against certain links in the chain by which globalization affects health outcomes. Essentially this entails working one's way through the framework, piece by piece rather than as a whole. Here we can encounter some evidence of health promotion effectiveness, two examples of which follow.

The International Framework Convention on Tobacco Control

The International Framework Convention on Tobacco Control (FCTC) was adopted by the World Health Assembly in May 2003 and is considered the first international health treaty – or, in health promotion jargon, the first global healthy public policy. As of September 2006, 168 countries had signed the agreement and 139 had become states parties to it following ratification. The FCTC requires these countries to enact bans on tobacco advertising, marketing and promotion, implement warnings on packages and implement measures to protect exposure to second-hand smoke, and "encourages" them (in multilateral parlance, a term that conveys intent without obligation) to raise tobacco taxes and consider litigation to hold the tobacco industry liable for its wrongdoings. The FCTC is not as strong a treaty as health and civil society organizations (CSOs) wanted. Several of these CSOs participated in the negotiating forum that led to the FCTC, and continue to lobby for amendments and compliance as a "Framework Conventional Alliance." They are credited with maintaining pressure against the continuous efforts of countries such as Germany, Japan, and the US – each with large tobacco industries – to weaken substantially the health provisions. Japan, whose government is a key stakeholder in its tobacco industry, played a particularly obstructionist role and successfully watered down the FCTC wording in several key sections (Assunta & Chapman, 2006).[*]

---

[*] The study by Asunta and Chapman is a good model for evidence-informed analyses of how "soft power" plays out in multilateral health negotiations. The study identified the pro-tobacco position of Japanese governments and officials during the FCTC negotiating rounds, the increasing number of negotiators sent by Japan to the different sessions (they had the largest number at the final round), texts of Japanese positions taken over the course of the negotiations and the extent to which these were embodied in the final treaty.

The FCTC, while nonetheless a positive start in the global control of the pandemics of tobacco-related diseases, is further weakened by its potential clash with multilateral trade treaties. In 1994 the Canadian government proposed the adoption of generic ("plain") packaging for cigarettes. Tobacco companies responded that such a measure would violate their intellectual property rights, i.e., their trademarks, which are protected by the World Trade Organization and NAFTA (North American Free Trade Agreement) agreements on intellectual property. The Canadian government abandoned this proposal. In March 2002, Phillip Morris International indicated that it believes proposed Canadian regulations to prohibit use of the terms "mild" and "light" on tobacco packages would again violate several provisions of NAFTA and WTO agreements (BRIDGES, 2002). Because the FCTC failed to get the use of these descriptors explicitly banned as part of the Convention (i.e., the wording of Article 11 of the Convention states that misleading terms "may include" such words as "light" and "mild"), it is unclear if this would preclude a future trade challenge by bans on their use. This has particular bearing on the names of certain brands, likely to be considered intellectual property rights under various trade treaties, such as the Japanese brand, "Mild Seven" and the Chinese brand "Long Life." A number of countries and regions have entered voluntary agreements with tobacco firms to eliminate the use of such terms, including Canada, Australia, Brazil and the European Union, but it is unlikely these voluntary pacts would hold out against a trade dispute, should one eventually be launched. It also leaves moot what a potential dispute settlement on such a trade/health conflict might be, since efforts to state that the FCTC would prevail should conflicts with trade agreements arise also failed leaving unresolved any explicit claim to which agreement should be superordinate. Would the dispute be heard by a trade treaty panel? Or by a special panel of the FCTC? Finally, Fidler (2002) points out that "whether the framework-protocol [such as the FCTC] provides an adequate foundation for such international legal evolution is still open to question" (p.56). Apart from the decline in nations participating in or ratifying the more demanding protocols that follow adoption of the generally worded framework treaty (and on which there is little reported development under the FCTC), there are presently no enforcement measures for countries that fail to abide by the protocols or their dispute resolution decisions. Trade agreements, however, have enforcement mechanisms in the form of sanctions or direct financial penalties.[*]

Treatment Action Campaign

The example of the FCTC is not meant to dissuade health promotion from tackling globalization-related health problems. While encumbered with future uncertainties, the FCTC still provides a normative framework supported by almost 170 ratifying

---

[*] On a more positive note, the International Union for Health Promotion and Education continues to play a role in lobbying for global tobacco control, and its materials on draft tobacco legislation for consideration by states parties to the FCTC is linked on the Framework Alliance website (International Union for Health Promotion and Education, 2003).

nations, and offers a different venue for negotiation than trade fora alone. The FCTC also owes much to the health advocacy of professionals and civil society organizations. Evidence of the (partial) effectiveness of this advocacy resides in the simple existence of the Convention; and in most areas of public policy, especially that entailing multilateral negotiations, partial success is all that can reasonably be expected. The example also underscores the pre-eminence of mobilization and advocacy as the principal health promotion tools in tackling globalization-related health issues. A clear example of this within a national context is the South African Treatment Action Campaign (TAC). TAC first mobilized around HIV treatment access in 1998 and grew to have branches in all South African provinces and most major cities. While TAC is only one of several popular social movements that arose in post-apartheid South Africa, it is credited with being the first "to enjoy huge popular support" (Endresen & von Kotze, 2005). It is also credited with galvanizing opposition to the court challenge brought by multinational drug firms against the South African government's attempts to import cheaper versions of antiretroviral treatments (ARTs) (a challenge later dropped due to mobilized global outrage); and with prodding its own government to move away from HIV-denialism to a belated (though still inadequate) ART roll-out. TAC consistently framed its advocacy as:

- A matter of human rights (the right to health is part of the South African Constitution, and was used by TAC in a successful court case that forced the government to dispense mother-to-child HIV transmission treatment).
- Part of a larger struggle for redistribution of wealth and resources (many of TAC's member organizations are involved in labour unions, anti-poverty movements and groups seeking to prevent poor people being cut off from access to water or electricity).
- A member of the "anti-globalization" global movement.[*]

In 2005 TAC commissioned an extensive independent evaluation of its work (Boulle & Avafia, 2005). It recommended a number of strategies that, if acted upon, would see TAC shift from being a social movement with fluid organization and a campaign-driven focus to a bureaucratic civil society organization with specified projects and outputs. This type of transition in "grassroots" community health organizing is well known and documented in the health promotion literature (cf. (Labonte, 1998) for examples), along with the potential loss of advocacy edge it might bring. However, unlike many social movement groups in Africa, TAC has attracted significant external funding and operates with a multi-million dollar budget and over 40 full time staff (Friedman & Mottiar, 2005). Its attributed successes include the treatment court challenges in which it participated, the de-stigmatization of HIV in South Africa (and beyond), and becoming a model

---

[*] There is a rich irony in a global movement that naively adopted the media's dismissive moniker of "anti-globalization." In more recent years, this term has been eschewed in favour of the more accurate "anti-neoliberalism" or "just globalization" movement, focusing attention on what is ethically wrong and population unhealthy about much of the present form of globalization, rather than with globalization *per se*.

for other movements defending socio-economic rights and monitoring government accountability. On this last account, however, there is conflicting evidence from a non-commissioned scholarly study (Friedman & Mottiar, 2005). While both evaluation studies relied upon detailed document analysis and qualitative interviews, the latter added a theoretical analysis of new social movement theory. TAC's reluctance to engage actively in a critique of the neoliberal economic contexts accepted by South Africa's government, and its willingness to use legal challenges to win single issue campaigns, *de facto* legitimized what other activist groups perceived as an illegitimate political order.

Admittedly from a weak evidence base of two studies, there are three other globalization/health promotion lessons that the TAC case presents. First, it is easier to mobilize around single, simple issues than multiple, complex problems. Second, it is easier to win policy change on medically defined problems than on those residing in the social determinants of health. Third, despite the powerful vested interests represented by pharmaceutical multinationals (and their governments), moral and political challenges to one sector of neoliberal globalization does not question the basic structure or rules by which it works. The same lesson can be drawn from the quarter-century experience of, first national and now global, campaigns against tobacco. It also explains why the "just globalization" movement has tended in its health advocacy to attend more to issues of treatment access, privatization of health care services and insufficient health workers than, for example, the global financial architecture that allows an estimated US$8 to $11.5 trillion in corporate profits and wealthy individual assets to sit untaxed in offshore accounts (Tax Justice Network, 2005; Utting et al., 2000). A nominal tax on the interest-growth of the smaller sum alone would raise over $US250 billion annually for redistribution, roughly twice the value of total development assistance and debt cancellation.

Polyphony of Current and Future Possibilities

These are two of many possible examples of where and how health promotion can intervene in globalization as a health determinant. Others include:

- An increasing number of academic and CSO groupings that engage in detailed analyses of globalization and health, ranging from fairer forms of aid, trade and debt cancellation to "fair trade" alternatives, north/south program and development partnerships and the renewal of the WHO's "Health for All" primary health care ideal. The combination of critical policy analysis and social movement advocacy emanating from Canada in the late 1990s, as one example, is credited with stalling OECD talks on a controversial "Multilateral Agreement on Investments." Health arguments were central in this campaign.
- The emergence of global networks of health activists concerned specifically and explicitly with globalization. The Peoples' Health Movement, a global umbrella of these networks, is one example. Founded in 2000, the PHM has held two global assemblies (Bangladesh, 2000; Ecuador, 2004); participated in producing the world's first "alternative health report," *Global Health Watch 2004–2005*;

launched right to health campaigns in various parts of the world (notably India); and contributed extensively to the formation of the WHO's Commission on the Social Determinants of Health. Health promoters throughout the world are contributing to the PHM's work and participating in its many national campaigns aimed at changing both national and global health policies.

- The WHO itself is becoming more engaged with the globalization – health dynamic, with a unit wholly dedicated to offering national governments advice on trade, human rights and intellectual property agreements such that global health equity is not compromised. In many countries, academics, civil society and professional health organizations enjoin with health ministry officials in debating more openly the implications of global economic and trade policies on health in an endeavour to create what is euphemistically called "greater policy coherence," and what in fact means holding finance and treasury departments to task for more than simply keeping the GDP on an up and up.

Few of these initiatives, however, have been evaluated. The evidence of their impact remains moot and, in the case of the "another world is possible" globalization "movement of movements"(Mertes, 2004), it is difficult to provide narrowly causal evidence. But, as Immanuel Wallerstein has argued, there is convincing inferential evidence of impact "in getting some states – perhaps all – to inflect their policies in the direction of human rights" (Wallerstein, 2004); p.269).

Health Promoting Globalization Interventions in Theory

The absence of a firm evidence base is no reason to avoid new effort. Health promotion has never been simply about knowing what causes health inequities (health inequalities that are unfair and changeable), but what policies and programs might reduce them. If we accept that evidence of impact will always be pluralistic and argumentative, rather than definitively causal, the intervention challenge posed by globalization is less about proving what works than deciding, in the first instance, where to intervene. Here we might consider a few of the strategy areas from the *Charter*.

Under *develop personal skills* globalization substantially alters the nature of what skills health promoters might seek to develop – in themselves, in others. While "skills" under this strategy are often taken as behaviour change or coping, analytical skills related to globalization quickly surface as important and was cited as another of TAC's major successes (i.e. creating a cohort of globally critical health analysts/activists in South Africa). Health promoters themselves need to learn more from the work of development economists and economic historians. It is also well within a health promotion rubric that at least some in the field become adept at trade policy analysis. There are public workers, academics and civil society organisations in most countries with (increasingly developed) trade analysis skills, but few of these take a broader social determinants approach to the trade/health relationship, focusing instead on agreements extending intellectual property rights and their impacts on access to essential medicines. Yet on-going trade negotiations on the lowering of industrial tariffs, or rules of government procurement (contracting out), or trade in services (and not just in health services) will have enormous health externalities that need to be understood, if not given precedence, by trade negotiators.

In *strengthening community action*, the first and most obvious challenge is defining what is meant by "community" under increasing globalization. Would we be seeking evidence, for example, of how health promotion work has strengthened global civil society networks and cross-national partnerships/alliances, in much the same way we now look to how our more locally-based programs have strengthened different facets of community capacity? This question does not imply that such alliances or networks *need* our support, at least in terms of analytical skill-strengthening; to presume so would in many instances be supreme acts of hubris. But they can often benefit by the financial or human resources and the health-specific legitimating networks that health promoters can bring to the globalization issue under scrutiny. A key health promotion research question here is the extent to which existing global health partnerships, such as the Global Fund and other global/international disease-based funding programs, integrate health promotion thinking within their disbursements and assessments. Evaluation studies of this question are only now commencing.

In related fashion, the call to *re-orient health systems* in the context of globalization raises a particularly critical question: To what extent have the past several decades of market-oriented and economic cost-effective approaches to health system reforms aided or hindered their ability to incorporate health promotion within their functions? We know one thing quite well about market-oriented health reforms: they tend to service those who can pay at the expense of those who cannot, and rely upon insufficient charity rather than cross-subsidized and risk-pooled entitlement to fill the equity gaps (Lister, 2005). (By one recent WHO estimate, as many people worldwide may be falling into medical poverty each year due to lack of insured coverage as are lifted from poverty by globalization's engines of economic growth.) We also know that the proliferation of disease-based aid or global funding programs often fracture what existing public health systems remain in many developing countries, with their differing requirements for reporting and program organization and staffing, and especially so in sub-Saharan Africa, which has suffered an enormous loss of its health workers to wealthier countries. We know less well the degree to which broader social determinants of health are considered within these programs, or empowerment/capacity-building goals that are now generally accepted as a "parallel track" in most health promotion programs (Labonte & Laverack, 2001a; Labonte & Laverack, 2001b). There is also a newfound global rush to increase the supply of health workers; the 2006 World Health Report estimates a present global deficit of over 1 million health workers in Africa alone (World Health Organization, 2006). But will efforts to close the gap privilege clinical workers (doctors, nurses) over community workers, health promoters, educators and the larger constellation of skills inherent in health promotion practice? For that matter, will the renewed call for comprehensive primary health care emanating from within and outside of the WHO default again to disease-based primary health care, and then to the even narrower project of simply improving access to primary *medical* care?

Finally, to *build healthy public policy* in a globalizing world is both a large and almost totalizing task. There is little in the realm of contemporary globalization's economic drivers that does not have some impact on health outcomes. One challenge – now being taken up by the Globalization Knowledge Network of the World Health Organization's Commission on the Social Determinants of Health – is to assemble a rich evidence base that indicates priority areas for intervention, as well as evidence (where such exists) of policies that have limited globalization's negative health impacts while allowing its positive health gains to be equitably shared. The somewhat belaboured issue of what constitutes evidence permeates this particular health promotion strategy. Attribution of intervention to outcome in any area of public policy change is difficult, and the more so when the policy domain is multilateral. A specific and more easily adduced evidence issue is whether efforts to use public policy levers within a country to reduce unhealthy practices (e.g. in food consumption or tobacco use) need to show that they do not simply displace these practices to another part of the planet. (As Canadian governments continue to outdo each other in restrictive tobacco legislation, its domestic tobacco industry is allowed to join its trade missions to developing countries, notably China.)[*]

An Apocryphal Summation

Interestingly, globalization (at least its dominant economic form) and health promotion both came into public discourse and policy practice around the same time (the late 70s and early 80s). The former, of course, is a bit of a Goliath to the latter's David, and I am not at all sanguine on the prospect of health promotion finding a magic sling shot with which to slay the toxic elements of much of globalization's present trajectory. Nor do I think it should. Health promotion (and those who mobilize under its conceptual umbrella) is one small player amongst many others concerned with steering globalization towards a future-fairer. We can learn to play our role more effectively, but gauging that effectiveness (since this is a chapter on evidence) will never be easy or complete.

I close by returning to one of my opening qualifications of contemporary globalization: the crisis of climate change (to which might be appended the related crises of resource depletion). The apocryphal environmental tale is that of the Easter Islanders, whose ideological enslavement to a belief in the ancients led to the erection of huge stone monuments, whose movement required skids of timber which, as competition amongst the families for more and bigger monuments

---

[*] I will leave the health promotion strategy to *create supportive environments* for another time, partly for brevity and partly because I never understood its distinction from the others since such environments are created through community action, public policy or both.

accelerated, denuded the island of every last tree (Wright, 2004). No trees, no birds, no insects, no mammals, no fresh water, no food. And by the time the Europeans bumped into the island, almost no people. The tragedy is that they likely knew what would happen even as they cut the last tree. Just as we know what will likely happen as we continue to fish our oceans to extinction, eliminate our carbon sinks and biodiversity, contaminate our sources of fresh water, grow our supposedly healthy economies with a continued addiction to toxic fossil fuels, and blind ourselves to the consequences with an ideological enslavement to growth as the only marker of progress.

The challenges our global environmental crisis poses for health promoters are many, to say nothing of the social crises (mass migrations, resource conflicts) that are its unsettling wake. But the most disturbing implication may be that it forces us to confront the fundamental fallacy of our field: Promoting the physical and mental health of individuals whose well-being rests, in part, on economic and consumption practices that are today's equivalent of logging the last Easter Island tree is morally unacceptable and, from an intergenerational health vantage, indefensible. This is not simply a matter of evidence – effectiveness. It is fundamentally one of equity, ethics and survival.

References

Assunta, M. & Chapman, S. (2006). Health treaty dilution: a case study of Japan's influence on the language of the WHO Framework Convention on Tobacco Control. *J Epidemiol Community Health, 60*, 751–756.

Bates, I., Fenton, C., Gruber, J., Lalloo, D., Medina Lara, A., Squire, S. B. et al. (2004). Vulnerability to malaria, tuberculosis, and HIV/AIDS infection and disease. Part I: determinants operating at individual and household level. *Lancet Infectious Diseases, 4*, 267–277.

Boulle, J. & Avafia, T. (2005). *Treatment Action Campaign (TAC) Evaluation.*

Breman, A. & Shelton, C. (2001). *Structural Adjustment and Health: A literature review of the debate, its role-players and presented empirical evidence* (Rep. No. WG6: 6). WHO: Commission on Macroeconomics and Health.

BRIDGES (2002, April 9). Phillip Morris Looks to Chill Canadian Plans to Ban Descriptors on Cigarette Packages. *Bridges Weekly Trade News Digest, 6.*

Cobham, A. (2002). Capital account liberalization and poverty. *Global Social Policy, 2*, 163–188.

De Vogli, R. & Birbeck, G. L. (2005). Potential Impact of Adjustment Policies on Vulnerability of Women and Children to HIV/AIDS in Sub-Saharan Africa. *Journal of Health Population and Nutrition, 23*, 105–120.

Endresen, K. & von Kotze, A. (2005). Living while being alive: education and learning in the Treatment Action Campaign. *International Journal of Lifelong Education, 24*, 431–441.

Fidler, D. (2002). *Global Health Governance: Overview of the Role of International Law in Protecting and Promoting Global Public Health* (Rep. No. Discussion Paper No.3). WHO.

Friedman, S. & Mottiar, S. (2005). A rewarding engagement? The treatment action campaign and the politics of HIV/AIDS. *Politics & Society, 33*, 511–565.

Goldstone, J. A. (2003). Comparative Historical Analysis and Knowledge Accumulation in the Study of Revolutions. In J.Mahoney & D. Rueschemeyer (Eds.), *Comparative Historical Analysis in the Social Sciences* (pp. 41–90). Cambridge: Cambridge University Press.

Gyebi, J., Brykczynska, G., & Lister, G. (2002). *Globalisation: economics and women's health*. London: Partnership for Global Health.

Held, D. (2004). Globalisation: the dangers and the answers. Open Democracy; http://www.opendemocracy.net/globalization-vision_reflections/article_1918.jsp

International Union for Health Promotion and Education (2003). Model Legislation for Tobacco Control; http://fctc.org/modelguide/.

Labonte, R., Schrecker, T., & Sen Gupta, A. (2005). *Health for Some: Death, Disease and Disparity in a Globalized Era*. Toronto: Centre for Social Justice.

Labonte, R. (1998). *A Community Development Approach to Health Promotion*. Edinburgh: Health Education Board of Scotland/Research Unit in Health and Behaviour Change.

Labonte, R. (1991b). Principles for sustainable development decision-making. *Health Promotion International, 6*, 147–156.

Labonte, R. (1991a). Econology: integrating health and environment. *Health Promotion International, 6*, 49–65.

Labonte, R. & Laverack, G. (2001b). Capacity building in health promotion, Part 1: for whom? And for what purpose? *Critical Public Health, 11*, 111–127.

Labonte, R. & Laverack, G. (2001a). Capacity building in health promotion, Part 2: whose use? And with what measurement? *Critical Public Health, 11*, 129–138.

Labonte, R. & Sanger, M. (2006a). Glossary of the World Trade Organisation and public health: part 1. *J Epidemiol Community Health, 60*, 655–661.

Labonte, R. & Sanger, M. (2006b). Glossary on the World Trade Organisation and public health: part 2. *J Epidemiol Community Health, 60*, 738–744.

Labonte, R. & Torgerson, R. (2005). Interrogating globalization, health and development: Towards a comprehensive framework for research, policy and political action. *Critical Public Health, 15*, 157–179.

Lee, K. (2002). *Health Impacts of Globalization: Towards Global Governance*. London: Palgrave Macmillan.

Lister, J. (2005). *Driving the Wrong Way? A critical guide to the global "health reform" industry*. London: Middlesex University Press.

Marmot, M. (2000). Inequalities in health: causes and policy implications. In A.Tarlov & R. St.Peter (Eds.), *The Society and Population Health Reader, vol. 2: A State and Community Perspective* (pp. 293–309). New York: New Press.

Mertes, T. e. (2004). *A Movement of Movements: Is Another World Really Possible?* New York: Verso.

O'Brien, R. (2002). Organizational politics, multilateral economic organizations and social policy. *Global Social Policy, 2*, 141–162.

Schrecker, T. & Labonte, R. (2006). Globalization and social determinants of health: A diagnostic overview and agenda for innovation. In *World Institute for Development Economics conference on Advancing Health Equity*.

Tax Justice Network (2005). Briefing Paper – The Price of Offshore. Tax Justice Network, UK; http://www.taxjustice.net/cms/upload/pdf/Price_of_Offshore.pdf

UNAIDS (2006). *AIDS Epidemic Update: December 2006*. Geneva: UNAIDS and World Health Organization.

United Nations Department of Economic and Social Affairs (2006). *World Economic Situation and Prospects 2006*. New York: United Nations.

Utting, P., Hewitt de Alcántara, C., Bangura, Y., Mkandawire, T., Razavi, S., Westendorff, D. et al. (2000). *Visible Hands: Taking Responsibility for Social Development, an UNRISD report for Geneva 2000* Geneva, Switzerland: UNRISD.

Wallerstein, I. (2004). New Revolts Against the System. In T.Mertes (Ed.), *A Movement of Movements: Is Another World Really Possible?* (pp. 262–274). New York: Verso.

Woodward, D., Drager, N., Beaglehole, R., & Lipson, D. (2001). Globalization and health: a framework for analysis and action. *Bulletin of the World Health Organization, 79*, 875–881.

World Commission on the Social Dimensions of Globalization (2004). *A Fair Globalization: Creating Opportunities for All* Geneva: International Labor Organization.

World Health Organization (2005). The Bangkok Charter for Health Promotion. World Health Organization;
http://www.who.int/healthpromotion/conferences/6gchp/bangkok_charter/ en/index.html

World Health Organization (2006). *World Health Report 2006: Working Together for Health.* Geneva: WHO.

World Health Organization (1986). Ottawa Charter for Health Promotion;
http://www.who.dk/ policy/ottawa.htm

Wright, M. W. (2004). From Protests to Politics: Sex Work, Women's Worth, and Ciudad Juárez Modernity. *Annals of the Association of American Geographers, 94*, 369–386.

13
Urbanization and Health Promotion
Challenges and Opportunities

ANDREA NEIMAN[*] AND MARY HALL

Urban areas provide tremendous opportunity for economic, social, political and technological growth; they are also creating truly congested regions where high rates of poverty, inequality, and challenges to environmental and public health are far-reaching and affecting persons of all ages, gender and economic status. While infectious diseases remain a critical public health priority for parts of the world, (Moore, Gould & Keary, 2003; WHO, 2002) many countries are grappling with a "double disease burden" (Yach, Hawkes, Gould & Hofman, 2004) as rates of non-communicable disease (NCDs), (i.e. diabetes, cardiovascular disease, obesity) reach epidemic levels worldwide, accounting for more than half of the global burden of disease[†] in both developing and developed countries (Ezzati, Lopez, Rodgers & Murray, 2004). As the global population continues to become more urbanized, with almost half currently residing in urban centers, this unique transition has tremendous public health impact and, more importantly, offers tremendous opportunity. Indeed, the health and vitality of global urban areas holds the promise of influencing the future health and strength of the global community. Therefore, understanding the evidence to effectively address the needs of an increasing urban population, and an increasingly older population, is a global public health priority (WHO, 2002).

Defining Urban and Urbanization Concepts

The urban environment includes a dynamic interaction between a population and its growth, the system of governance and city management, as well as the natural environment or ecological system in which the built environment and urban area is developed and located. There are many different ways to define the urban. The critical issue is that the meaning of urban is one of constant redefinition. Like health

---

[*] The views and opinions in this chapter are those of the authors and do not necessarily reflect the views of the Centers for Disease Control and Prevention of the Department of Health and Human Services.

[†] Disability-Adjusted Life Years (DALYS) is the sum of years of potential life lost due to premature mortality and the years of productive life lost due to disability.

promotion, the urban studies field does not have any agreed upon definition of urban or urbanization. For example, the United Nations Department of Economic and Social Affairs, Population Division (2005), does not use the word "urban" in and of itself but uses the term "urban agglomerations," which it defines as comprising the city or town proper as well as the suburban fringe or thickly settled territory lying outside of, but adjacent to, the city boundaries. Others define the urban in terms of the population density, or the number of persons living in a proscribed area (UN, 2006); or alternatively, in terms of the geophysical boundaries for which governance is made that also provide services and facilities. Urbanization is seen by some as the social and physical process by which a country's population changes from primarily rural to urban or the expansion of a city or metropolitan area, namely the proportion of total population or area in urban localities or areas (cities and towns), or the increase of this proportion over time. Urbanization can thus represent a level of urban relative to the total population or area, or the rate at which the urban proportion is increasing (Satterthwaite, 2005). Both can be expressed in percentage terms, the rate of change as a percentage per year, decade or period between censuses (Wikipedia.com, 2006). Causation and by-products of this process are often offered as part of the definition. The World Bank describes urbanization as "the process by which a country's population changes from primarily rural to urban. It is caused by the migration of people from the countryside to the city in search of better jobs and living conditions" (World Bank, 2005). Nonetheless, it is quite clear to anyone perusing these following sources that a lively effort to describe the urban phenomena is taking place.

Beyond these and many other attempts at defining urban, a number of popular urban concepts are part and parcel of many discussions now taking place. For example there is debate about what is urban, suburban, exurban and rural. What may be considered by some as patently obvious is never so simple. In antiquity, and even in recent history, most urban areas were defined by a perimeter wall, often for protection and one knew when one was inside what was known as the city. Gradually these external walls were breached by development and generally seen as the "old" city. Even until the end of the 19th century most urban areas were dense and very circumscribed. Modern transportation, particularly the automobile, has drastically changed the shape and scope of the "city." While some ancient cities retain their dense core and original layout even today, most urban areas throughout the world now spread across wide areas, often making it impossible to tell where the urbanized area ends. Thus we are more likely to think of metropolitan urban areas today rather than "cities." Cities tend to be defined by political boundaries that do not relate well with the built up agglomeration or urbanized areas around them. Many major metropolitan areas today may have less than 10 percent of their population living in the named central city.

In a similar fashion "cities" have changed their overall structure considerably in the past century. Many metropolitan areas have diffuse "downtowns" or multiple "business" districts. The old pattern of political center, market center, religious center being at the heart or center is a disappearing idea, though many nostalgically search for the "city center" (Lang & LeFurgy, 2003). The pattern is further complicated by the emergence of "edge" cities and "edgeless" cities; these are patterns that particularly characterize the most recent urbanization patterns in advanced industrialized countries. For example, more and more offices and businesses once seen as belonging to a central business district are now spread throughout a metropolitan region. The impact of these new patterns is enormous and affects every function of the urban area's complexity and thus affects how health promotion interventions have to be framed.

As a result of these rapid changes, new concepts such as "urban sprawl" have emerged. Urban sprawl is an important issue and can potentially have tremendous health and economic impact (Sheehan, 2002). Urban sprawl is a complex pattern of land use and development that is typified by the spread-out, single-use nature of peripheral growth beyond traditional urban boundaries. There are many negative impacts on health and quality of life that sprawl is reported to affect and may potentially continue to impact in the future. It is reported to have many negative consequences on health and quality of life and may continue its negetive impact in the future (Ewing, Frank, & Kreutzer, 2006). In the various components of this chapter it will be seen that many health promoting and other interventions are dedicated to addressing the reputed deleterious effects of sprawl. At the other end of the urbanizing spectrum is the popular assertion that increasing density is a solution to many of the problems of sprawl and population growth.

Finally the whole area of urbanization cannot be separated from other large conceptual ideas, notably globalization. In the most obvious sense urbanization is one major outcome of globalization. It is a global phenomenon and is driven by major forces and trends in the global economy (please see Labonté chapter in this book). Urban areas have always been the centers of markets, trade and industry, thus it is hardly surprising that globalization is relevant to urbanization. Within the ongoing discussions of urbanization in this context, there is debate about the nature of urban areas in terms of their role as world cities, regional cities, local cities and their governance. Some researchers, economists, journalists and practitioners have reported that the contexts in which these urban areas continue to grow, develop and become interconnected for economic growth and development will continue to intensify and promote a "flat world" (Friedman, 2005). The demographic transformations related to these classifications affect greatly health consequences and the social determinants of health, as discussed elsewhere in this monograph (please see Metzler et al. chapter in this book). For our purposes, part of the urbanization concept is the further development of advanced, electronic based, financial and communication networks that put cities at the forefront of communicating health promoting messages and providing a platform from which the health of the population can be addressed.

Historical Context of Health in Urban Environments

Throughout history, cities have been sources of creativity, catalysts of change, innovation, and engines for economic growth and development. However, compared with their non-urban counterparts, urban populations have also been victims of the disproporticnate growth and spread of infectious disease, poverty, and inequality (Marsella, 1995; McMichael, 1999). From Imperial Rome's famous aqueducts (Frontinus, 1961) to London's heroic water sanitation efforts (Snow, 1855), public health shares a common history with the development and growth of urban areas and has been greatly affected by the policies and environmental interventions in the urban context (Pinkney, 1958; Mumford 1961).

Efforts to improve the urban environment were also happening in Paris, Chicago, and New York City. For example, Louis Napoleon and Baron Haussmann in the rebuilding of Paris in the 1850s and 1860s created great, wide boulevards, or "the sanitary street": the sewer was placed under the street which was, supported and skillfully engineered into what is termed as the "civilized street" (Griscom, 1845; Pikney, 1958; Kostof, 1991; Grob, 2002).

At the same time, demographers, anthropologists and sociologists were observing the dynamics of urban conditions and the affect on people's health and well-being. In London, Graunt (1662) carried out an analysis of the social distribution of mortality rates by sector of built-up areas. Virchow (1851) and Engels (1973) worked on social class and working conditions and illness rates. Durkheim (1897) in Paris, in the late 19th century, was interested in and studied social integration and suicide.

In these early efforts to intervene in the growth and development of the city, infrastructure preceded overstructure and housing (Fishman, 1993). The water systems improved, sewers were built, factory laws and housing were adopted, parks were created and it was implied that the health, well-being and prosperity of the urban population was linked to and affected by the land use and built environment. Healthy cities were envisioned to be utopias (Richardson, 1876; Fields, 1999). If one looks at the development of urban areas and the health of the populations that were a part of this pre-20th century history, the following common themes emerge: sanitation, education, housing, health care, infrastructure, public spaces. These all became part of the urban fabric as well as part of the public health legacy shaping urban areas and cities for centuries. In *The Death and Life of Great American Cities*, (1961) Jane Jacobs discusses the critical impact of the built environment on social, mental and physical health. Out of this heritage, one sees the charge of health promotion to ensure that the health of urban populations is protected and able to thrive. But prior to health promotion, however, it was the collective effort and insight of urban planning, land use development, zoning regulation, municipal leadership and rational thinking that established the way to accomplish prosperity and health. By the late 19th century, the death rate in cities dropped to rural levels or below (Fields, 1999).

Modern Urbanization – Western / Post-Industrialized Cities

The 20th century brought increased wealth and prosperity to more city centers as investments in public health infrastructure, education systems, housing, sanitation and waste management increased and became standardized throughout western societies.

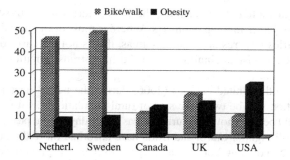

FIGURE 13.1. Trips walking or biking and obesity rates

Source: Compiled by Jacoby ER, 2004 and based on data from the Victoria Transport Institute, 2002; WHO, 2000.

This has led some to conclude that an urban advantage exists (Vlahov, Galea & Freudenberg, 2005; Marshall, 2004) when it comes to health (i.e., increased resources for health, education, social interaction). While this may be true, the problem of urban sprawl may have deleterious health impacts that, in many ways, balance out this view, including air pollution, automobile crashes, pedestrian injuries, water quantity and quality, sedentary lifestyles, mental health and social capital (Frumkin, 2002; Handy, 2005; Butterworth & Duhl, 2006). Putnam (2000) for example, found that for every ten minutes of commute time there is a 10 percent decrease in social capital. Ewing, Schmid, Killingsworth, Zlot and Raudenbush (2003) reported that people living in sprawling urban areas are more likely than people who live in more campact urban areas to walk less, weigh more and suffer from hypertension. And while these studies are mainly based on data in the United States, similar findings have also been seen globally (Martorell, Khan, Hughes, & Grummer-Strawn, 2000; Uauy, Albala, & Kain, 2001; Bell & Popkin, 2002; WHO, 2005). In places in which more integrated planning exists, meaning an integration of non-motorized transportation and public transit, rates of obesity are lower than those countries in which sprawl is much more of a phenomenon. (Figure 13.1) It is important, therefore, to learn what works in the context of promoting health, preventing disease and increasing sustainable development.

Modern Urbanization – Emerging Economies / Developing Countries

That urbanization represents a global challenge is unquestionable. One-half of the world's population, or 3 billion people, reside in urban areas compared to only about 2% in 1800 and 17% in 1950. (UN, 2006)

In sharp contrast to the 20th century, the 21st century will see most urbanization taking place in lower income countries. Whereas most of the population in high-income countries now resides in urban areas, this is not the case for low-income countries that are just beginning to see the huge transformation from rural to urban (Figure 13.2).

According to the United Nations (2006) during the next 3 decades the world's urban population will be twice the size of rural populations, as it is estimated that almost 180,000 people move into urban areas every day. In the past 25 years, mega cities, such as Bangkok, Cairo, and Lima have absorbed more than twice as many people as London or New York did at the peak of their growth at the end of the 19th century through the middle of the 20th century (Brockerhoff & Brennan, 1998). The pace of urbanization and the implications of national and local governments to plan and meet the needs of their growing population, given the relatively low level of available resources to adequately provide even the most minimal level of services, is unprecedented. As a result, new forms of urban poverty have emerged, seen in overcrowded, poor housing conditions, homelessness, limited access to (healthy) nutrition, urban crime and lack of basic services, such as clean water and sanitation. With the exception of South Asia and Sub-Saharan Africa, this rapid growth is expected to concentrate in burgeoning urban areas and towns of the Global South (i.e. Latin America, Asia, and Africa) (UN, 2006). The dire poverty that so sorely afflicted much of the rural developing world is now being transferred rapidly to urban setting. The implications of this transformation on health are great, and they are also present significant challenges to health promotion and public health.

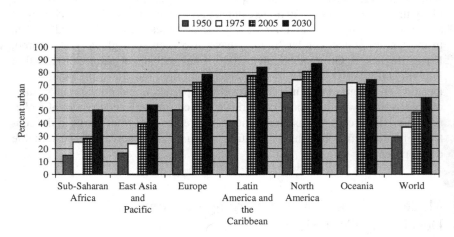

FIGURE 13.2. Percent of Global Urban Population: 1950–2030

Source: United Nations, Department of Economic and Social Affairs, Population Division (2006). World Urbanization Prospects: The 2005 Revision. Working Paper No. ESA/P/WP/200.

Certainly this great transformation has to be addressed by health promotion and effective health promotion interventions. Yet in this chapter we have given only limited attention to urbanization in the developing world. This is not because of a lack of concern, but rather the lack of significant research on this relatively new phenomenon in the developing world that prohibits the timely analysis that we could hope to carry out. Only recently (National Research Council, 2003) have scholars begun to carefully examine the urban transformation that is occurring in the developing world. Places like Jakarta, Indonesia, Shanghai, China, and Curitiba, Brazil provide interesting and important examples about common challenges faced in the rapidly urbanizing world. For example, in Curitiba, a model public transportation has been developed that accommodates and supports the mobility of more than one million people each year, while encouraging walking and cycling and reducing air pollution (Rabinovitch & Leitman, 1996). From urban areas in other countries, we have examples of interventions that adversely impact health. In China, the rates of vehicle-ownership are estimated to grow by about 12,000 additional cars per day. This tremendous shift from predominantly active transport (biking and public transit) to increased private, motorized transport has dramatically increased the rates of pedestrian accidents, air pollution, as well as seen a rise the rates of childhood and adult overweight and obesity (Bell & Popkin, 2002). Between 1995 and 2000, the number of motorized vehicles in Indonesia increased by almost 7 million with air pollution levels reported to be almost three times above the safe limits specified by the World Health Organization. Estimates indicate that air pollution costs the Indonesian economy at least $400 million (USD) every year, and is linked to the sixth leading cause of death in Indonesia (World Bank, 2003)

Because much of the information is empirical, one can find very little evaluation from a health perspective. Consequently the authors of this chapter felt that the major issues of urbanization in the developing world, particularly issues around interventions, are topics that need considerably more research and constitute an important topic for Volume II of this monograph. Nonetheless, the lessons of the industrialized world during the past 2 centuries of urbanization should not be lost in facing this new transformation in the developing world. The major challenges will clearly mirror those of the North and West in regard to health promotion: the environment (Hardoy, Mitlin, & Satterthwaite, 2001), governance (McCarney, Halfani, & Rodriquez, 1995), inequity (Davis, 2006), infrastructure (Lund, 2005), the economy, and the impact on health (Galea, Freudenberg & Vlahov, 2005).

Why this is Important in a Global Context

First, the health and quality of our cities will largely determine the health and quality of life for most people in the future. The increase in demand for finite resources, such as food, housing, fuel, water and health services, coupled with increases in motor vehicle crashes, pedestrian injuries, and mental health diagnoses, will have magnified their influence and vulnerability in global urban areas and mega cities. Furthermore, there is a high potential for impact if proper measures are taken to address the issues of rapid urbanization, modernization, and industrialization in countries with developing economies.

Second, while non-communicable disease have been most commonly associated with high-income societies, recent findings from the *World Health Report* demonstrate that the epidemic is indiscriminate and far-reaching (WHO, 2002). The risk factors and the chronic conditions associated with them, are now also increasingly dominant in developing countries. Finding best practices that may effectively address and prevent or delay these conditions is a public health priority.

Lastly, cities and mega cities are increasingly viewed as mechanisms of social and economic development. Herein lies the opportunity to provide innovative approaches to manage the demographic changes seen in societies; the mobilization, urbanization, the growing population; and burden of disease associated with these dramatic shifts.

Urbanization and the Challenge to Health Promotion

Urbanization is a dynamic process. Essentially it is the transformation of a given area of land from rural to non-rural over a period of time. In the first consideration, an area goes either from non-use by people or agricultural use to an area of settlement characterized by non-agricultural use. Urbanization is a global phenomenon that has been occurring since early civilizations. However in the past few centuries this phenomenon has increased in tempo and importance. In essence the world has shifted most rapidly in the past century from being largely rural in nature to being urban. The phenomenon continues and United Nations (2006) estimates that within the next 5 years, the majority of the global population will be predominantly urban. Some areas of the world, notably the country of Singapore, have reached a point of being totally urban; undoubtedly this is an exceptional case as many countries will always have a dedicated portion of population and land to agricultural and non-urban use. However, it is the dynamics of urbanization globally that presents the major challenge for interventions aimed at improving the health of urban populations. Thus, most health promoting inventions relate to addressing the changes in urban settings over time.

Many consider that the rapidly urbanizing world mainly presents a problem with what some term the "developing world". While the countries with emerging or developing economies have unique challenges posed from this phenomenon, nothing could be further from the truth. The problems of urbanization cut across socio-economic considerations. The major areas that are affected by and affect urbanization, (i.e. migration, suburbanization, changes in the role of government and globalization), all have a major impact on both countries with developing and developed economies (see chapter 12 in this book). The urbanization taking place in highly economically developed countries often has profound environmental impact such as, loss of green space, long commuting times, impact on water and energy systems and the financial stability of regional agricultural economies (McMichael, 2000). It is also quite obvious that health care infrastructure is heavily compromised by the phenomenon of urbanization (Burchell, Downs, McCann & Mukherji, 2005).

The complexity associated with urbanization is another key challenge for health promotion. Urban areas are a composite of complex systems such as to name a few: water and sewer management, refuse and waste handling, electric and gas power, transportation, medical care, education, communities, fire and police management. In addition, urban areas are centers of politics, culture, arts, education and the media. Indeed, it is always a marvel that huge metropolitan areas such as New York, London, Tokyo, Sao Paulo, Mexico City, Mumbai and Shanghai manage to function so extraordinarily well on a day by day basis. From a social determinants perspective urban areas are a laboratory for assessing the etiology and role of social determinants, on health and disease, as is discussed in Chapter 14 of this book.

Finally, urban areas are both containers of multiple "settings" and are in themselves "settings". All the classical settings-based interventions in health promotion-namely schools, workplaces, hospitals, and communities-are found in the urban context. Two important points to keep in mind are the following: First, urban settings, because of their sheer size, may have profound implications for health promotion interventions that encourage a settings approach. For example, schools may become very large or very specialized. Clearly there are profound differences between schools in small towns and rural areas from those in large metropolitan areas. Second, urban areas as a totality are a setting in and of themselves, thus being contextually unique. Even with relatively similar metropolitan populations, most would not consider Paris to be the same kind of setting as London, Tokyo the same as New York despite having similiar metropolitan populations.

Consequently, one sees that the broad concept of urbanization critically represents most of the areas of interest for health promotion practice. The challenge to health promotion is to work within this broad framework and make a difference on population health. Obviously, health promotion took on this challenge to some degree in the development of the Health Cities Programme (HCP) in the 1980s. This chapter discusses some of the work that has now been carried out globally for nearly three decades throughout the globe. Other fields have taken up the challenge and relate highly to the interests of health promotion. Movements such as New Urbanism and Smart Growth are examples of some of these efforts.

Health Promotion Relevant to Urbanism

Health promotion shares many common and classical interests associated with issues in the urban context. To begin with is the underlying concern with the built environment, which not only shapes the "look" of an urban area but also, and more importantly, defines communities both spatially and socially. Urban communities often refer to themselves by their location within a metropolitan area—for example, "east enders", "westsiders," "riverside,"— and "uptown." People living in the same geographic area often believe that they share common interests and values with regard to their city. The urban area may be seen as a collection or amalgamation of communities that share the general commonality of belonging to a larger metropolis. This idea is extended further in the way in which suburban areas of central cities define themselves as either belonging to a large metropolitan agglomeration or as being distinct geographic entities. Thus, the urban context as a critical idea in urban interventions resonates fully with the idea of contextualism in health promotion.

Policy and governance are key areas of health promotion work as discussed in the chapters by de Leeuw and Wise, Chapters 5 and 16 respectively. These broad ideas serve important roles in intervention activities pertaining to urbanization with regard to health promotion. In its early stages, WHO's Healthy Cities approach embraced the concept that interventions in cities should be conducted while maintaining a close connection with the system of governance (Butterworth & Duhl, 2006). Thus the mayor of a city was seen as a key partner in any Healthy Cities approach. Not only was the mayor important, but also the whole office of the mayor was seen as a way to show political involvement in the Healthy Cities project. In a later section of this Chapter space will be devoted to attempts to assess the healthy cities effort and frame those in terms of evidence of healthy cities as an intervention.

Finally, health promotion emphasizes certain principles and perspectives relating to efforts to improve the global impact of urbanization. In terms of principles, some people have argued that health promotion practice should be empowering, participatory, holistic, inter-sectoral and multidisciplinary (WHO/EURO, 1988). Certainly, many of these principles are shared by those active in addressing the issues of urbanization, in particular the ideas of multi-disciplinarity and inter-sectorality. With regards to health promotion perspectives the generalized idea of the importance of context resonates firmly with efforts of Smart Growth, New Urbanism and the Healthy Cities Programme. The idea of context is often discussed in terms of other important concepts such as lifestyle, life conduct, life conditions, life situations and life chances (Ruetten, 1995). For example, life chances deals with the structural-based probability of the correspondence of lifestyle (the collective pattern of life conduct) and life situation (the collective pattern of life conditions). Coincidentally, this quasi-Weberian sociological approach to analyzing context brings to play many theoretical issues related to health promotion practiced in the context of urbanization.

Intervention Concepts in Urbanization

Many health promoting interventions occur within urban areas; however, these are not necessarily interventions related to urbanization. Our concern in this chapter is to focus on interventions that are designed to address the broad concept of urbanization itself. Interventions that primarily focus on single topics, such as transportation, or communities, or schools, are not the concern here but we recognize the important contributions that these areas have on health and well-being.

With regard to urban intervention concepts there are several types, including urban renewal, New Urbanism, Smart Growth, Healthy Cities, Healthy Municipalities and Healthy Communities. We will focus on two that relate highly to health promotion and the general health of urban areas, namely Smart Growth and New Urbanism, followed by a more critical discussion of the urban intervention most associated with health promotion, namely Healthy Cities and its related interventions. One will note the similarities among these intervention approaches; however, there are subtle differences in their underlying strategies. The health promotion approach of Healthy Cities, Healthy Municipalities and Healthy Communities has, in general, used a social and political based strategy, addressing problems through government structures (e.g. mayors) and communities. Smart Growth has generally been concerned with the control of growth and may be seen as historically related to environmental issues. New Urbanism has been more concerned with the built environment and has a stronger legacy from urban planning and architecture. Of course, all of these intervention approaches share many common concerns - for example the concern with conservation, housing, density, transportation, zoning issues promoting active, healthy living.

Evidence, Effectiveness and Urbanization

Obviously, when it comes to judging the effectiveness of interventions in the urban context all the issues associated with evidence in health promotion come to bear. Three methodological aspects are critically highlighted. First, the design of an intervention approach is greatly challenged by urban interventions. Much has been written, both pro and con, about the applicability of the randomized-control trials (RCTs) to evidence research. With regard to interventions on urban areas or urbanization, it is difficult to imagine examples where RCTs would be either appropriate or feasible. One could, of course, imagine a broad community-based intervention taking place in a city, say Hamburg, Germany, but what city would be the "control" city? Could it be another German city such as Munich, or a city of somewhat similar size in a neighboring country, say Amsterdam or Lyon? However, the more one thinks about the many differences, both culturally and demographically, between say Hamburg and Lyon, the more one would question whether this would be a legitimate "control" city. Furthermore, the possibility of contamination would be ever present. For example, Lyon, upon discovering it was the "control" city might run a series of articles and commentaries in the local press. In any case, at best comparison type studies seem to be the only reasonable possibility, but even these are fraught with methodological challenges.

A second major methodological challenge is that of indicators. This topic is taken up in Chapter 18, Campostrini however it is not a new topic by any means. The search for indicators that could relate to urban areas has gone on for some time and has been pursued by health promoters as well as many others. Indeed a popular approach of the international press is to rate cities as "best" to live in, "best" to work in, "best" to visit and so forth. The ranking of cities globally, regionally and nationally by various indicators is a common practice. However, few of these indicators provide the kind of validity and reliability that serious researchers rely on for evidence. Earlier attempts to provide sound standardized indicators to assess the Health Cities Programme were deemed unsuccessful (Noack & McQueen, 1988) and O'Neill and Simard (2006) in their important paper on evaluation reject the idea of universal indicators for health cities.

Finally, both methodological challenges and opportunities lie in the future use of social and behavioral monitoring systems to assess the dynamics of change in urban areas. The opportunity, of course, is the possibility to see into the effects of broad health promoting interventions in their dynamic setting. As outlined by Campostrini in Chapter 18, surveillance offers the possibility to assess effectiveness of programs and interventions over time. Such applications of surveillance data tied to urbanization have started with the Smart Behavioral Risk Factor surveillance system (BRFSS) in the United States. The fruits of this approach are just beginning to appear, but offer many interesting possibilities (Centers for Disease Control and Prevention, 2006).

Some Major Interventions

Researchers, practitioners, and both governmental and non-governmental organizations have long been interested and involved in efforts to address the unique social, political, economic and health challenges of concentrated urban populations. Often times, these efforts are seen as networks of people with a common purpose however, critical and careful evaluation of these efforts has been lacking or not well-documented; even less has been discussed regarding the effectiveness of these efforts, particularly with regard to health promotion.

These movements or interventions come under many banners: New Urbanism (NU), Traditional Neighborhood Development (TND), Transit Oriented Development (TOD), Smart Growth, and Adaptive Re-use are most often tools for new development but as Landis, Deng & Reily write (2002) " . . . growth is like toothpaste. Squeezed out of one location, it must go somewhere else." Fundamentally, all of these efforts are broadly trying to make more efficient, sustainable use of the (limited) urban space and address the continued growth.

Multiple reasons exist as to why many of these initiatives have taken root. Increased car dependency, longer commute times and increased traffic injuries and fatalities which are considered to be some of the results of urban sprawl have encouraged discussions that focus on efforts to reduce these trends and the high levels of resource consumption associated with them. A changing market demand for community diversity and widening of personal choices in lifestyle, travel and vocational options and preferences have also encouraged new development patterns that focus on the community, increase quality of life, and social capital

(Handy, 2005; Centre for Transit-Oriented Development and the Centre for Neighborhood Technology, 2006); something that is a challenge in more diffuse communities (Putnam, 2000). Most recently, active living and health concerns have become integrated aspects of urban planning and development, and transportation (Handy, 2005). In all cases, there is a renewed interest to address the growing issue of urban sprawl and the increased rates of chronic disease and to promote environmental sustainability and stewardship; evidence of effectiveness, however, has yet to substantiate some of these approaches to mitigate and prevent some of the adverse affects.

Smart Growth is a Western-based conceptual idea in urban design, community and transportation planning used to encourage policies that revitalize neighborhoods and promote economic development while balancing and preserving the natural environment. Smart Growth promotes land use patterns that are compact, transit-oriented, walkable, bicycle-friendly, and include mixed-use development with a range of housing choices (Handy, 2005; SmartGrowth.com, 2007) and are based upon 10 principles that address the community in 7 broad "issue" areas. This philosophy keeps density concentrated in the center of a town or city, combating urban sprawl. It is a conceptual idea in urbanism arising largely from what some people have termed a "vicious cycle" in urban planning. Cervero (2006) discusses the need to improve and alter the so-called "vicious cycle" in which urban planning and urban development have been caught during the last four to five decades. Urban sprawl begets high levels of road investment and car dependence, which gives rise to pollution, increased sedentary living, increased premature morbidity and mortality, thus continually fueling the cycle. In contrast to the so-called vicious cycle, there is a discussion to promote a more "virtuous cycle". A virtuous cycle would create a different form, more walkable, mixed-use neighborhoods, which would induce higher transit use, and encourage more active living. Experiences demonstrate that increased demand results in increased investment; a more virtuous cycle provides more transportation options to the private car, potentially giving rise to increased demand for transit which also encourages mixed-use development, creates more affordable housing options and thus creating a market, which, on its own, sustains a more virtuous cycle (Cervero, 2006), as illustrated in Figure 13.3.

New Urbanism was introduced in 1998 as a "design philosophy that focuses development in compact, pedestrian-oriented town centers, and often looks to historic towns and urban areas for inspiration" which emphasizes the multi-layered approach at regional, city and street level (SmartGrowth.com, 2007). Many New Urbanist designs include features that characterize urban areas in the pre-automobile age, such as mixed land use and walkability. This is sometimes recognized as traditional neighborhood design or transit-oriented design (TOD).

Some common elements of New Urbanism design and Smart Growth are parallel to what may be seen as health promotion, although not labeled as such. Architects, urban planners, legislators and community developers promoting the New Urbanism and Smart Growth principles seek to create neighborhoods that are walkable, diverse, affordable and well-connected, thereby creating a sense of

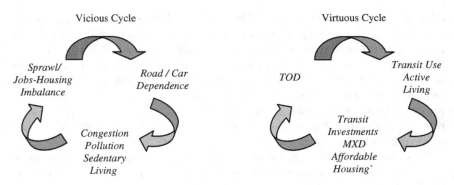

FIGURE 13.3. Breaking out of the Vicious Cycle Smart Growth: Transit-Oriented Development

Source: Cervero, R. presentation at International Union for Health Promotion and Education Meeting: Urbanization and Health Promotion, Atlanta, GA August 16–17, 2006

community while increasing social capital and promoting collective social interaction as well as integration and economic development. While mostly focusing upon a more micro-environment of the neighborhood scale, New Urbanists encourage and support regional efforts for open space, balanced development of jobs, housing and planning. They believe these strategies are the best ways to reduce the time that people spend in traffic, increase the supply of affordable housing, and temper urban sprawl.

What is the State of our Current Knowledge about Evidence and Effectiveness of New Urbanism and Smart Growth as it Relates to Health?

Within New Urbanism and Smart Growth thus far, most of the evaluation is based on the success in the marketplace or evaluation from discrete perspectives (i.e. impact on energy consumption, congestion, land value, or policy implementation) (Handy, 2005; Talen, 2006a). For example there are over 600 towns, villages, and neighborhoods in the US that have incorporated the New Urbanism and Smart Growth principles. Metropolitan regions are looking to the principles of New Urbanism and Smart Growth to link transportation and land-use policies, while using the neighborhood, and community, as the fundamental building block of a region (Landis et al., 2002). Some promising case studies have been conducted; however, many of the principles, such as affordability and diversity, are matters that have yet to be shown as being effective (Center for Transit-Oriented Development and the Centre for Neighborhood Technology, 2006). In fact, this point seems to be one of the major criticisms of New Urbanism (Talen, 2006b). However, the significance of both of these movements' ambitions

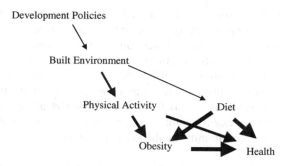

FIGURE 13.4. Causal Pathways (showing level of research)

Source: Ewing, R (2006) presentation at International Union for Health Promotion and Education Meeting: Urbanization and Health Promotion, Atlanta, GA August 16–17, 2006

in terms of public health may be the shift from instituting change at the scale of the single project to instituting change more systemically, both at the scale of regional transportation and ecosystems and in terms of legal regulations and codes. While yet to be seen, this shift appears to be the direction and hope for the future (Handy, 2005).

Many gaps remain in our knowledge on the evidence and effectiveness of these urban interventions as they relate to health and this may be due to methodological, definitional, and sector-specific constraints of studies in the urban context. Ewing, Frank, and Kreutzer (2006) outline challenges and provide a summation on the state of knowledge in specific areas as it relates to urban growth management, Smart Growth principles, and health outcomes (Figure 13.4) The width of the arrows in Figure 13.4 demonstrates how much literature and evaluation exist, with the lighter arrows showing areas in need of further inquiry. There are limited or no conclusive data (Turbov & Pitvin, 2005) available on the social, mental, and physical benefits to health as a result of Smart Growth and New Urbanism. The dilemma is that the pursuit of evidence is approached from distinct sector perspectives, thus making the analysis of health impact studies limited. For example, transportation engineers analyze safety and congestion-relief benefits, but to properly evaluate societal benefits, there needs to be some way to conduct a comprehensive accounting of cost versus benefits, which is a difficult task. Using tools such as health impact assessment (Dannenberg et al., 2006), which approaches evaluation from a much broader perspective, will enable more comprehensive understanding of the health, social, and economic impact of New Urbanism and Smart Growth.

An additional challenge in understanding the effectiveness of New Urbanism and Smart Growth on health and health promotion is that *The Charter for the New Urbanism* and information on Smart Growth are seen to be more principle than action oriented (SmartGrowth.com, 2007; CongressforNewUrbanism.com, 2007) therefore, implementing them might pose challenges. While both movements acknowledge the connection between community environments and quality of life, as well as promote policies and practices that can lead to improvements in community well-being, subtle differences exist in terms of effectiveness from a public health standpoint. The primary difference is the unit of analysis used: for Smart Growth or New Urbanism, it is the idea of physical place or the environment *per se*, whereas in public health, the impacts of individual and community health as a result of the environment are the variables of interest.

This is a subtle but important distinction and can be further explored using the principles outlined for Smart Growth and in *the charter for New Urbanism* to the seminal health promotion charters-namely, the Ottawa Charter for Health Promotion (1986) and the recent Bangkok Charter for Health Promotion in a Globalized World (WHO, 2005). Many similarities exist regarding the overarching principles of these documents; however, the Bangkok Charter was developed in conjunction with strategies, actions, commitments and signed pledges representing a consensus of experts in multiple sectors, from international, national and local health agencies. Furthermore, an important aspect of the Health Promotion Charters emphasizes the need to have cooperation and collaboration between multiple sectors, including but not limited to: local and national governments, non-governmental organizations, civic associations, private sector, and public health. Indeed, the importance of political support to promote sustained action, together with broad civic participation is seen as paramount in promoting health and well-being and is outlined in 5 principles of actions in the Bangkok Charter: 1) advocacy for health based on human rights; 2) investment in sustainable policies, actions and infrastructure to address the determinants of health; 3) build capacity for policy development, leadership, knowledge dissemination and research; 4) regulation and legislation to ensure equal opportunity for health and well-being of all people; and 5) partnerships with public, private, non-governmental organizations (NGOs) and international organization to create sustainable action. The primary components of the Ottawa Charter that proposed health promotion action were to build health public policy, create supportive environments, strengthen community actions, develop personal skills, and reorient health services.

New Urbanism and Smart Growth show encouraging signs of a healthier, balanced development through implementation of local governance, public policy, and increased community involvement. Yet we have limited evidence that this type of development philosophy impacts positively on social, environmental, mental and physical health. Moreover, in a global context, some of these principles may be viewed as universally adaptable, meaning that there are limited examples from countries and cities with emerging and developing economies.

Healthy Cities Programme

Healthy Cities Programme (HCP) is a long-term development program that places health on the agenda of cities around the world, and builds a constituency of support for public health at the local level (Tsouros, 1995). Recognizing that social, physical and mental health are affected by and a result of how our environments are built, it is necessary then to promote public policies that support and promote healthy, sustainable places to live, work and play. The initiative is based upon the principles outlined in the Ottawa Charter for Health Promotion (1986) whose goal is to improve those physical and social environments and expand those community resources which enable people to mutually support each other in performing all the functions of life and in developing to their maximum potential (Hancock & Duhl, 1988; Kickbusch, 1989; de Leeuw, Abbema & Commers, 1998).

Healthy Cities promotes the development of comprehensive healthy public policies at the local level to address the physical, social, environmental, and mental well-being of communities. With over 7,000 communities involved, some have argued that it is not a program but a process (Duhl, 2006). The reason for this argument is due to the unique nature of each program, meaning that there are no two quite the same. The goal however, is the same: ensuring quality of life and improving conditions of housing, education, recreation, and the physical environment.

HCP is also a process that involves the participation of many people in many different settings in order to bring unique and non-traditional community members to local partnerships. It is through public policy and services that the Healthy Cities process holds the promise of being able to address these imperatives of public health. That is to say, a clean and safe physical environment; an ecosystem which is stable now and sustainable in the long run; a strong, mutually supportive and non-exploitative community; a high degree of participation and control by the public over the decisions that affect their lives and their well-being; the meeting of basic needs, like food water, shelter, income, safety, and work for all the people; and the access to a variety of experiences and resources with a chance for a wide variety of contact, interaction, and communication; a diverse, innovative city economy (Duhl, 2006). Overall, major themes that the HCP promotes are participation, a systemic approach, and equity.

Growing out of the Healthy Cities movement, the Healthy Municipalities and Communities (HMC) approach has burgeoned largely across Latin America and the Caribbean. Similar to Healthy Cities, the HMC movement strives to place health promotion at the highest level of the political agenda by building support through political structures. A public declaration of commitment to HMC by local government is considered a key feature in gaining political support for health at the highest levels. Multi-sectoriality, participation and empowerment are key health promotion features, and are often main targets for evaluation.

What is the State of our Current Knowledge about Evidence and Effectiveness of Healthy Cities, Healthy Municipalities and Healthy Communities?

The HCP is a comprehensive approach to promoting health in urban areas that embraces the political, social, environmental, physical and mental health of the community. This strength, at times serves as a challenge when attempts are made to evaluate the direct health impact of the HC program or policy. Healthy Cities Programmes are not amenable to conventional epidemiologic techniques, often posing a challenge in the evaluation itself, as the application of reliable and valid methods, agreed upon indicators, scales and uniform approaches are seen as some of the major obstacles (de Leeuw & Skovgarrd, 2005). Moreover, the outcomes of many HCPs are based upon independent efforts of municipal leaders, community groups, as well as emerging new actors that provide a dynamic approach but also focus on specific outcomes desired.

For example, de Leeuw (2001) assessed the (healthy public) policies that were developed within the context of Healthy Cities in the EU and found that social entrepreneurship in the context of the policy change model adopted by participating cities was seen to influence the local policy agendas. Donchin, Shemesu, Horowity & Daoud (2006) conducted an evaluation to address the level of implementation and the process of development of Healthy Cities in Israel. And in Curitiba, Moysés et al. (2006) found that the Healthy Cities Programme policies are significantly more effective in the prevention of dental trauma. Healthy Cities has created increased awareness of the need to collaborate and encourage decision makers and non-traditional partners to incorporate language and efforts in healthy public policies. (de Leeuw, 2001).

An examination of the Healthy Cities experience in developing countries revealed much about their similarities to those in developed countries, as well as highlighted the challenges to producing generalizable evidence from such a framework. In examining the experiences of four WHO-funded HCPs in developing countries, Harpham, Burton & Blue (2001) found little evidence of municipal policy change, not unlike earlier experiences in Europe. Also similar to the European experience, the development of the municipal health plan, a key feature of HCPs, was not completed in most of the developing countries evaluated. Authors cited limited capacity for assessment, limited stakeholder participation, and reluctance of non-health sectors to integrate the HC goals, experiences similar to those in developed countries. As has been described earlier, the complex and variable (top-down vs. bottom up, for example) nature of the policy making process makes HC difficult to evaluate (Curtice, Springett & Kennedy, 2001) It is a dynamic process with multiple actors with varying power and varying concerns. Though the ultimate outcome of policy change may be easier to assess, evidence regarding elements that lead to success or failure to change policy does not yet exist. This phenomenon may be even more complex in rapidly urbanizing areas, where sectors are constantly changing and consequent turnover in key personnel makes sustainable policy change even more challenging.

The evaluation of processes and the documentation of strategies, structures and experience are important for providing an evidence base, but thus far, has accomplished little to demonstrate the evidence of HCP's effectiveness. At the local and international level, the Healthy Cities Programme has limited information uniformly available of the progress thus making it difficult to discern what is being done and how best to evaluate these efforts. Though there are scattered attempts to do so, there is no universal repository of information regarding all, or even a cross-section of experiences, making it difficult to determine the scope of activity taking place, and even less so, to determine the extent of success. De Leeuw & Skovgaard (2005) states that, "after 20 years of the HCP there is very little evidence that in substantial ways, makes a difference when dealing with urban health." However, they continue to state that there is "evidence" that Healthy Cities works ... but the evidence is fraught with mainly three overarching issues: 1) Evidence – How is a healthy city defined? How is the evidence generated? What are the outcomes measured and for what purpose? 2) If one is assessing the original intent of the HCP, meaning building political support to place health and health promotion on the political agenda, then perhaps one can conclude the program to be a success. The limitation being that the programs grew too fast and thus limited the parameters to explore the success of the different elements of the concept. Thus, this has left the HCP as a program characterized by more action than reflection for it has also moved from being a specific approach to public health to an integrated approach to urban management (De Leeuw & Skovgaard, 2005). 3) Somewhat similar to the evidence question is that HCP are not easily framed in theoretical or methodological terms. Broad-based efforts in health promotion yield more effects and sustainable effects on a variety of health indicators rather than a definitive conclusion from a more limited focus, (i.e. positive health, improved beliefs and attitudes regarding health, increased capacity for health promotion, and increased capacity for policy-making to improve health).

Political support appears to be the one of the defining elements for having a sustained and promoted the HCP since its inception. With evidence available, although limited in quantitative research, it appears that the HCP has gained wide appeal and acceptance among diverse community and civic leaders in cities and towns throughout the world. One may conclude that there appears to be an enlightened perspective that the HCP works; from a problem-solving perspective, it is more difficult to ascertain the evidence for decision-making in urban health. Despite local and international examples of practice-based approaches to HCP available, there is limited information uniformly available of the progress thus making it difficult to both discern what is being done and how best to evaluate these efforts, and to quantify the direct health impact of these efforts difficult, if not impossible (Baum, 1998).

In Closing

We have examined much of the available evidence of effectiveness related to health promoting intervention efforts in an urbanizing world. We have outlined the historical context and advances that have resulted in effective health promotion in the urban context. In addition we have identified some of the recent approaches to address emerging and increasingly complex issues in the rapidly expanding urban environments globally. With regard to health promotion and urbanization we need more interventions based on the best theory of practice and we need comprehensive and systematic reviews that account for urban change efforts, particularly in countries with emerging economies. Most of the available knowledge base that we have is based on Western literature from the most economically developed, high-income countries.

Despite urbanization being a key area of challenge for health promotion interventions, we conclude that there is insufficient evidence at this time to make any solid recommendations to the health promotion community. It seems to be too early to provide the practicing health promoter interested in cities a comprehensive list of what is best practice. Having said that, it is clear that health promotion will continue to work in this area and provide, on a case-by-case basis, many sound examples of how to approach the generic problems of urbanization. The city as a concept along with its urbanized region remains a key setting for health promotion action. It is also clear that many other groups concerned with urbanization share many of the core values, principles and concepts of health promotion and that the development of closer partnerships with these groups will undoubtedly yield better, and hopefully, more effective practice.

Acknowledgments. The authors would like to recognize the valuable contributions of the participants who presented and participated in an expert meeting on Urbanization and the Effectiveness of Networks in Health Promotion. Participants included: Lauretta Anash, Robert Cervero, Leonard Duhl, Ellen Dunham-Jones, Linnea Evans, Reid Ewing, Robert Fishman, Mary Hall, Enrique Jacoby, Catherine Jones, David McQueen, and Andrea Neiman. This discussion meeting on evidence and effectiveness related to the Global Programme on Health Promotion and Education (GPHPE) was held on August 16–17, 2006 and resulted in a base of presentations and dialogue to provide insights for this chapter.

In addition, there are two individuals who provided tremendous support and guidance with the development and completion of this chapter and the authors are most appreciative: Catherine Jones for helping to organize and participate in the initial meeting in August 2006, and Linnea Evans for her significant contribution to helping complete the chapter. The authors are most grateful for their essential advice and assistance.

References

Baum, F. (1998) Measuring effectiveness in community-based health promotion. In Davies, J. and Macdonald, G. (Eds.), *Quality, Evidence, and Effectiveness in Health Promotion: Striving for Certainties*, Chapter 4. Routledge, London, UK, pp. 68–91.

Bell, K. & Popkin, B. (2002). The Road to Obesity or the Path to Preservation: Motorized Transportation and Obesity in China. *Obesity Research.* 10 (4):277–83.

Brockerhoff, M. & Brennan, E. (1998). The Poverty of Cities Developing Regions. *Population and Development Review*, 24,1:75–114.

Burchell, R., Downs, A., McCann, B., Mukherji, S. (2005). Sprawl Costs; Economic Impacts of Unchecked Development. Washington: Island Press.

Butterworth, I. & Duhl, L. (2006) Healthy cities and the built environment: Documenting program impacts on psychological conceptions of place and community. (*In press*).

Curtice, L., Springett, J. & Kennedy, A. (2001). 14. Evaluation in urban settings: the challenge of Healthy Cities. In I. Rootman & M. Goodstadt & B. Hyndman & D. V. McQueen & L. Potvin & J. Springett & E. Ziglio (Eds.), *Evaluation in Health Promotion: Principles and Perspectives* (pp. 309–334). Denmark: World Health Organization.

Center for Transit-Oriented Development and the Center for Neighborhood Technology (2006). The Affordability Index. A New Tool for Measuring the True Affordability of a Housing Choice. The Brookings Institution, Urban Markets Initiative, Market Innovation Brief. Brookings Metropolitan Policy Program. Washington, DC. (http://www.brookings.edu/metro/umi/20060127_affindex.pdf) Accessed on March 16, 2007).

Centers for Disease Control and Prevention, BRFSS, (2006). Available at: http://apps.nccd.cdc.gov/brfss-smart/index.asp, Accessed on December 28, 2006).

Cervero, R. & Gorham, R. (1995). Commuting in transit versus automobile neighbor-hoods. *Journal of the American Planning Association*, 61, 210–225.

Cervero, R. (2006). *Urbanization*. Unpublished material presented at *Urbanization and Effectiveness of Networks in Health Promotion* meeting hosted by the International Union for Health Promotion and Education, August 16-17, 2006 in Atlanta, GA.

Congress for the New Urbanism, 2007. Charter of the New Urbanism. http://www.cnu.org/sites/files/Charter.pdf (Accessed on March 16, 2007)

Dannenberg AL, Bhatia R, Cole BL, Dora C, Fielding JE, Kraft K, McClymont-Peace D, Mindell J, Onyekere C, Roberts JA, Ross CL, Rutt CD, Scott-Samuel A, Tilson HH. (2006). Growing the Field of Health Impact Assessment in the United States: An Agenda for Research and Practice *American Journal of Public Health*. 96(2): 262–270.

Davis, M. (2006). Planet of Slums *New Perspectives Quarterly*, 23(2): 6–11.

De Leeuw, E., Abbema E. & Commers M. (1998). *Healthy Cities Policy Evaluation – Final Report*. Maastricht / EU DG V, Luxembourg: WHO Collaborating Centre for Research on Healthy Cities.

De Leeuw, E. (2001). Global and local (global) health: the WHO Healthy Cities Programme. *Global Change and Human Health*, 2(1): 34–53.

De Leeuw, E. & Skovgaard, T. (2005). Utility-driven evidence for healthy cities: Problems with evidence generation and application. *Social Science & Medicine*. 61, 1331–1341.

Donchin, M., Shemesh, AA., Horowitz, P., Daoud, N. (2006). Implementation of the Healthy Cities' principles and strategies: an evaluation of the Israel Healthy Cities Network. *Health Promot Int*. 21(4): 266–273.

Duhl, L. (2006). *Urbanization*. Unpublished material presented at *Urbanization and Effectiveness of Networks in Health Promotion* meeting hosted by the International Union for Health Promotion and Education, August 16-17, 2006 in Atlanta, GA.

Durkheim, E. (1897) *Suicide: A study in sociology* (JA Spaulding & G. Simpson, Trans.) – Glencoe, IL: Free Press.(Original work published 1897) 1951.

Engels, F. (1973). The condition of the working class in England in 1844. Moscow: Progress Publishers.

Ewing, R., Frank, L. & Kreutzer, R. (2006). Understanding the Relationship between Public Health and the Built Environment, a report prepared by Design, Community & Environment. A Report to the LEED-ND Committee.

Ewing, R., Schmid, T., Killingsworth, R., Zlot, A., Raudenbush, S. (2003). Relationship between Urban Sprawl and Physical Activity, Obesity, and Morbidity. *American Journal of Health Promotion*, September/October. 18(1): 47–57.

Ezzati, M., Lopez, A. D., Rodgers, A., & Murray, C. J. L. (2004). Comparative quantification of health risks: global and regional burden of disease attributable to selected major risk factors. World Health Organization: Geneva, Switzerland.

Fields, G. (1999). City systems, urban history, and economic modernity: Urbanization and the Transition from Agrarian to Industrial Society. *Berkeley Planning Journal*, 13, 102–128.

Fishman, R. (1993). The Decline of Megalopolis as a Cultural Center. In T. Barker & A. Sutcliffe, (Eds.), *Megalopolis: The Giant City in History*. London: Macmillan.

Friedman, T. (2005) *The World Is Flat: A Brief History of the Twenty-first Century*. New York NY: Farrar, Straus, Reese, and Giroux.

Frontinus, SJ. (trans. Charles Bennett). (1961). Stratagems and the Aqueducts of Rome. Cambridge, Massachusetts: Harvard University Press.

Frank, LD., (2000). Land use and transportation interaction: Implications on public health and quality of life. *Journal of Planning Education and Research*, 20, 6–22. (Review Article)

Frumkin, H. (2002). Urban sprawl and public health. *Public Health Rep*. 117, 201–217.

Galea, S., Freudenberg, N. & Vlahov, D., (2005). Cities and population health. *Soc Sci Med*. 60, 1017–1033.

Graunt, J. (1662). Natural and Political Observations made upon the Bills of Mortality. London, UK: Martyn.

Griscom, J. (1845). Sanitary condition of the laboring population of New York. New York: Harper & Brothers.

Grob, GN. (2002). The deadly truth: a history of disease in America. Cambridge: Harvard University Press.

Jacobs, J. (1961). *The Death and Life of Great American Cities*, New York: Random House.

Hancock, T. & Duhl, L. (1988). Promoting Health in the Urban Context. WHO Healthy Cities Paper No. 1 Copenhagen: FADL. 55.

Handy, S. (2005). Smart Growth and the transportation-land use connection: what does the research tell us? *International Regional Science Review* 28(2): 146–167.

Hardoy, J.E., Mitlin, D. & Satterthwaite, D. (2001) Emvironmental Problems in an Urbanizing World. London: Earthscan.

Harpham, T., Burton, S. & Blue, I. (2001). Healthy city projects in developing countries: the first evaluation. *Health Promotion International*. 16(2): 111–125.

Kickbusch, I. (1989). Healthy cities: a working project and a growing movement. *Health Promot*. 4, 77–82.

Kosof, S. (1991). *The City Shaped. Urban Patterns and Meanings Through History*. Bullfinch Press, London: Thames and Hudson Ltd.

Landis, J. D., Deng, L. & Reilly, M., (2002). Growth Management Revisited: A Reassessment of its Efficacy, Price Effects and Impacts on Metropolitan Growth Patterns. Working Paper 2002–02. University of California: Institute of Urban and Regional Development.

Lang, R & LeFurgy, J. (2003). Edgeless Cities: Examining the Noncentered Metropolis. *Housing Policy Debate* 14:3; 427–460.

Lund, V.K. (2005). The healthy communities movement: Bridging the gap between urban planning and public health.
http://www.design.asu.edu/apa/proceedings99/LUND/LUND.HTM (Accessed on March 16, 2007).

Marsella, AJ. (1995). Urbanization, mental health and psychosocial well-being: some historical perspectives and considerations. In: T. Harpham & I. Blue (Eds.), *Urbanization and mental health in developing countries* (pp. 3–14). Aldershot: Avebury.

Marshall, SJ. (2004). Developing countries face double burden of disease. *Bull World Health Organ*; 82(7): 556.

Martorell, R., Khan, L. K., Hughes, M. L., Grummer-Strawn, L. M. (2000). Obesity in women from developing countries. *Eur. J. Clin. Nutr.* 54, 247–252.

McCarney, P., Halfani, M.& Rodriquez, A. (1995) "Towards an understanding of governance: the emergence of an idea and its implications for urban research in developing countries," In, R. Stren & J. Bell (Eds.), *Urban Research in the Developing World. (Vol.4). Perspectives on the City*, (pp 91–141). Toronto: Centre for Urban and Community Studies, University of Toronto.

McMichael, AJ. (1999). Urbanisation and urbanism in industrialised nations, 1850-present: implications for health. In LM. Schell & SJ. Ulijaszek (Eds.), *Urbanism, health, and human biology in industrialised countries* (pp. 21–45). Cambridge: Cambridge University Press.

McMichael, AJ. (2000). The urban environment and health in a world of increasing globalization: issues for developing countries. *Bull World Health Organ*; 78(9), 117–126.

McQueen, D.V. and Noack, H. (1988) Health promotion indicators: current status, issues and problems. *Health Promotion*. An International Journal, 3(1): 117–125.

Moore, M., Gould, P. & Keary, BS. (2003). Global urbanization and impact on health. *Int J Hyg Environ Health*. Aug:206;4–5, 269–78.

Moysés S.J., Moysés ST., McCarthy M., Sheiham A. (2006). Intra-urban differentials in child dental trauma in relation to Healthy Cities policies in Curitiba, Brazil. *Health Place*. 12:48–64.

Mumford, L. (1961). The City in History: Its Origins, Its Transformations, and Its Prospects. A Harvest Book, Harcourt, Inc. New York, NY.

National Research Council. (2003). *Cities Transformed: Demographic Change and its Implications in the Developing World*. Washington: The national Academies Press.

Noack, H., & McQueen, D.V. (1988) "Towards health promotion indicators," *Health Promotion*, 3(1): 73–78.

O'Neill, M & Simard, P. (2006). Choosing indicators to evaluate Health Cities projects: a political task. *Health Promotion Intenational*, 21(2): 145–152.

Ottawa Charter for Health Promotion (1986). Available at:
http://www.who.int/hpr/NPH/does/ottawa_charter_hp.pdf Accessed on April 25, 2007.

Pinkney, DH. (1958). *Napoleon III and the Rebuilding of Paris*. Princeton, NJ: Princeton University Press.

Putnam R.D. (2000). *Bowling Alone: The Collapse and Revival of American Community* New York: Simon & Schuster.

Rabinovitch, J. & Leitman, J. (1996). Urban Planning in Curitiba. *Sci. Am.*, 274(46): 53.

Richardson, B.W. (1876). Modern Sanitary Science – A City of Health *Van Nostrand's Eclectic Engineering Magazine* 14: January:31-42. Reprinted from *Nature* 12 (October 14, 1875):523-25 and (October 21, 1875):542–545.

Ruetten, A. (1995) The implementation of health promotion: a structural perspective. *Social Science and Medicine*, 41(2): 1627–1637.

Satterthwaite, D. (2005). The scale of urban change worldwide 1950–2000 and its underpinnings. Available at http://www.iied.org/urban/Urban_Change.html (accessed November, 2006)

Sheehan, M. (2002). What Will It Take To Halt Sprawl? Washington, DC: World Watch Institute. http://www.worldwatch.org/pubs/download/EP151A/ (Accessed on March 16, 2007).

SmartGrowth.com, (2007). About Smart Growth. http://www.smartgrowth.org/Default.asp?res=1024 Accessed on March 16, 2007.

Snow, J. *On The Mode Of Communication Of Cholera.* London: Churchill, 1855. Reprinted in Frost WH (ed.). *Snow on Cholera.* New York: The Commonwealth Fund, 1936.

Talen, E. (2006a). New Urbanism and American Planning: the Conflict of Cultures (Routledge, 2006)

Talen, E. (2006b). Design for Diversity: Evaluating the Context of Socially Mixed Neighborhoods, *Journal of Urban Design* 11(1): 1–32.

Tsouros, A.D. (1995). The WHO Healthy Cities Project: State of the art and future plans. *Health Promotion International*, 10, 133–141.

Turbov, M. & Piper, V. (2005). Hope VI and Mixed-Finance Redevelopments: A Catalyst for Neighborhood Renewal: A Discussion Paper Prepared. Washington, DC: The Brookings Institution Metropolitan Policy Program.

Uauy, R., Albala, C. & Kain, J. (2001) Obesity trends in Latin America: Transiting from under- to overweight. *J Nutr.* 131(3):893S–899S.

United Nations Department of Economic and Social Affairs, Population Division (2005). *Principles and Recommendations for Population and Housing Censuses*, Revision 1. Series M, No. 67, Rev. 1 (United Nations publication, Sales No. E.98.XVII.1). (para. 2.51).

United Nations, Department of Economic and Social Affairs, Population Division (2006). World Urbanization Prospects: The 2005 Revision. Working Paper No. ESA/P/WP/200.

Virchow, R. (1851). "Die epidemien von 1848." Archiv für Pathologische Anatomie und Physiologie 3: 1-12.

Vlahov, D., Galea, S. & Freudenberg, N. (2005) Urban Health: Toward an Urban Health Advantage. *J Public Health Management Practice*, 11(3): 256–258.

Wikipedia.com (2006). Urbanization. http://en.wikipedia.org/wiki/Urbanization Accessed on January 10, 2007.

World Bank. (2003). Indonesia Environment Monitor: Special Focus: Reducing Air Pollution available at: http://wbln0018.worldbank.org/eap/eap.nsf/Attachments/062403-EnvMonitor2003/$File/indo + monitor.pdf. Accessed on January, 5, 2007.

World Bank. (2005). *World Development Indicators, 2005.* Washington, DC: The World Bank.

World Health Organization (EURO). (1998) *Health promotion evaluation: recommendations to policy-makers: report of the WHO European Working Group on Health Promotion Evaluation.* Copenhagen (Document EUR/ICP/IVST 05 01 03).

World Health Organization. (1990). Healthy Cities Project: A Project becomes a Movement. Review of Progress 1987–1990. Geneva, Switzerland: World Health Organization.

World Health Organization. (2002). *The World Health Report 2002–Reducing Risks, Promoting Healthy Life.* Geneva, Switzerland: World Health Organization.

World Health Organization. (2005). The Bangkok Charter for Health Promotion in a Globalized World Available at: http://www.who.int/healthpromotion/conferences/6gchp/bangkok_charter/en/print.html. Accessed on January 6, 2007.

Yach, D., Hawkes, C., Gould, CL. Hofman KJ. (2004). The Global Burden of Chronic Disease. *J. Am. Med. Assoc.* 291: 2616–2622.

14
Community Interventions on Social Determinants of Health:
Focusing the Evidence

MARILYN METZLER[*], MARY AMUYUNZU-NYAMONGO,
ALOK MUKHOPADHYAY AND LIGIA DE SALAZAR

Public health has been described as "what we as a society do to collectively assure the conditions in which people can be healthy" (IOM 1989, 2003). The Ottawa Charter for Health Promotion identifies eight essential preconditions to health (Ottawa Charter for Health Promotion, 1986). Over the past decade-and-a-half, the term "social determinants of health" has been used broadly to refer to social and economic factors that influence health, including income, food, housing, education, safety, social relationships, and health care. Social determinants have also been described as " . . . life-enhancing resources and opportunities that effectively determine the length and quality of life by their distribution across populations" (James, 2002), pointing to the need to consider not only what the conditions are, but also *for whom*. Joining conditions needed for health to questions of distribution locates the realm of social determinants within the health promotion arena, where equity has always been emphasized, at least conceptually, if not always in practice.

Mounting scientific evidence consistently and strongly supports the need to address social conditions to improve health outcomes. The emergence of new theories, methods, frameworks, and tools, in addition to the convening of commissions on the social determinants of health by WHO (WHO, 2005a) and by multiple countries and cities, all demonstrate a growing understanding of this need. Despite this and despite more than twenty years of health promotion activities, little is known about how to effectively intervene on social determinants, either at a broad policy scale, locally, or at other points on a continuum. This lack of evidence is largely due to the paucity of interventions concerned with conditions for health compared to the number of those focused on access to health care or individual risk factor reduction. The lack of evidence is also possibly an unintended casualty of the ongoing health promotion effectiveness debate. That debate – about what constitutes effectiveness in health promotion – may detract from the issues and challenges posed by interventions on social determinants. Given the growing demands for evidence by policy-makers and others, and the interest expressed by communities and

---

[*] The views and opinions in this chapter are those of the authors and do not necessarily reflect the views of the Centers for Disease Control and Prevention of the Department of Health and Human Services.

other geopolitical entities for public health activities that seek to ameliorate inequality in the conditions for health, this is a critical question for health promotion. One way to explore it is to examine concrete examples of interventions in social determinants, a task we undertake in this chapter. We begin with a very brief overview of the current health promotion effectiveness debate. We then present three case studies of interventions addressing social determinants of health in three different community settings. Following this, we return to the question of evidence to see how adequately current effectiveness strategies capture concerns raised by these interventions. Finally, we pose a series of questions intended to help orient the effectiveness discussion in the direction of community interventions explicitly focused on social determinants of health.

Framing this discussion in terms of community-level approaches to social determinants does not negate the need for national and international policies on social conditions that impact health. It is widely recognized that although community is an appropriate and important focal point for health promotion activities, community health is fundamentally tied to macro and micro policies that affect individual and collective behaviors and opportunities. Nor do these three case studies represent the range of community interventions on social determinants. However, individually and collectively they provide inspiration for possible courses of action as well as illustration of key issues related to effectively intervening on social determinants of health at the community level.

The current health promotion effectiveness debate is rigorous, multifaceted, and not easily summarized. It is generally agreed that health promotion is an emerging, multidisciplinary field that encompasses a wide range of research, programs, and interventions informed by a profound ideology and broad theoretical underpinnings (McQueen, 2001). It is also generally agreed that the community is a primary point of entry or "center of gravity" for health promotion research and practice (Green, 1996). Multidisciplinarity, plus the acknowledged complexity of communities and community life, gives rise to questions about what counts as evidence and who gets to decide. Questions center on research design, types and sources of evidence and, importantly, knowledge development, given an eminently Western bias, which values quantitative data over qualitative, outcomes over process, and professional opinions over those of community members.

Few would argue in favor of limiting evidence to that gleaned from randomized controlled trials given the complexity of community interventions, although some still use this framing. The lack of control groups, on the other hand, limits generalizability. The contextual nature of community interventions shifts the emphasis to principles, frameworks, and empowerment strategies to guide the development, adaptation, and evaluation of locally relevant interventions (Goodstadt, Hyndman, McQueen, Potvin, Rootman, Springett, & Ziglio, 2001). The complexity of community interventions thus gives rise to the need for evaluation designs that combine methodologies, use a diverse range of data and sources, and assess a range of both outcomes and processes (Nutbeam, 1998). For example, the growing use of community-based participatory approaches has expanded the range of evidence to include assessment of *how* the intervention was implemented (Please see, for e.g., Hills, O'Neill, Carrott & McDonald, 2004; Roussos & Fawcett, 2000). For a more thorough discussion of the health promotion effectiveness debate, please refer to relevant chapters in this volume and also to *Evaluation in Health Promotion: Principles and Perspectives* (Rootman, Goodstadt, Hyndman, McQueen, Potvin, Springett & Ziglio, 2001).

To explore the relevance of this discussion to community interventions that explicitly deal with social determinants of health, we turn our attention to three projects currently being implemented in communities in Kenya, India, and Colombia. To determine that they are indeed addressing social determinants, we referred to a set of previously-established criteria that identified community interventions on social determinants of health as those with one or more of the following: 1) people, organizations, and communities working to directly change social determinants of health such as poverty, discrimination or discriminatory institutional policies, or the physical environment; 2) efforts that focus beyond individuals to, for example, develop community cohesion, institutional processes, and/or social policies that reduce disparities or inequities in health, or alter environmental conditions; 3) efforts to increase community or organizational capacity, such as restructuring a health or other governmental department or other organization; or 4) developing measures of effectiveness for projects working in marginalized communities (adapted from SDOHD, 2003). Using these criteria, these three projects are indeed addressing social determinants of community health, and case studies were developed for presentation and discussion here.

Creating Healthy Child Development at the Mitumba Informal Settlement Nairobi, Kenya

Urban informal settlements, more commonly referred to as "slums," are home to almost one billion people globally, including one-third of those living in cities in developing regions (UN-Habitat, 2005). Such settlements provide some of the harshest conditions found in any collective living arrangement due to overcrowding, poor sanitation, and minimal access to essential resources (Gulis, Mulumba, Juma & Kakosova, 2004). These conditions also result in stigmatization, social isolation, and discrimination (APHRC, 2002). In Africa, people in urban settlements experience higher rates of morbidity and mortality than rural residents and have less access to health services (Amuyunzu-Nyamongo & Taffa, 2004; Zulu, Nii-Amoo Dodoo & Ezeh, 2002). Children are hit hardest by these conditions, with under-five mortality 35% higher among children in Nairobi settlements than among children in rural Kenya (Amuyunzu-Nyamongo & Taffa, 2004; APHRC, 2002).

Mitumba, a Kiswahili term meaning "second hand" or "used," is a Nairobi settlement of approximately 18,000 people established in 1992. Mitumba is smaller than other Nairobi settlements and consequently has received little attention or support from governmental or other organizations. In 2006, the African Institute for

Health & Development (AIHD), with support from the U.S. Centers for Disease Control and Prevention, established a partnership with residents of Mitumba to undertake a pilot project to promote healthy child development. AIHD is a Nairobi-based non-governmental organization (NGO) with multidisciplinary staff including anthropologists, sociologists, economists, and education specialists established in 2004 to conduct research, training, and advocacy on health and development issues.

The goal of the Mitumba project is to facilitate empowerment processes with mothers of under-five children to improve health; these include increased access to health information, safety, and early child development opportunities. The project follows general principles of community-based participatory research (CBPR), fully engaging mothers of under-five children, community health workers, and community leaders throughout the entire project period (Israel, Schulz, Parker & Becker, 1998). CBPR expands beyond the education and awareness paradigm, which usually involves interventions imposed on communities by outsiders, to an approach inspired by Freire (1968), in which the process actively involves community members and organizations in developing the capacity to improve their health and well-being (Labonte, 1997). Communities are encouraged to take control of their situations and to collectively improve them through cycles of planning, action, and evaluative reflection, on the rationale that the beneficiaries must drive the improvement and promotion of their own health with effective and sustainable strategies (Loewenson, 2002; Macfarlane, Racelis & Muli-Musiime, 2000).

To generate collective understanding about living conditions in Mitumba, baseline data were collected over a 10-day period through social mapping with youth and adults to understand community resources and boundaries. Surveys and focus group discussions were held with mothers to identify community conditions and norms affecting maternal and child health. Interviews were obtained with key informants to gain insight on community issues and challenges. Participatory processes informed the design of the questionnaires as well as efforts to assure respondents of confidentiality.

The findings revealed that Mitumba has three narrow roads passable by car during non-rainy seasons, six narrow paths for foot traffic, four churches, one school, and no health facilities.

Housing structures are small and crowded: in 68% of the households, 3 to 5 people share a single 10' × 10' room for both cooking and sleeping; occasionally, it also includes a toilet. Most houses are made of metal sheeting and plastic, and have dirt floors. Water, available from community taps, is purchased at high prices and is mostly unclean because the vendors who supply the water use low quality pipes. Toilets, constructed by landlords, are shared by large numbers of people, poorly maintained, and often full. Children are not allowed to use them because of these conditions and because the holes are too big, creating safety concerns. Consequently, most children eliminate their waste on the open ground causing serious sanitation problems. The sole community school in Mitumba has six classrooms, none of which has doors, windows, desks or books. The nearby city council school does not accept children from settlements. Some children attend private schools but most families cannot afford the fees.

Some 65% of the mothers in Mitumba have received primary education and 35% a secondary education. Most residents engage in casual labor in industrial areas or construction sites. Women work in nearby wealthy households, although more than half were unemployed at the time of the baseline study. Poor economic conditions limit access to safe, affordable child care when mothers work or run errands. Young children (0–3 years) are usually left with neighbors who are not obligated to feed or clean them; older children (3–5 years) are usually left outside of the locked house. Children are often seen looking for food, loitering around neighboring houses, or sleeping on the ground when their mothers are away. Mothers reported that the major concerns facing young children include lack of food (20%) and diseases (42%), including malaria, respiratory infections, and diarrhea and vomiting. Due to lack of access to health services and limited economic resources, mothers stated that when their children are sick they frequently rely on chemists and drug vendors who often sell inadequate or inappropriate remedies (Amuyunzu-Nyamongo & Nyamongo, 2006). Thus, 20% of households reported at least one child having died.

With this information, a consensus-building forum was held with mothers to identify and prioritize their needs and to enable them to think of homegrown, practical approaches they could adopt and implement without stretching their scarce resources. Three initiatives were decided upon by the community: establishing a day care center (the core project), soliciting support for the community school, and working with youth to enhance their ongoing activities and to open new horizons for them. Together, these initiatives support the overall goal of improved child health while also increasing skills and capacities among various groups in the community.

For example, the mothers stated that they wanted their children nurtured in a home-environment staffed by older mothers with experience and training in child care and development. They identified two such mothers from the community, potential venues, and determined the cost per child they could afford per child. The community members and AIHD jointly planned the intervention, including defined roles and responsibilities for each group, in a signed memorandum of understanding, to develop commitment and to safeguard against potential misunderstandings.

They constructed the day care by refurbishing and expanding an existing facility. The floors were cemented, fences added, and walls painted with bright colors and murals of story book characters. Fifteen mothers attended a training session to learn how to make toys and other items needed for the center. Additional sessions focused on nutrition, developmental needs and health and safety issues. Within a few weeks, the day care center reached full capacity, with 20 children, and the partnership began discussing the development of additional centers.

Additional Activities

Community members also stressed the importance of education for the growth of individuals, communities, and the nation at large. Current educational conditions in Mitumba make it difficult for the children to learn and thus fully participate in the world. During meetings with community members, the school chairman, and teachers, the partnership identified the need to: construct a fence around the school to ensure safety; obtain access to desks, textbooks, and writing materials; secure windows and doors; and pipe water in for personal hygiene and food preparation. The group developed a proposal to seek city council sponsorship.

Another serious problem in Mitumba is the lack of employment for youth, which contributes to alcoholism, drug abuse, prostitution, and single parenthood. Using an approach similar to that adopted by the mothers, a partnership was established with Tuff Gong, a community youth group in existence since 2004 that has been involved in environmental cleanliness, HIV and AIDS education, and football activities. Members started monthly cleanups but no longer have the equipment necessary to continue, and the partnership is seeking funds to support their activities.

Evaluation activities for the pilot phase of the Mitumba project will include review of the registers used to record implementation activities, before and after photography, periodic informal discussions with the community members, and end-of-project surveys.

Addressing Health and Social Determinants of Vulnerable Communities Delhi and Shivpuri, India

Since achieving independence in 1947, India has made remarkable progress toward improving health. From a situation of sociopolitical and economic degeneration, with hunger and malnutrition universal, half of all children dead before the age of five, primary health care nonexistent, and nine-tenths of the population illiterate, India has doubled life expectancy and halved infant mortality rates over the past five decades (Mukhopadhyay & Choudhury, 1997). However, all people have not shared equally in these achievements. Life expectancy ranges from a high of 68 years in richer states to a low of 53 years; infant mortality ranges from 16 to 98 per 1,000 live births. With a population of more than one billion people, of which nearly one-third, or 300 million, live below the poverty line, India faces many challenges as it seeks to achieve its "Health for All" goals. The health needs of those who are poor remain underserved, with primary and public health measures only rarely reaching them. Poverty is the underlying factor behind many conditions that contribute to poor health including malnutrition, lack of education, and few livelihood opportunities.

Since independence, India has experienced marked declines in urban poverty rates, yet rural poverty remains essentially unchanged. People living in areas difficult to access are more susceptible to disease, yet receive fewer services, than those who live in more developed areas. The annual government per capita expenditure on health care is estimated to be 10 times greater in cities than in rural areas. Highlighting the relationship between poverty and health is the poverty disparity between states with better and worse health outcomes: in Punjab, 6% of the people live in poverty and the infant mortality rate (IMR) is 45/1,000; in Madhya Pradesh, 37% live in poverty and the IMR is 79/1,000 (Mukhopadhyay & Choudhury, 1997).

Voluntary Health Association of India

The Voluntary Health Association of India (VHAI) is a federation of 27 state-level health associations that links more than 4,000 Indian health and development organizations and is the largest such alliance in the world. For the past three decades, VHAI has pursued a vision of social justice and human rights by "making health a reality for all the people of India," and has placed priority on the provision and distribution of health and health services to the less privileged millions. A primary strategy for achieving this vision is to assist existing health and development initiatives with establishing participatory efforts in remote communities. To ensure that programs have a lasting impact, VHAI emphasizes sustainability as an essential feature of its projects by supporting grassroots organizations in collaborations with existing organizations and government resources and infrastructures.

The "KHOJ" Initiative

Khoj is a Hindi word meaning "to search." The philosophy of the Khoj initiative, begun in 1993 with funding from the German foundation Evangelischer Entwicklungsdienst e.V., is to search for new methods and strategies to improve community health related problems in remote areas, including alternatives to existing health care and development models followed by many government and voluntary organizations. Khoj seeks to realize the untapped potential of smaller projects that have shown promise of moving toward effective, self-sustaining community health and development programs, but which have been hindered from attaining excellence by a paucity of resources or capabilities.

The potential for Khoj to be successful was enhanced by an emerging climate within the national government to strengthen Panchayats, locally elected councils that take decisions on issues key to a village's social, cultural, and economic life. When Khoj began, district officials sought to establish effective partnerships between local government health officials, representations of development organisations, NGOs, the private sector, and communities to optimize the health community for the purpose of improving people's health and development status. This opened the potential for community residents and elected village leaders, of whom many are women, to be integrally involved in community development strategies.

With this backdrop, VHAI coordinated the development of Khoj projects in 17 remote areas in 160 villages, despite the fact that social and economic strata and gender status are extremely rigid and society continues to be organized feudally. Key approaches included developing projects based on local needs as expressed by the community; identifying local partners in the volunteer sector; the use of existing government infrastructure; emphasizing sustainableinitiatives, including financial and human resources; and, ensuring improved health and development status through capacity building with members of the community.

One of the 17 Khoj projects was initiated in the Shivpuri district in Madhya Pradesh for the benefit of Saharia tribes living in 20 communities. People in Shivpuri identified health as a major concern, with their first priority, access to health services and health education. Using participatory approaches, village development committees, youth groups, and self-help groups were formed and trained to increase community ownership and confidence. Access to health services, including medical visits, prenatal care, lab tests, and health screenings, was improved by partnering with local government health programs. Planning and management systems were developed to support project implementation, monitoring, and evaluation.

Community members also identified the need to improve their living situations in order to improve community health. VHAI staff trained village residents in community assessment, problem identification and prioritization, and action planning. Resulting activities included the development of multiple income-generating activities that emphasized sex equality and the overall empowerment of women. These included kitchen gardening, livestock farming, and Mahila Mandals or women's savings clubs. The Mahila Mandals, in addition to improving economic conditions for participating members, provide support to community development activities such as improved sanitation, purchase of seeds, and school enrollment by village children. Ongoing community assessment activities include monitoring prenatal care among pregnant women; sex ratio among children (given problems with female feticide); school attendance; housing and sanitation conditions; and morbidity and mortality data.

Since 1993, the 20 Shivpuri Villages have created and sustained 64 self-help groups, 20 Mahila Mandals and 20 Village Development Committees, resulting in multiple education and health programs that have improved school attendance, increased access to health services, and improved housing and environmental conditions. Shivpuri now has 15 village health workers and 21 trained birth attendants; prior to 1993 there were none. Between 1993 and 2003, the IMR decreased from 124 to 50/1,000, prenatal care increased from 16% to 79%, and annual maternal deaths decreased from 15 to 0.

The Khoj project recently completed its 10-year commitment to the 17 project areas and similar achievements were found in health and community development throughout the areas. Sustainability is supported through the organizational structures that have been established, increased capacity among village health workers, resources generated from the self-help groups and various projects, and ongoing collaboration with the local government and Panchayats.

In a large, complex, vibrant country like India, local health promotion is challenging but critical to improving well-being. Solutions to complex problems clearly exist in many innovative, successful experiments across the country; unfortunately, but most programs continue to operate in unimaginative ways. Collaborating with local communities to restructure and revitalize the health sector increases its effectiveness and sustainability and improves the overall conditions for community health.

The School Nutritional Strengthening Program
Valle de Cauca, Colombia

The Department of Valje de Cauca (DVC), located in southwestern Colombia, is home to approximately 4.4 million people. In 2000, 52% of them lived at the poverty line and an additional 15% lived in destitution (less than the equivalent to US$1 per day) (Plan De Desarrollo Departamental, 2004). In Latin America, as elsewhere, poverty often sets into motion a vicious cycle. Poor families frequently cannot afford to send their children to school, but poor children who attend school often under-perform because of inadequate nutrition and poorly educated children have fewer opportunities to move out of poverty.

The Colombian School Nutritional Strengthening Program (SNSP) is a national policy to provide free meals to all children attending public elementary schools. Each department, or state, is charged with implementing the policy according to guidelines established by departmental and local governments. In the DVC, implementation of the SNSP is part of the official governmental strategy to promote social well-being equably, assuring that children and others in the community have access to nutrition, health services, education and improved living conditions (DVC 2004).

Prior to the SNSP, school breakfasts had been provided by the national Colombian Institute of Family Wellbeing (ICBF), but coverage had reached less than one-third of the children. In 2004, the new DVC governor reformulated the program to increase coverage, reduce school desertion, and encourage community and economic development. The current program is conceived as a response to previous failed local development efforts and is coordinated with other programs related to the social determinants of health, including poverty, unemployment, and the internal conflict and displacement resulting from Colombia's longstanding civil war. Institutional participants in the intersectoral partnership include the national government; the DVC governor and ministries; mayors of the 42 DVC municipalities and their respective secretaries of health, education, social development, agriculture, etc.; education and health care institutions; citizens' watch offices; community action boards; NGOs; and, the Financial Institute for the Development of Valle del Cauca.

Three levels of decision-making guide the program: the DVC management committee; the technical committees (one departmental and 42 municipal); and municipal operations committees, which bring together the education community, citizens, and local suppliers. Resources are provided by the national government, the DVC, decentralized public entities such as the Industria de Licores del Valle and the Worker's Welfare Funds, and contributions from DVC managerial staff. Agreements pertaining to development and resource management are secured through inter-administrative covenants between the various partners.

In 2005, the University of Valle's Center for Development and Assessment of Policies and Technology in Public Health was contracted to assess SNSP conceptualization, methodological, and implementation activities through a systematization exercise. This is a qualitative research approach that simultaneously assesses and builds processes to empower social change initiatives (De Salazer, 2004). It encourages all actors to participate in learning to deepen understanding and interpretation of the processes used to implement action, to critically analyze actions, and to build on the knowledge of communities and social groups to establish the conditions needed for sustainability.

In the assessment, partners agreed on the main goal of the SNSP and had a common understanding that improving the situation of children and communities requires making decisions within the context of cultural and environmental conditions, including understanding community attitudes and beliefs about food, the benefits of nutrition, local agricultural practices, and land use. They agreed that this requires integrated actions across governmental and other entities and identified the key roles and responsibilities of the various partners as follows:

Health sector: establish baseline information to identify critical issues, conduct nutritional surveillance in schools, monitor nutritional development, provide nutrition programs for students and families, develop guidelines to train teachers on nutrition, and improve environmental sanitation in the schools.

Education sector: monitor program coverage, design and implement nutritional courses for teachers, and monitor participation of school principals and teachers.

Agriculture and fishing sector: provide information about associations of producers that may be involved in the program, support processes for food production, provide information about harvest products and purchase alternatives, monitor and support increased availability and use of organic products.

Social development sector: monitor the inclusion of small producers as program suppliers, develop the capacity of associations and small businesses to participate in the program, assess the economic impact on associations and small businesses.

Financial Institute for the Development of VDC: manage the financial resources.

Colombian Institute of Family Wellbeing: provide technical guidelines to monitor nutritional quality and compliance with the menus.

To implement the SNSP, collaborations and contracts were developed with small community-based organizations for food preparation, transportation, and distribution, generating local employment opportunities and encouraging use of local foods. Family mothers participate through special meetings with government and school officials. Public hearings and other activities designed to monitor government actions have been redirected to facilitate interaction between citizens, mayors, and those in charge of the SNSP in the municipalities.

Across the DVC, communities tailor general guidelines to implement, and in some cases build upon, the SNSP program. In La Cumbre, a community of 10,000 people located at an elevation of 6,600 feet in the Andes Mountains, early discussions focused on food as more than a substance for consumption but as also being important to the cultural, environmental, and economic life of the community. The people agreed they wanted their children to have a school menu based on traditional foods, especially given concerns about the increasing availability of "fast food" and the rise in obesity in developing countries. They also saw the program as an opportunity to grow more food locally and to rethink their relationship to the surrounding land and local agricultural practices, agreeing to limit the use of pesticides and other chemicals in favor of more organic approaches. Two years into the SNSP program, 50% of the food grown in La Cumbre was considered "clean" – an intermediate designation for food grown on land that has not yet been without chemicals for the three years required to be labeled "organic." In the third year of the program, the community partnership was discussing how to build upon their many successes to create additional opportunities for income generation, having realized that the SNSP was a very good program but that much more needed to be done to eliminate local poverty.

Successes and Challenges

Under the reorganized SNSP program, 100% of DVC's 400,000 public school children are now receiving school lunches. In addition to this major achievement, other successes include increased communication between government and citizens, as well as the participation of civil society organizations in public management. Factors facilitating these successes include the commitment and political will of the governor and the mayors, commitment of most of the government entities involved, execution of agreements that guarantee the activities, availability of departmental and municipal resources, existence of a development plan, community acceptance, emphasis on a local development approach, and, the support of the educational sector, which increases legitimacy, strength and leadership.

SNSP partners also identified many challenges including lack of a generalized approach that can be locally adapted, as well as political, administrative, cultural, and geographic differences between municipalities that can adversely affect overall program achievements. Tensions also exist around resource management, which affects efficiency is implementing the agreed upon strategies. For example, participants noted the need to improve the timeliness of government payments to suppliers because small businesses find it difficult to go long periods of time without being paid for their services. The scope of the alliances and the complexity of the program require greater capacity to negotiate, manage implementation, and to determine program impacts. The people involved need increased visibility in order to generate positive public opinion and to appropriately position governmental institutions in support of the SNSP. Bridges between small farmers and local producers of processed food must be strengthened.

Community partners also emphasized the health value of traditional foods over the highly processed foods gaining popularity among children. New opportunities for food production and agricultural development must be explored in every municipality to meet the needs of the SNSP. Suppliers need to be trained in food storage, preparation, and preservation; and site owners and persons responsible for handing food need training in basic sanitation. Finally, information must be systematically consolidated to monitor program activities, to recover the knowledge produced, and to empower partners to adjust and transform the program.

Planned future assessment of the SNSP will includes a cost-effectiveness evaluation, and strategies will be developed to continuously rebuild and reorient the program. Other contributions to be assessed include reductions in school desertion, increased educational coverage, improved nutrition among school children, the generation of employment, and improved agricultural practices. Making the SNSP sustainable will require institutionalizing it within the policies, structures, and resources of each of the partners. Making the successes of the SNSP visible to citizens is also critical to assure sustainability.

Discussion

These three case studies demonstrate that interventions to alter social determinants of health can be implemented in multiple settings: a single community, a network of villages, or the schools and communities in a governmental jurisdiction. Community partnerships that address social determinants of health can also be implemented between a variety of agencies, e.g., a small NGO, a large volunteer organization, or a public administrative unit. Finally, the range of available resources can vary widely – from seed money to bureaucratic budgets – athough this will obviously impact the range of outcomes that might be expected.

These case studies also show that familiar health promotion theories, methods, and tools, including social support, health education, partnership development, capacity building, community assessment, and structural change are useful when implementing such interventions to address social determinants. However, the emphasis shifts from efforts to change the individual characteristics to those that seek to change the characteristics of communities and their environments, including a community's ability to influence factors beyond its environment. This presents a challenge in measuring impact as change is not always obvious and often takes longer than the intended life of the intervention to be understood.

In its simplest form, the health promotion evidence debate is about the question, "How will we know if our actions are improving health and the conditions for health?" We bemoan the paucity of health promotion evidence overall but know even less about what works to improve the social factors that influence health. Yet most of us would agree that providing supervised day care to a child in an urban settlement or feeding poor school children and creating jobs in their communities will improve health in the short term, and recent studies in life course epidemiology suggest the effects may be lifelong (Kuh & Ben-Shlomo, 2004). So while we might agree on the goal – improving social factors to improve health – in the face of little or no evidence, we differ on ways to reach it.

In the search for evidence, although it is often not possible to see changes in terms of morbidity or mortality in short periods of time, it may be feasible to assess intermediate outcomes, such as improvements in social conditions. Using a variety of qualitative and quantitative evaluation methods, these communities provide evidence that some conditions have changed: a daycare center where there was none, women's savings clubs, lunches for students. In large part, the processes used to make the changes will determine whether they last. The participatory approaches used to develop these interventions certainly suggest that the changes are integral to the life of the communities.

Much of the health promotion evidence discussion on processes relates to community organizing and participation. Interventions that seek to improve the social determinants of health suggest that additional processes warrant examination. Many of the questions such an examination might raise are related broadly to health promotion and are discussed elsewhere in the literature. We here present questions intended to focus the discussion on community initiatives that are explicitly concerned with social determinants of health. Whether a social determinants intervention can be considered "effective" may depend on how these questions are answered, although they are not exclusive or exhaustive. Other questions will be raised as the number and type of such community interventions increase.

1) How does this intervention seek to alter the social determinants of health?
Although this may seem like a rhetorical question, especially given that the foundation of health promotion rests on the ecological model, the "default mode" of most health promotion activities is an emphasis on individual behavior change. Reasons for this range from the wealth of behavioral theories and the dearth of social theories to guide activities (McQueen, 1996), to priorities established by policy-makers, and the connections between these. No common or explicit social theory or theory of change cuts across the three communities discussed, yet each demonstrates that improving social conditions improves community health. Activities sometimes include individual change, but the primary emphasis is on social conditions. Maintaining a focus on social determinants requires a clear definition and a set of criteria by which to assess the intervention's effectiveness.

The increase in scientific analyses establishing relationships between social conditions and health is stimulating interest in improving social conditions. As the number of activities intended to change social conditions increases, the knowledge gained can be used to identify and develop new theories of social change, including those that help to explain relationships between conditions and health (Potvin, Bilodeau & Chabot, 2005). Methods are needed to help unravel the effects of various components of multifaceted interventions. For example, systems thinking and modeling are well suited to capturing the complexities of interventions based on multifaceted, ecological approaches (Homer & Hirsch, 2006), but given this field's infancy in the public health arena, much is yet to be learned about how it can be used to develop and evaluate community level interventions.

2) How does this intervention seek to achieve health equity?
Health equity is achieved when all groups in a society enjoy the standard of health enjoyed by the most socially advantaged group within that society (Braveman, 2006). Each of these projects places priority on improving the health of those who experience the poorest health in their societies. Those who experience the worst health are usually the same people who are socially disadvantaged due to

economic conditions, racism, and other forms of discrimination (versus being disadvantaged, for example, due to genetic endowment) (Giles & Liburd, 2007). Emphasis on equity raises issues of fairness and the distribution of health and resources for health and is undoubtedly an issue of societal values and political will (Raphael, 2006a). Health equity is of great importance to health promotion researchers and practitioners because lack of attention to equity can actually increase health gaps, and broad-based interventions often improve health for those who are already relatively healthy but fail to reach those who live at the margins of society (Baum, 2005). Overall health status has improved in most countries over the past century, yet tremendous gaps continue and, in many situations, are widening. In some African countries, life expectancy is declining after a century of increases. Broad-based, generalized health promotion strategies will not close the gaps or increase life expectancy.

Public health needs an ethical imperative to focus efforts and resources on those who experience the worse health outcomes. This requires the development of definitions and notions of equity in concert with communities (Houston, 2006), access to multiple sources of reliable data, and the development of tools to assess the effectiveness of our efforts (See, for e.g., Tugwell, O'Connor, Anderson, Mhatre, Kristjansson, Jacobsen, Robinson, Hatcher-Roberts, Shea, Francis, Beardmore, Wells & Losos, 2006). Many would claim such an imperative already exists, yet this shift in approach means a shift in resources from broad-based strategies to those that seek to alter especially the fundamental conditions, experienced by those with the poorest health. Although the three initiatives presented here are located in developing countries, the need to consider health equity is important for all countries, given that one-half of the world's 6 billion people live in poverty, including significant and growing numbers in developed countries.

3) How have empowerment approaches been facilitated?
One of the main tenets of the Ottawa Charter is the strengthening of communities so they can actively work on their own behalf to create conditions for health. Community participation in health promotion activities is the backbone of empowering strategies but by itself is insufficient (Wallerstein, 2006). Empowerment begins with a community versus outsider definition of need, including preliminary community assessment and ongoing efforts to uncover and build upon community strengths (Minkler, 2002). Assessment of community strengths shifts the perspective from the often prevailing "we need to empower the community" to an appreciation of the critical nature of local knowledge and capacity that embraces the question, "how can we facilitate empowerment processes?" Community-based participatory research is both the foundation of and the point of departure for empowerment processes that move beyond collective decision-making to, for example, explicit principles of participation in data gathering, interpretation, dissemination, and ownership, as well as the sharing of resources (Schulz, Israel, Selig, Bayer & Griffin, 1998; Detroit Community-Academic Urban Research Center, 1996). In Colombia, the national government established the school lunch policy, but the Department of Valle del Cauca chose an implementation strategy specifically designed to support community empowerment even though

contracting the program to a series of large businesses may have been more expedient. The systematization approach used to assess project implementation was specifically designed to simultaneously uncover inherent tensions and to use that information to build knowledge useful to program development and community empowerment. Additional ideas and framing for unpacking tensions and encouraging empowerment by "bottom-up" versus "top-down" approaches have been proposed (Laverack, 2000), as have tools for measuring community empowerment (Laverack & Wallerstein, 2001).

4) How have innovative alliances been developed and how have they functioned?
The social determinants literature is rife with calls for multi-sectoral partnerships, understandable given that conditions conducive to health cut across all aspects of our collective arrangements for living, working, socializing, and so on. Yet as seen in Mitumba and to some extent in the Khoj project, multi-sectoral partnerships are not always possible because many of the world's poorest people live outside the domain of influence sought by policy makers, administrators, and other professionals.

The types of collaborations often proposed – within, across, and in partnership with government sectors – are unfamiliar to most public health practitioners and move beyond our experiences of partnerships with community-based organizations. Many government entities, presumably accountable to a common leader and populace, compete with each other for resources and recognition. Common goals and incentives to collaborate are rare. In Colombia, despite governmental support for the SNSP, its implementation was challenged by lack of cooperation across various administrative units, a problem identified and being worked on through the assessment process. Using lessons from community-based approaches, initiatives focused on social determinants can articulate the need for and help define how these multi-sectoral partnerships can function effectively.

5) How is sustainability conceptualized and approached?
The sustainability of any community social determinants intervention involves three important considerations. First, early and broad strategic planning is required to increase the possibility that changes in conditions for health can continue beyond the project's initial funding period (Minkler, 2002). The three interventions discussed here began with the premise that sustainability was key and used strategies to integrate their activities into existing systems. In Mitumba, sustainability was approached by initially relying on available community resources, limited though they were. In India and Colombia, sustainability was conceptualized as requiring program integration into community and larger governmental systems.

Second, the question of whether all projects should be sustained must be asked. Presumably, some should come to an end if they have met their goals; others should grow to meet growing needs (St. Leger, 2005). In Mitumba, achieving full capacity at the daycare center led to questions about the need for additional centers, suggesting a sort of "dynamic sustainability." This requires thinking beyond the "routinization" of activities, which can imply a certain stagnancy or loss of momentum, to assessing organizational routines to determine if and how activities can be sustained and, when appropriate, further developed (Pluye, Potvin, Denis & Pelletier, 2004).

Finally, and perhaps of greatest importance, are the questions of how the intervention fits into a sustainable community development and its impact on natural systems. Traditionally within the domain of environmental health, if considered at all, the issue of sustainable communities is one that public health must begin to embrace. Health promotion, with its emphasis on community systems and holistic approaches to health and development, is well positioned to take a leadership role in this endeavor (Brown & Ritchie, 2006), especially with the growing interest in the social and physical conditions for health. Evidence that embedding sustainable community goals into existing interventions is possible as seen in La Cumbre, where a school lunch program grew into a community economic development program focused on the health of the land as well as the health of the people.

6) What is the role of professionals?

Community participatory approaches are grounded in critical reflection, capacity building, and other strategies to increase community involvement and ownership. Professionals must also reflect on their role in these approaches, particularly because researchers trained in Western traditions primarily determine what counts as evidence. Other voices must be included in the evidence discussion, especially those of people from developing countries (McQueen, 2001). Those trained in Western approaches are accountable to colleagues and others to meet certain professional and scientific standards, which can lead to "scientific conservativism" when faced with limited or non-traditional forms of evidence (Rychetnik & Wise, 2004), even though educating policy makers and others about the importance of social determinants has been suggested as a key role for health promotion professionals (Raphael, 2006b).

It is important that we consistently look for innovative and more efficient ways to improve conditions for health. This may include, as seen with the Khoj project, building on the successes of existing activities. It may also include questioning the assumptions we hold about how health promotion activities are framed. For example, macro policies and community level interventions are often seen as opposites. However, as seen in Colombia, a national policy took on far greater significance and had a much larger impact precisely because it was implemented using community-based approaches. In India, a group of rural villages using community development strategies has the potential to develop regional capacities that improve health and social conditions for large numbers of people as well as possibly limiting migration to crowded urban areas to search for opportunity.

Professionals must also approach social determinants of health interventions with an orientation toward the future. Improving conditions for health is warranted on ethical, scientific and economic grounds. We must also consider the long-term implications of our approaches given the goal of sustaining changes. A future orientation can include, for example, discussions that anticipate the needs of new generations of students who complete primary or secondary school and who will subsequently look for opportunities to continue their educations. In Mitumba, children learning their ABCs in the day care center are better prepared for primary education, leading to community interest in improving educational opportunities for current and future students. Unintended outcomes also need to be considered. For example, in one Khoj initiative, following a successful educational intervention, suicide rates increased among young men because they were unable to find jobs after developing new skills and who did not want to return to "the old ways." Systems modeling is one approach to exploring potential, as well as unintended consequences, and can contribute to the development of theories and strategies that provide prospective analysis of plausible futures (Sterman, 2006) by, for example, thinking critically about "what if" scenarios (Leischow & Milstein, 2006).

Closing Thoughts

Raising yet more questions about effectiveness increases concern about contributing to a rhetorical debate that, due to the complexity of the endeavor, can lead to "paralysis analysis" and the wait for more convincing evidence before moving to action (Nutbeam, 2004). However, a tangible value of the evidence debate is that the acknowledged complexity of community interventions has broadened the discussion about appropriate evaluation strategies (McQueen, 2002). It is hoped that these questions, as viewed through the lenses provided by these case studies, will help sharpen the focus on effectiveness and move the discussion forward. Lack of attention to these issues could result in the proverbial problem of developing right answers to the wrong questions.

For many, these interventions and the questions they raise will seem familiar because of historical attempts to improve health by improving the underlying conditions. Yet what is retained from past efforts, primarily in the era immediately following the signing of the Alma-Ata Charter, is mostly anecdotal (Kelly, Bonnefoy, Morgan & Florenzano, 2006; Baum, 2006). Little evidence remains from that period to guide us in the present, which contributes to the erroneous assumption that the current emphasis on "social determinants of health" is new. Scientific evidence of the relationships between social determinants and health is growing exponentially, but the effort to improve health by altering the underlying conditions is at least as old as the public health endeavor itself.

These three case studies demonstrate pragmatic approaches to improving the conditions for health but may be less than convincing to many researchers, funders, policy makers and others who require evidence that individual behavior has changed. Our task then, in partnership with communities and as stewards of public and private resources, is to contribute to the development of credible, practical, and culturally appropriate theories and methods to assess the effectiveness of community health and development interventions. The ability to do this rests on our willingness to shift our attention and resources in that direction and to approach the current generation of social determinants of health initiatives with a future orientation that is relentless in its pursuit of health equity.

Acknowledgments. We greatly appreciate the many contributions of those who made the development of this chapter possible. These include Rahel Oyugi, Sushil K. Vasan, Jenny Andrea Vélez, Norma Liliana Campo, Martha Perry, Catherine Jones, Marie-Claude Lamarre, Mary Hall, Linnea Evans, Andrea Neiman, Angel Roca, David McQueen, Marilyn Wise, Maurice Mittlemark, and Susan Chu, as well as families and friends who provide feedback, wait patiently, or otherwise encourage our work. Support for site visits, data collection, and collaboration between the co-authors was provided by the Centers for Disease Control and Prevention. For this we are equally appreciative.

References

African Population and Health Research Centre (APHRC). (2002). Population and health dynamics in Nairobi's informal settlements. Nairobi: African Population and Health Research Centre.

Amuyunzu-Nyamongo, M. & Nyamongo, I.K. (2006). Health seeking behaviour of mothers of under-five-year children in the slum communities of Nairobi, Kenya. *Anthropology & Medicine*, 13(1), 25–40.

Amuyunzu-Nyamongo, M. & Taffa, N. (2004). The triad of poverty, environment and child health in Nairobi informal settlements. *Journal of Health & Population in Developing Countries*. Available at:
http://www.jhpdc.unc.edu accessed on December, 15, 2006.

Baum, F. & Harris, L. (2006). Equity and the social determinants of health. *Health Promotion Journal of Australia* 17(3), 163–165.

Baum, F. (2005). Who cares about health for all in the 21st century? *Journal of Epidemiology and Community Health* 59, 714–715.

Braveman, P. (2006). Health disparities and health equity: Concepts and measurement. *Annual Review of Public Health* 27, 167–194.

Brown, V.A. & Ritchie, J. (2006). Sustainable communities: What should our priorities be? *Health Promotion Journal of Australia* 17(3), 211–216.

De Salazar, L. (2004). Efectividad en Promoción de la Salud. Guía de Evaluación Rápida. Capítulo 8: La Sistematización de Experiencias en Promoción de la Salud. CEDETES – Universidad del Valle. Cali, Colombia.

Department of Valle del Cauca. (2004). Development Plan. 2004–2007. Ordinance 182.

Detroit Community-Academic Urban Research Center. Community-Based Public Health Research Principles. Adopted July 1996.
Available at http://www.sph.umich.edu/urc/research/accessed 12/15/2006.

Freire, P. (1968). Pedagogy of the oppressed. New York: Seabury.

Giles, W.H. & Liburd, L. (2007). Achieving health equity and social justice: Prevention is primary. In Cohen, L., Chavez, V. & Chehimi, S. (Eds.), *Prevention is primary: Strategies for community well-being*. San Francisco: Jossey-Bass.

Goodstadt, M.S., Hyndman, B., McQueen, D.V., Potvin, L., Rootman, I. & Springett, J. (2001). Evaluation in health promotion: synthesis and recommendations. In Rootman, I., Goodstadt, M.S., Hyndman, B, McQueen, D.V., Potvin, L., & Ziglio, E. (Eds) *Evaluation in health promotion: Principles and perspectives* (pp. 517–533). Copenhagen: World Health Organization.

Green, L.W. & Kreuter, M.M. (1996). *Health promotion planning: an educational and environmental approach*. 2nd ed. Mayfield: Mountain View.

Gulis, G., Mulumba, J., Juma, O. & Kakosova, B. (2004). Health status of people of slums in Nairobi, Kenya. *Environmental Research* 96, 219–224.

Hills, M., O'Neill, M., Carroll, S. & MacDonald, M., on behalf of the Canadian Consortium for Health Promotion Research (2004). Effectiveness of community initiatives to promote health: An assessment tool. A report submitted to the Public Health Agency of Canada. 3/31/04.

Homer, J.B. & Hirsch, S.M. (2006). System dynamics modeling for public health: Background and opportunities. *American Journal of Public Health* 96(3), 452–458.

Houston, S. (2006). Equity, by what measure? *Health Promotion Journal of Australia* 17(3), 206–210.

Institute of Medicine (IOM). (1989). *The future of public health*. Washington, DC: National Academy Press.

IOM. (2003). *The future of the public's health in the 21st century*. Washington, D.C: National Academy Press.

Israel, B.A., Schulz, A.J., Parker, E.A. & Becker, A.B. (1998). Review of community-based research: assessing partnership approaches to improve public health. *Annual Review of Public Health* 19, 173–202.

James, S.A. (2002). Social Determinants of Health: Implications for Intervening on Racial and Ethnic Health Disparities. Keynote presentation University of North Carolina Minority Health Conference, March 1, 2002. Available at:
http://www.minority.unc.edu/resources/webcasts/ accessed 11/04/06.

Kelly, M.P., Bonnefoy, J., Morgan, A. & Florenzano, F. (2006). The development of the evidence base about the social determinants of health. World Health Organization Commission on Social Determinants of Health Measurement and Evidence Knowledge Network.

Kuh, D. & Ben-Shlomo, Y. (Eds). (2004). *A life course approach to chronic disease epidemiology*. (2nd ed.) New York: Oxford University Press.

Labonte, R. (1997). Community, community development, and the forming of authentic partnerships: Some critical reflections. In M. Minkler (Ed.), *Community organizing and community building for health* (pp. 88–101). New Brunswick, NJ: Rutgers University Press.

Laverack G. & Wallerstein, N. (2001). Measuring community empowerment: A fresh look at organizational domains. *Health Promotion International* 16(2), 179–185.

Laverack G. & Labonte, R. (2000). A planning framework for community empowerment goals within health promotion. *Health Policy and Planning* 15(3), 255–262.

Leischow, S.J. & Milstein, B. (2006). Systems thinking and modeling for public health practice. *American Journal of Public Health* 96(3), 403–404.

Loewenson, R (2002). Participation and accountability in health systems: The missing factor in equity? Equinet Discussion Paper, UN AIDS. Available at:
www.equinetafrica.org accessed 12/9/2006.

Macfarlane, S., Racelis, M. & Muli-Musiime, F. (2000). Public health in developing countries. *Lancet,* 356 (9232), 841–846.

McQueen, D.V. (1996). The search for theory in health behavior and health promotion. *Health Promotion International,* 11(1), 27–32.

McQueen, D.V. & Anderson, L.M. (2001). What counts as evidence: issues and debates. In Rootman, I., Goodstadt, M.S., Hyndman, B., McQueen, D.V., Potvin, L. & Ziglio, E. (Eds.), *Evaluation in health promotion: Principles and perspectives* (pp. 63–81). Copenhagen: World Health Organization.

McQueen, D.V. (2001). Strengthening the evidence base for health promotion. *Health Promotion International,* 16(3), 261–268.

244   Marilyn Metzler et al.

McQueen, D.V. (2002). The evidence debate. *Journal of Epidemiology and Community Health.* (56), 83–84.

Minkler, M. (2002). *Community organizing and community building for health.* New Brunswick, NJ: Rutgers University Press.

Mukhopadhyay, A. & Choudhury, A.R. (1997). Report of the independent Commission on Health in India Voluntary Health Association of India, New Delhi, India.

Nutbeam, D. (2004). Getting evidence into policy and practice to address health inequalities. *Health Promotion International* 19(2), 137–140.

Nutbeam, D. (1998). Evaluating health promotion – progress, problems, and solutions. *Health Promotion International.*13(1), 27–44.

Ottawa Charter for Health Promotion. (1986). *Health Promotion,* 1(4), iii–v.

Plan De Desarrollo Departmental 2004–2007 "Vamos Juntos Por el Valle Del Cauca". Departamento del Valle del Cauca – Colombia. Gobernación. ORDENANZA No. 182 de Junio 11 del 2004. Page 3.

Pluye, P., Potvin, L., Denis, J.L. & Pelletier, J.P. (2004). Program sustainability: Focus on organizational routines. *Health Promotion International* 19(4), 489–500.

Potvin, L. Bilodeau, A. & Chabot, P. (2005). Integrating social theory into public health practice. *American Journal of Public Health* 95(4), 591–595.

Raphael, D. (2006a). Social determinants of health: Present status, unanswered questions, and future directions. *International Journal of Health Services,* 36(4), 651–677.

Raphael, D. (2006b). The social determinants of health: What are the three key roles for health promotion? *Health Promotion Journal of Australia* 17(3): 167–170.

Rootman, I., Goodstadt, M.S., Hyndman, B., McQueen, D.V., Potvin, L., & Ziglio, E. (Eds.) (2001). *Evaluation in health promotion: Principles and perspectives.* WHO Regional Publications, European series, No.92. Copenhagen: World Health Organization.

Roussos, S.T. & Fawcett, S.B. (2000). A review of collaborative partnerships as a strategy for improving community health. *Annual Review of Public Health* 21, 369–402.

Rychetnik, L. & Wise, M. (2004). Advocating evidence-based health promotion: Reflections and a way forward. *Health Promotion International* 19(2), 247–257.

Schulz, A. J., Israel, B.A., Selig, S.M., Bayer, I.S. & Griffin, C.B. (1998). Development and implementation of principles for community-based research in public health. In R.H. MacNair (Ed.), *Research strategies for community practice* (pp. 83–110). New York: Haworth Press.

Social Determinants of Health Disparities: Learning From Doing (SDOHD) (2003). U.S. Centers for Disease Control and Prevention. October 29–30, 2003.

St. Leger, L. (2005). Questioning sustainability in health promotion projects and programs. *Health Promotion International,* 20(4), 317–319.

Sterman, J.D. (2006). Learning from evidence in a complex world. *American Journal of Public Health* 96(3), 505–514.

Tugwell, P., O'Connor, A., Anderson, N., Mhatre, S., Kristjansson, E., Jacobsen, M., Robinson, V., Hatcher-Roberts, J., Shea, B., Francis, D., Beardmore, J., Wells, G. & Losos, J. (2006). Reduction of inequalities in health: assessing evidence-based tools. *International Journal for Equity in Health.* 5–11.

United Nations Center for Human Settlement (UN-HABITAT). (2005). Global report on human settlements. London and Sterling, Va.

Wallerstein, N. (2006). What is the evidence on effectiveness of empowerment to improve health? Copenhagen, WHO Regional Office for Europe (Health Evidence Network report; http://www.euro.who.int/Document/E88086.pdf accessed November 10, 2006.

World Health Organization. (2005a). Commission on Social Determinants of Health. http://www.who.int/social_determinants/about/en/Accessed March 24, 2006.

World Health Organization. (2005b). Action on the social determinants of health: Learning from previous experiences. A background paper prepared for the Commission on the Social Determinants of Health. Available at:
http://www.who.int/social_determinants/resources/action_sd.pdf. Accessed 10/20/06.

Zulu E., Nii-Amoo Dodoo, M.F. & Ezeh, A.C. (2002). Sexual risk-taking in the slums of Nairobi, Kenya, 1993–98. *Population Studies* 56, 311–323.

15
Strengthening Peace-Building Through Health Promotion
Development of a Framework

ANNE W. BUNDE-BIROUSTE AND JAN E. RITCHIE

The concept of health itself has been considered an entry point for working to improve the determinants of well-being in a society, and decrease areas of vulnerability in pre-conflict states.

(The Journal of Humanitarian Assistance, 2000).

In September 2003, the Australian Agency for International Development (AusAID) provided support to a team based at the School of Public Health and Community Medicine (SPHCM) at the University of New South Wales (UNSW) in Sydney, Australia to explore how health sector and health promotion action might effectively contribute to peace building. This chapter will provide the rationale for this work and describe how a tool was developed that would assist those working in fragile settings to consider their work in relation to promoting peace, such that they could incorporate peace-building principles into their efforts (Zwi, Bunde-Birouste, Grove, Waller & Ritche, 2006). It will conclude with a short discussion on the results of the tool's field pilot testing in regards to the effectiveness debate in health promotion.

Setting the Scene for Health Promotion and Peace-Building

The Ottawa Charter clearly recognizes the link between health promotion and peace building in recognizing peace as a determinant to health (Ottawa Charter for Health Promotion, 1986). At the same time, in the realm of peace-building work, optimising health is considered a means to contribute to peace building (MacQueen, & Santa Barbara, 2000). In the sense of reciprocal determinism, health then becomes a determinant for peace building or, in other words, peace ultimately becomes an outcome of health promotion action.

But what does this mean exactly, and how can we know if indeed our work is effective in contributing to building a peaceful environment? How can we design and implement our programs in fragile and vulnerable communities so that they will have a maximum chance of contributing to building peace rather than risking exacerbation of tensions?

These questions provided the basis for the UNSW Health and Conflict team's work as we undertook to design a framework that could provide a foundation to guide health sector contributions to peace building through health initiatives in fragile settings (UNSW Health and Conflict Project, 2004).

Attempting to Measure Peace-Building Impact

It is quite clear that the challenge of measuring the impact of health promotion on peace-building will be as difficult and nebulous as that experienced in measuring any worthwhile health promotion practice. This challenge results primarily because worthwhile health promotion should meet the complexity of criteria as succinctly compiled by IUHPE (1999) and reiterated and reinforced by McQueen (2001), with measurement of this complexity therefore needing to be drawn from multiple sources of evidence (McQueen, 2002, 2003; McQueen & Anderson, 2001).

This complexity means that it is virtually impossible to identify any one factor as the direct cause or determinant of peace. Rather, we propose that it can be feasible to determine indicators of peace-building by identifying factors which act as markers towards a peace-building outcome. These indicators will more likely demonstrate a trend in the favored direction rather than a definitive causal pathway, yet this demonstrated change can be highly indicative of desired results (Zwi, Bunde-Birouste, Grove, Waller & Ritchie, 2006).

Health in Fragile Settings: From Exploration to a Framework

Health development work in fragile settings involves different approaches from that provided in more stable situations. Fragile communities or states are those where resources are strained or lacking, services are sporadic or failing, and communities have become fragmented (Bunde-Birouste, Zwi et al., 2004). The overall result of these weaknesses is that society tends to break down. Conflicts often result during this societal breakdown, which can occur at multiple levels – political, economic, social, cultural, ethnic, religious, resource-based etc – and can often involve multiple actors with different agendas. Although conflict is not necessarily negative or destructive, problems can arise when non-violent conflict becomes violent. Violent conflicts and war are often the results of social breakdown that may have been building over time (Darvill, 2004; Gutlove & Thompson, 2003; Human Security Center, 2005; Zwi & Grove, 2006).

Our research supports previous studies suggesting that impacts of violence can be addressed through health sector action generally and health promotion practice specifically, with some positive effects. Our research also strongly supports the caution that the best intentioned actions can harm or make things worse rather than better when attention has not been given to a series of criteria that we found needed to be considered. Care here must be the very essence of our actions (Anderson, 1999; The Journal of Humanitarian Assistance, 2000).

The learning on health and peace-building that has occurred in the past two decades has drawn in particular from a critical analysis of the human security, emergency and health, and peace building literature. In reviewing the context of relief and development work in post-conflict settings, we discovered numerous frameworks of assessment proposed as integral steps for effective aid interventions in conflict-prone societies (Anderson, 1999; Bush, 1998 & 2003; Gaigals & Leonhardt, 2001; MacQueen & Santa Barbara, 2000; Silove, 2000a). Conflict-impact assessments and conflict sensitivity tools of various sorts have become increasingly popular with international donor agencies; conflict vulnerability assessments have aimed to identify the risks and drivers of violence. We found that few of these explicitly addressed health or health sector work as part of their analysis (Bunde-Birouste, Eisenbruch, Grove, Humphrey, Silove, Waller, Zwi, 2004; UNSW Health and Conflict Project, 2004). As such, the extent to which health initiatives consistently and consciously include the necessary elements which facilitate a potential contribution to preventing violent conflict or promoting peace-building in post-conflict settings, remained elusive. Our hypothesis was that combining a conflict impact analysis assessment with a health assessment could generate a more informed understanding of how health initiatives could be designed and/or monitored to enhance their input to contribute effectively to peace-building. This learning has provided the basis for the development of the tool which we have termed the Health and Peace-building Filter.

Development of the Framework

Fundamental Concepts

The team's objective was "to develop an innovative tool that would provide for rapid assessment of the peace-building/conflict prevention components of health initiatives in precarious, unstable settings." An ideal Filter would be multi-purpose allowing:

i. monitoring/assessment of the conflict prevention/peace building potential of existing health service and health promotion activities;
ii. program conception guidance to ensure that new programs are developed with peace-building elements included.

Our early research also resulted in identifying impacts of violence specifically related to health, and how they could be addressed by health sector and health promotion action. These preliminary findings highlighted recurring "human rights" concepts that figure as essential underlying principles to peace-building and conflict resolution (UNSW Health and Conflict Project, 2004). We initially classified these into thirteen points, however for the tool to be effective, it needed to be manageable. These 13 elements were thus consolidated into a more succinct grouping of five broad categories which included sub-components that reflected the thirteen original principles. See Box 15.1 for a list of the 13 original principles.

Box 15.1. Original 13 peace-building principles

1. Conflict Management
2. Trust
3. Non-violence
4. Cultural competence
5. Equity
6. Non-discrimination
7. Human rights
8. Social justice
9. Social cohesion
10. Psycho-social
11. Transparency
12. Good governance
13. Capacity building and community empowerment

The next step in the framework development process required validation of these concepts (Zheng, 2000).

A questionnaire for this purpose was developed with support from qualitative research experts in the School of Public Health and Community Medicine. Respondents were asked to provide their own definition of the five concepts, to rank them in order of importance, and to reflect on a variety of sub-components that they considered essential and related to each concept. The questionnaire was distributed to a reference group of 66 recommended experts in April 2005. Responses were consolidated into a form that could allow those planning, implementing, overseeing or evaluating programs or projects in fragile societies to check and reflect on the extent to which they had considered the peace-building concepts in their work. This became the first version of the Filter.

Preliminary Trials of Draft Tool and Further Validation of Concepts

The early version of the Filter contained a number of indicators for each guiding principle. The indicators were designed to provide specific health-related points of action for the principles which are generic in the sense that they can be interpreted across a number of disciplines. In essence they are fundamental principles of humanitarian behaviour.

The validation and refinement of the actual draft Filter was carried out in a variety of settings:

a) an international workshop
b) two key informant interviews
c) international field research.

The consolidation and validation process resulted in a framework with the following five focused areas: cultural sensitivity, conflict sensitivity, social justice, social cohesion and good governance. The essential meanings of these five domains, as they could be applied in fragile and vulnerable situations, are summarized in the words of the Filter's Companion Manual, as follows:

Cultural Sensitivity

A culturally sensitive approach recognises and respects cultural diversity, and demonstrates awareness of the range of beliefs, customs, rituals, and religious practices of groups and communities. Cultural sensitivity is particularly important in areas where conflict has been about political independence, self-determination, the maintenance of particular cultures and traditions.

Conflict Sensitivity

A number of factors may influence the occurrence of violent confrontation: these include ethnic, religious or other disputes over resources and their distribution in society. Knowing different reasons for tensions and understanding how they play out in the community is important when considering intervention options, and the implications of acting, or not acting, in a particular way, with particular partners, at a particular point in time.

Social Justice

In the context of this work, social justice includes promoting human rights, responding to inequalities in the determinants of health and in access to services, and opposing discrimination on the basis of gender, race, ethnicity, political affiliation and other social or economic characteristics. Health promotion programs have the opportunity to promote social justice, human rights, and dignity by respecting community members, responding to inequalities and discrimination. This issue is perhaps one of the trickiest due to its complexity.

Social Cohesion

Social cohesion reflects the quality of social relationships, mutual obligations and respect within communities and the wider society. At a societal level, violent conflict disrupts social networks and destabilises the political, social and economic life of a community. Considering how the tensions might have harmed relationships and understanding what could help repair them will contribute to the development of more responsive community and health services.

Good Governance

Governance refers to the processes and means through which groups and organizations manage their resources and run their programs. Good governance in the health and social sector involves ensuring sound approaches to project design

TABLE 15.1. Examples of indicators within Health and Peace-Building Filter core concepts

Cultural sensitivity	• integrate traditional, local and western interventions for health and community development; • modifying clinic hours to respect local needs and practices
Conflict sensitivity	• training to assist staff to deal with issues related to the armed conflict • building trust is important when attempting to bring communities together for service delivery
Social justice	• assuring equity of access to services with particular attention to the most vulnerable in the community; • particular attention to engaging women in all phases of project activity
Social cohesion	• health programs offer an avenue to repair fractured social relations and build new ones by proposing mechanisms for dialogue and joint activities
Good governance	• purposeful involvement of range of community members • base action on agreed priorities to avoid suspicion concerning collusion or corruption

and implementation. Good governance includes a number of characteristics such as transparency, accountability, opportunities for community participation, contributing to building capacity, and ensuring cooperation and coordination with other stakeholders, with other sectors, equitable distribution of services and information, and effective mechanisms of accountability (Zwi, Bunde-Birouste, Grove, Waller & Ritchie, 2006). An example of each indicator in a health-related context is presented in Table 15.1.

The tool gained the name "Health and Peace-building Filter" (Filter) as the original scope requested by the funding agency was to design a framework to monitor and assess the peace-building potential or elements of a program. Although the trials of the Filter has indicated a much wider potential application for the tool, the name has been retained, given that it provides as its initial emphasis that it is not a recipe for a way of functioning, but more a screen through which to view one's proposed or actual work.

Learning from the Field

The final phase of the Filter's development entailed application of the framework in three countries which have recently experienced severe conflict situations: Sri Lanka, East Timor and the Solomon Islands. The field trials provided the opportunity to validate the pertinence of the concepts upon which the Filter was founded, and provided important learning about its use as a tool. Some illustrations follow.

Assessing Cultural Sensitivity

Cultural sensitivity includes sensitivity to context-specific concepts, even when they may clash with alternative viewpoints. In order to contribute to peace building and minimize harm, decisions about language and importing "foreign ideas" need careful consideration. A story illustrating this point was shared with us while we were in Sri Lanka. It involved a donor funded school-based mental health healing and promotion program, which included preparing and providing meals during the workshops. Certain castes in Sri Lanka do not eat the same food as others. The project team, comprising Sri Lankans with their ex-patriot project leader, discussed this at length and decided that they needed to respect local cultural practices, and not push for all of the children to eat the same. Pushing a different and, in the Western sense, more "equitable" practice of everyone getting the same meal, would have, at that time, disrupted community cohesion rather than built it. The team considered that, in this instance, the caste system provided grounding to the displaced population and that trying to change things too fast was unrealistic and potentially damaging. In that difficult atmosphere of a post-conflict situation, meddling in local culture could have negative consequences and be more destabilizing than if one tried to work with current understanding.

At the same time, new ideas can give people a common language, a space to learn and work with each other, and provide a new common approach and procedure to enhance community well-being and services. Sensitivity is the key here – it is essential to take the time to examine the context, consider the implications of how best to act and at what point in time. This concept of examining context cannot be stressed enough and is particularly important in the second principle: Conflict Sensitivity.

Appraising Conflict Sensitivity

An example of the importance of conflict sensitivity arose during our field trials in an East Timor water project. The project team was considering enabling two villages to share their water source. These villages had managed to co-exist peacefully on the surface, but previously had had a history of tensions between them. Without knowing and taking into account the reasons for the tensions, implementing this project, where a vital life source is to be shared, could have made the tensions resurface. A major point in conflict sensitivity, which has already been referred to here, is that of trust. Mistrust contributes to suspicion and may exacerbate tensions in situations prone to violence and instability.

Considering Social Justice

A striking example of social justice issues is illustrated in post-tsunami housing in Sri Lanka. The tsunami hit Sri Lanka in an area that had long been impacted by the civil war. Post-tsunami aid was thus being delivered in an area that was already facing the needs of post-conflict resettlement, with the displaced people being given a monthly stipend to assist them resettling after the hostilities. In the influx of post-tsunami aid, affected community members were also given support – except that the level of support was significantly higher than that of those nearby who had been impacted by the conflict, but not the tsunami. In addition, these non tsunami displaced communities were still in just as much need, as illustrated in the poignant testimony "We watched the aid trucks roll right by us".

In conflict-affected settings, pressure to improve social justice and human rights may be considerable. It is important to realize that building social justice and human rights will be progressive, and will take time, rather than happen overnight. Projects must be careful not to seek change at a rate that cannot be absorbed by communities.

Ensuring Social Cohesion

An illustration of the importance of ensuring social cohesion was made clear to us in post-tsunami Sri Lanka where, prior to the tsunami, different fisher-people had had different roles. Some fished with nets, others with boats. After the tsunami, donations of boats were wide-spread and most received one. This meant that the former boat people, who depended on net-fisher people and others, found themselves without the labor they had previously had for support. This generosity of donors thus destabilized the community cohesion and economic structure rather than contributing to building it.

It is important to consider ways in which people identify themselves and potentially establish differences between themselves and other groups. In some circumstances health promotion programs can provide an opportunity to bring people together around a common cause. Much care is needed, however when attempting to build bridges between groups which have been violently divided, as new services can easily become another source of contention in the community. Here again cultural sensitivity also comes into play.

Psychosocial well-being is of course an important part of rebuilding social and community cohesion. People's perceptions of their safety, their future, their community, their sense of control over their lives and of hope significantly affect their individual and collective well-being. The Butterfly Garden in Sri Lanka is an innovative program of accompaniment and healing for war-affected children, and reconciliation at community level. It builds on research from multi-country studies on psychological distress in war-affected children.

Assessing Good Governance

An excellent example from our field research of the need to consider the quality of governance involved an expatriate health advisor, and his transformation to a more peace-promoting approach to his work. One of the communities where he was to support rebuilding of health services wanted to develop a healthy communities' project and seek funding from the government. He assisted the community to prepare and submit its proposal, but no communication was forthcoming regarding what had happened to the proposals; initially in discussions with our project team he rather shrugged and indicated that this was par for the course, and that people accepted it as "the way it is". After working with the Filter, however, he came to realize that without a clear process to let communities know how proposals are evaluated, and without communication about what is happening to the proposals, tensions can rise; in particular if some communities are seen to get returns and others not. The health advisor taught his colleagues how to develop ways to follow the dossier through the hierarchy and advocate for its support from the Ministry. The group eventually got the support they sought and are on the way to building their health promoting community.

This example makes clear that, under the principle of good governance is included community capacity-building and empowerment. A project that contributes to peace building is one that is inclusive and involves community members in all key aspects of its design and implementation, including decision-making, and particularly supporting marginalized groups to have their voice heard.

Consolidating for Maximum Impact

Just as the most effective HP involves a combination of strategies, the most effective health and peace building efforts consolidate all the different fundamental principles. Individually each principle is important, but their collective integration into a project will provide an environment more conducive to peace-building.

There is an inspiring example of bringing the principles together during our work in the Solomon Islands. On the island of Malaita, issues over land have been rising; there are distinct communities living in the mountains from those living on the coast. Culturally land ownership is in a sense sacred as people have a holistic ecosystem consideration of life. The mountain people at times need to come down off their own lands because there are no services in the highlands. When they have to stay for prolonged periods of time, this puts pressure on land on the coast, owned by others. While they are on the coast, the mountain people live where they have no land rights and no access to means of support. In addition, ethnic and cultural tensions run throughout as the bush people from the mountains are feared and misunderstood. Pressures rise, and there are risks of violence. To avoid the increasing tensions, a mountain village leader has worked with the local hospital to build a culturally appropriate housing ward for the mountain people on the grounds of the hospital. The housing ward recognizes the specific gender cultural practices and also offers an equitable access to care for the bush people from the highlands. Included in the land donated are spaces for the bush people to garden, thus reducing the strain on them and their coastal relatives. These different initiatives should contribute to lessening tensions, and over time, build social cohesion. In addition the chief has designed a plan to rebuild a local clinic in the mountains to provide services for the 3000 plus people who live in villages scattered among the mountain heights. His strategic plan is designed to address the cultural specificities of the different tribes in the highlands. He has involved the villagers and bush people in the design and development thus far, and has now come to the point where he needs appropriate certification from government. In addition they need resource support, as these people live off the land and have very little need for hard currency.

It is likely that bureaucratic obstacles and lack of communication will occur when the village tries to get information and support from necessary authorities.

These governance issues may have the capacity to undermine the fragile peace that is building among the two communities. This is also an example of the importance of conflict sensitivity as previous tensions in the country have been sparked by land issues. Support from local and regional health officials is crucial. If the decision makers along the way have been sensitized to peace building principles, there is hope that the initiative will contributes to maintaining and building the currently fragile state of peace.

Contributing to the Evidence Debate: Future Directions

Throughout the field trials, the Filter has proved to be an engaging "tool" with which to consider the interface between health and peace-building (Zwi, Bunde-Birouste, Grove, Waller & Ritchie, 2006). An example of a section from the Filter can be viewed in Figure 15.1. The development process coupled triangulation of learning from the pilot applications with a creative design that evolved following pilot users' feedback. The resulting Filter has high potential as a useful tool for the planning, design, monitoring and evaluation of health promotion initiatives in fragile settings. Although its newness precludes confirmation of its widespread value, all indications lead to it being able to contribute to health promotion practice with the desired impact of intervention being achieved effectively. Learning from the trials indicated that one of the most valuable aspects of the Filter is likely to be to be its ability to provide a simple framework for discussions – to support managers in mapping out the areas of concern and ensure that the implementing agency is given some clear guidance as to the issues that need addressing. The Filter complements and extends traditional modes of assessment and monitoring by ensuring attention to less quantifiable dimensions of project activity, and shedding light on the relationships and processes underpinning health-related activities in fragile settings. In so doing, debate and response to issues such as building trust, promoting social cohesion and social justice, or assuring cultural and conflict sensitivity, is legitimised, normalised and enabled (Zwi, Bunde-Birouste, Grove, Waller & Ritchie, 2006).

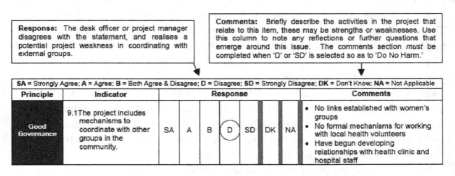

FIGURE 15.1. Example from Health and Peace-Building Filter

The Filter focuses on health, and was initially designed to be used by the project management staff of a donor agency working in development. However, feedback indicated that the principles and approach taken make the Filter adaptable to more widespread use, in other sectors, and with other stakeholders, including the non-governmental, and possibly the governmental sector itself. The Filter is not a prescriptive tool; rather, it can be either descriptive, diagnostic, or analytic. It can identify areas where projects already apply peace-building principles, or highlight where such principles might be included in project design. In addition it draws attention to where health-related activities might make matters worse and provides suggestions for further actions and resources.

The project team seeks to promote further use and reflection on the Filter, and to stimulate debate on the underlying context in which the benefits to be derived from its application may be maximised. The Filter should probably be used early in the design and planning of projects and programs. It is a tool to be used with sensitivity, by an intelligent practitioner to assist in enhancing the quality and value of a project or program, to facilitate reflection, and careful design and implementation. The Filter offers opportunities to open out space in which critique and reflection can be legitimised and enabled.

In closing we would like to reiterate that the complexity of health promotion action makes it improbable that one can actually "measure" the full impact of this practice on peace-building activities. We propose that measurement is not the essential element; what is important is that the concepts are systematically considered, and built into any project or program design and implementation, and monitored throughout to maximise positive impact, and to ensure that harm is not inadvertently done in the field (Zwi, Bunde-Birouste, Grove, Waller & Ritchie, 2006).

References

Anderson, M. B. (1999). *Do No Harm: How Aid Can Support Peace – Or War*, Lynne Rienner Publishers, Boulder, Co.

Bunde-Birouste, A., Eisenbruch, M., Grove, N., Humphrey, M., Silove, D., Waller, E. & Zwi, A. (2004). *Background Paper I: Health and Peacebuilding: Securing the Future*. The School of Public Health and Community Medicine, University of New South Wales, Sydney. Available from http://healthandconflict.sphcm.med.unsw.edu.au.

Bush, K (2003). PCIA Five Years On: The Commodification of and Idea. In A. Austin, M. Fischer & O. Wils (Eds.), *Berghof Handbook Conflict and Dialogue Dialogue Series No. 1 Peace and Conflict Impact Assessment (PCIA)*. Berghof Research Center for Constructive Conflict Management. Available from: http://www.berghof-handbook.net/index.htm.

Bush, K (1998). Peace and Conflict Impact Assessment (PCIA) of Development Projects in Conflict Zones. *Working Paper No.1 – The Peacebuilding and Reconstruction Program Initiative & The Evaluation Unit*, IDRC: International Development Research Centre, Available from http://www.idrc.ca.

Darvill, S. (2004). Economic Strategies for Conflict Resolution: From Development Economics to Peacebuilding Economics. *International Symposium on Resources and Conflict in the Asia-Pacific*, Metcalfe Auditorium, NSW State Library, Sydney, Australia.

Gaigals, C. with Manuela Leonhardt. (2001). Conflict-Sensitive Approaches to Development: A Review of Practice. *International Alert, Saferworld, IDRC*: London, UK. Available from http://www.bellanet.org/pcia/documents/docs/conflict-sensitive-develop.pdf.

Gutlove, P. &. Thompson, G. (2003). Human Security: Expanding the Scope of Public Health. *Medicine, Conflict & Survival* 19(1): 17–34.

Human Security Center. (2005) University of British Columbia. *Human Security Report 2005*. New York: Oxford University Press.

IUHPE (1999). *The Evidence of Health Promotion Effectiveness: Shaping Public Health in a New Europe*; A report for the European Commission by the International Union for Health Promotion and Education, © ECSC-EC-EAEC, Brussels – Luxembourg, 1st edition. Paris: Jouve Composition & Impression.

The Journal of Humanitarian Assistance (2000). *A Health-to-Peace Handbook.* http://www.jha.ac/Ref/r005.htm.

MacQueen, G. & Santa Barbara, J. (2000). Peacebuilding through Health Initiatives, *British Medical Journal*, 321, 293–296.

McQueen, D. V. (2003). "The evidence debate broadens: three examples," Editorial, Social and Preventive Medicine, 48(5): 275–276.

McQueen, D.V. (2002). "The evidence debate," invited editorial in Journal of Epidemiology and Community Health, 56, 83–4.

McQueen, D.V. (2001). "Strengthening the evidence base for health promotion." Health Promotion International, 16(3): 261–268.

McQueen D.V. & Anderson L. (2001). "What counts as evidence? Issues and debates," Chapter 4 in Rootman, et al., pp. 63–83. Reprinted in Debates and Dilemmas in Promoting Health: A Reader, 2cd. Ed., Edited by M. Sidell, et al., Milton Keynes: Open University Press, 2002.

Ottawa Charter for Health Promotion (1986). WHO/HPR/HEP/95.1 http://www.who.int/hpr/Santa Barbara, J. & MacQueen, G., (2004). Peace through Health: Key Concepts, *The Lancet* 364, 384–386.

UNSW Health and Conflict Project (2004). *Issues Paper I: Health and Peacebuilding: Securing the Future.* AusAID, Canberra. Available from: http://healthandconflict. sphcm.med.unsw.edu.au.

WHO (2003). *Mental health of refugees, internally displaced persons and other populations affected by conflict.* Available from: http://www.who.int/hac/techguidance/pht/mental_health_refugees/en.

Zheng, B., Hall, M., Dugan, E., Kidd, K. & Levine, D. (2002). Development of a Scale to Measure Patients' Trust in Health Insurers. *HSR-Health Services Research*, 37(1): 187–202.

Zwi A., Bunde-Birouste A., Grove N., Waller E. & Ritchie J. (2006). *The Health and Peacebuilding Filter* and *The Health and Peacebuilding Filter: Companion Manual.* Sydney, School of Public Health and Community Medicine, University of New South Wales. Available from http://healthandconflict.sphcm.med.unsw.edu.au.

Zwi, A., & Grove, N. (2006). Challenges to Human Security, Reflections on Health, Fragile States and Peacebuilding. In A. Melbourn (Ed.) *Health and Conflict Prevention*, (pp. 119–137). Sweden: Gidlunds forlag.

16
The Role of Governance in Health Promotion Effectiveness

MARILYN WISE

Governance

Governance refers to the various ways in which social life is coordinated. Government can be one of the organisations involved in governance – but not the only one (Heywood, 2000; p. 19). Governance is the process whereby societies or organisations make important decisions, determine whom they involve and how they are held accountable (Plumptre, 2006). Governance is the means by which societies and organizations harness, legitimise and use power to set goals, to identify problems and solutions, to create and manage assets and resources; to design and deliver services and programs, to ensure accountability to constituents or members; to ensure that the rights and interests of all residents/citizens/customers are represented and protected; and to build partnerships to enable people/organizations/governments to work together to achieve mutually beneficial objectives (Dodson & Smith, 2003).

The principal modes of governance are markets, hierarchies and networks. Markets coordinate social life through a price mechanism which is structured by forces of supply and demand. Hierarchies include bureaucracy and thus traditional forms of government organisation, and operate through "top-down" authority systems. Networks are "flat" organisational forms that are characterised by informal relationships among essentially equal agents or social agencies (Heywood, 2000 p. 19).

In the 21st century one of the principal challenges for health promotion is to bring about changes in societies and individuals so that all people have equitable access to the conditions needed to achieve and maintain good health. Health promotion, as a field, has long understood the relationship between social conditions and personal health choices, and has understood the need for all sectors in society to contribute to good health. Considerable scientific effort has been invested by the health sector (in particular) to identify policy instruments (and programs or services) that will contribute, effectively, to improving the health of populations (or at least to reducing specific behavioural or environmental risk factors). More recently, there has been investment by the health sector in the development of assessment tools to assist the health and other sectors to identify the actual or potential population health impact of policy decisions. Health Impact Assessment and the Equity Gauge are two examples of tools developed to assist policy makers in all sectors to assess, a priori, the potential effects of their decisions on the health of populations, with particular focus on the equity of the distribution of these effects.

However, health promotion has devoted much less time to understanding the politics of social decision making and has been slow, or perhaps, reluctant, to recognise that the distribution of power within society and organisations to make social decisions is an independent social determinant of health.

Governance is about power, relationships, and processes of representation and accountability – about who has influence, who decides, and how decision-makers are held accountable (Plumptre & Graham, 1999; Dodson & Smith, 2003). Governance determines the quality of social decisions about **what** policy instruments and programs or services or products are considered to be desirable or effective, and **how** the most effective of these are adopted and implemented.

Multiple organisations at local, state, national and global levels make decisions that affect the health and well-being of individuals and societies. The concepts of "good" governance, from the perspective of promoting health, apply to each of these organisations (as structures) and to the processes used by each to make decisions. Ensuring that organisations responsible for health promotion as their core business adopt the standards of good governance is necessary for the future of the field, itself, as a discipline or component of the health sector. In addition, working with other sectors to develop standards of good governance in relation to health promotion will be necessary as evidence of the relationship between governance and the decisions made by organisations (relevant to health) evolves.

What are the Elements of "Good" Governance?

Systems of governance should be assessed by their consequences. (Arneson, 2004, 40). The United Nations Development Programme (1997) put forward a set of principles that guide much subsequent work in the area of monitoring governance. (Graham et al, 2003). The principles are not only about the results of power but about how well power is exercised. This approach deems that good governance exists where those in positions of power are perceived to have acquired their power *legitimately*, and there is appropriate *voice* accorded to those whose interests are affected by decisions. Further, the exercise of power results in a sense of overall *direction* that serves as a guide to action. *Performance* is a fourth criterion: governance should result in performance that responds to the interests of citizens or stakeholders. In addition, good governance demands *accountability* between those in positions of power and those whose interests they are to serve. Accountability cannot be effective unless there is *transparency and openness* in the conduct of the work being done. And, finally, governance should be *fair*, which implies conformity to the rule of law and the principles of equity (Graham et al, 2003).

The World Bank identified six measures of good governance (as pre-requisites for the reduction in poverty within nations) and conducted analyses of these in 213 nations over the last decade. (Kaufmann, Kraay & Mastruzzi, 2005). These criteria include indicators that reflect the extent to which countries have been able to implement "good governance" going beyond the normative statements of the UNDP and IOG's principles (Graham et al, 2003) above.

- Voice and accountability
- Political stability and the absence of violence
- Government effectiveness
- Regulatory quality
- Rule of law
- Control of corruption

Indigenous organisations seeking to codify rules for effective self-governing organisations in Australia defined governance as having four main attributes (Institute on Governance (IOG), 1999; Plumptre & Graham, 1999; Sterritt, 2001; Westbury, 2002; cited in Dodson & Smith, 2003).

legitimacy – the way structures of governance are created and leaders chosen, and the extent of constituents' confidence in and support of them;

power – the acknowledged legal and cultural capacity and authority to make and exercise laws, resolve disputes, and carry on public administration;

resources – the economic, cultural, social and natural resources, and information technology needed for the establishment and implementation of governance arrangements; and

accountability – the extent to which those in power must justify, substantiate and make known their actions and decisions.

Including the concept of "voice" overtly with accountability, as the World Bank has done, is an important refinement, implying that good governance requires a high order of participation on the part of the people being "governed" in deciding on agendas, in deliberating on issues, and in taking the decisions – for which the organisation and its members are to be held accountable. The groups and organisations responsible for establishing these criteria have determined that the quality of governance is a prerequisite to ensure that societies, communities and organisations have transparent, secure, and fair means of social decision making, and hence, of creating the social, economic, and environmental conditions necessary for good health – and for its equitable distribution.

There are no universally agreed upon measures or indicators of "good governance" that apply to health promotion, in particular. Nor has there been a significant body of research to affirm the positive relationship between good governance, the implementation of effective, efficient policies, services, and programs and the health of populations. However, Navarro and colleagues (Navarro, Muntaner, et al, 2006) have verified the relationship between politics, government and health outcomes at national levels; Wallerstein's review (2006) confirms the positive relationship between empowerment and health at local levels, in particular; and globally, the World Bank's work appears to affirm that those countries which meet the criteria for good governance are more likely to experience (using their outcome measure of poverty) lower levels of poverty.

As a field, health promotion has taken steps toward the definition of criteria of "good governance" – most often described as "organisational capacity to promote health" – but it has applied these, most fully, to organisations within the health sector responsible for promoting health and to specific health promotion projects. Important though these steps have been, the achievement of equitable population health outcomes implies that it is necessary to expand the scope of ambition to include all the organisations and structures responsible for social decision making – including governments and private sector organisations.

Pathways Between Governance and Population Health

"Only countries (or communities) led by their own people and their own governments can ultimately make the decisive changes that are needed to fight poverty" (Benn, 2006) and, it might be added, to create conditions in which all citizens can become healthy and sustain positive health and well-being throughout their lives. Further confirmation of the relationship between the means of governing and health is provided by the experiences of First Nations communities in Canada, where self continuity (expressed as self government) has been found to result in reduced rates of suicide among young people in some communities (Chandler & LaLonde, 1998). Taking a long-term view, Szreter (2003) found that widespread improvements in the life expectancy of populations in newly industrialising countries in Europe in the 19th and early 20th centuries occurred only when an expansion of the political voice of the growing urban masses began to influence public policy, particularly with respect to the distribution of social resources, through their voting power from the late 1860s onwards. While Sen has famously pointed out that there has been no famine in India since the implementation of representative self-government (Sen, 1999).

Empowerment, expressed as participation and engagement, has been shown to contribute to the effectiveness of health promotion interventions directly and indirectly (Wallerstein, 2006), although most of the evidence is built on action at local community levels.

On a nation-wide level, Frey and Stutzer (2005) found evidence of a positive relationship between participating in social decision making and self-reported well being. Their study found a positive relationship between self-reported well-being and participation rights in the political mechanisms of decision-making (in Switzerland) – ranging from voting in elections, launching and voting on referenda, to running for a seat in parliament. These elements of participation may provide a feeling of being involved and having political influence, as well as a notion of inclusion, identity and self-determination. With the rights to participate, the decision to participate is left up to the individual whether to actually participate or not. Persons may value the right to participate even if they rarely exercise it themselves.

But at national and global levels, in particular, the right to participate in social decision making as it has evolved in some modern democracies has not translated into universal social engagement. The power to make or at least to influence, social decisions and their outcomes is highly differentiated across class, race, and, often, gender (Schlozman, 2004; Bartels, 2002).

One of the challenges for health promotion in the 21st century is to reclaim the focus of the work to place greater emphasis on the political and social determinants of health – to return to the roots of modern public health, with the added wisdom of historical analysis (Szreter, 2003) that highlights the need not only to empower and build the capacity of people and populations that have been excluded by current public policies and practices (and discrimination) from social decision making, but also to change the structures and processes through which the social decisions that shape our societies are made.

Based on the values of social justice, fairness, the application of democratic principles, and a sense of collective responsibility with the aim of achieving "health for all", (Minkler, 1998; p. 6), health promotion has understood the need to combine good process and a high level of technical knowledge and skill to bring about the widespread social change that is necessary to enable all citizens of all countries to achieve and sustain good health. Evidence has grown of the impact of democratic, participatory decision making on positive health outcomes.

Pathways between good governance and the health of populations are still being mapped and evidence is still evolving. However, there is some evidence that points to the role of "good governance" and the health and well-being of populations. Societies or communities in which there is a high level of trust among citizens and between citizens and the organisations and agencies responsible for designing and delivering services or programs or products tend to be healthier (Putnam, 1993; O'Hara, 2004). Trust of this kind is built on a base of respect and tolerance for diversity, transparent decision-making processes combined with transparent reporting procedures to account for progress (or not), and on the extent of the legitimacy given to organisations or individuals to speak on behalf of (to advocate for) groups or communities or society. The implementation of measures to prevent or control corruption, to ensure that the rule of law prevails everywhere and to all citizens equitably has also been found to contribute to the health of populations – directly and indirectly. The availability of, and fair, just distribution of social resources (including, but not only, financial resources) is a further critical element of "good governance".

Good governance is defined by the extent to which the structures and processes used to make social decisions in any context (local, state, national or global) actively engage all citizens (or their representatives) in decisions affecting their health – not only in the personal sense of making positive personal choices, but in the social sense of making positive social choices to create conditions for health – ensuring equitable access to the social determinants of health.

It means, too, ensuring that the processes established to self-govern are deliberate, transparent, and committed to the achievement of equity, and that they enable direct actions to be taken to ensure accountability, to eliminate corruption, and to ensure that the rule of law supports fairness and equity, and is enforced impartially.

The criteria proposed in this paper to assess the quality of governance for promoting health are:

- participation and power
- legitimacy
- appropriate *voice* accorded to those whose interests are affected by decisions
- transparency
- accountability
- competence, including control of corruption
- respect for and fair application of the rule of law

Governance and Health Promotion

Health promotion as a discipline is based on values of social justice and equity that in turn, imply that all people have the right and opportunity to participate actively in the decisions affecting their own lives and their societies. Active participation in social decision making is essential to good health. Conversely, one of the most powerful ways in which to deny people the opportunity to achieve and maintain good health is to deny or exclude people from participating in the decisions that affect their health – that is, in all decisions about the creation and distribution of societies' resources.

On one level, it is possible to find overlaps between elements of good governance and the concepts, practice and indicators of organisational capacity for health promotion that have been developed by the field over the last decade, in particular. (Crisp et al, 2000; Laverack & Wallerstein, 2001; Jackson et al, 2003; Hawe et al, 1999). There is, now, evidence of the organisational infrastructure and processes that constitute good governance within the field. There is evidence, too, that this capacity does result in more effective programs and services, and in empowered people and communities and that it does, also, have positive impacts on health outcomes (Wallerstein, 2006).

However, the persistence and scale of inequalities in health status that exist within economically developed societies, and between the populations of economically developing nations and developed nations, necessitate further investigation of the concept of governance – to identify the components of governance that are critical to the health of populations and to identify standards and indicators that can be used to improve practice by and within the field.

Power

Power to shape and make social decisions is at the heart of governance and it is the effective use of such power that is the focus of the evaluation of "governance" in health promotion.

Lukes and Gaventa identify three levels of power in society (Lukes, 1974; Gaventa, 1980). They describe three levels of political power that people and populations must be able to access if they are to be able to influence social decision making. The first level is a simple form of pluralism where various forums exist for the expression of concerns, which are then discussed and hammered out by the actors and players involved in the community. At this level of power equal access to the decision making table is assumed, (Hess, 1999) but Schlozman et al's work (2004) highlights the fact that access to the table is highly skewed in most countries, including democracies.

The second dimension of power realises that to benefit from the pluralist level you have to have enough power to get your items on the agenda. Following on Schattschneider (1960) and Bachrach & Baratz (1970), Lukes observes that the rules within any decision-making system inherently bias the mobilization of resources for formulating agendas against some individuals and groups versus others. Furthermore, because only a few issues can be handled on any agenda at a time, many items simply never make it on the agenda (Hess, 1999).Those that do make it to the agenda are addressed from the perspectives of groups that are likely to be more advantaged and hence are more likely to be resolved in their favour.

The third face of power relies upon the ability of communities to create their own set of issues for the agenda. Lukes and Gaventa believe that traditionally weak or minority communities have difficulties defining what issues they wish to see on the agenda. Like Gamsci, Luke and Gaventa are concerned that weak communities may have their aspirations manipulated. In other words, patterns of relations within a community may be so weakened (or oppressed) that issue identification may not develop (Hess, 1999).

Recent experience has demonstrated the power of civil society in challenging the policy agendas and outcomes of governments and global organisations – on issues such as the environment, HIV/AIDS, and women's rights, for example. These movements have reframed political agendas, have engendered high levels of support within some groups in civil society, have provided high quality evidence of alternative policy choices, and have persisted in their efforts across considerable time. There is much to be learned from such experiences.

However, for health promotion to succeed in the 21st century, for the redistribution of the resources necessary for equitable health outcomes across the globe, more evidence is needed. Political inclusion is necessary – to enable all social groups to participate in and influence decision-making not only from the "outside" (civil society) but also from the "inside" – from within government, the private sector and the non-government sector (Gaventa & Valderrama, 1999).

Political inclusion is necessary not only because it is the right of all citizens to participate fully in their societies' decision-making, but also because "only through close, empathetic engagement with the concerns of others can we gain the sort of perspective that we really require to do true justice to them, their needs and interests, aspirations and anxieties" (Tronto, 1992). Ober (2006) points out that Athenian democracy (the most successful of the ancient Greek democracies) was designed to organise the dispersed knowledge of citizens – to enable an active exchange of useful social and technical knowledge among diverse teams of citizens, to promote learning, and to improve the chances of developing and implementing innovative and effective policies. In this, Athens succeeded for 300 years.

What public officials hear clearly influences what they do. Because citizens differ in their opinions and interests, the level playing field of democracy requires that we take seriously the fact that citizens differ in their capacity, and desire, to take part politically (Schlozman, 2004).

Schlozman et al, in a US study found that a relatively small proportion of the population was active in politics, a group that is anything but a random sample of the population as a whole. The politically active differ from those who are politically quiescent along a variety of dimensions that are germane to politics: in their demographic characteristics; in their needs and preferences for government action; in their policy priorities (Verba, Schlozman & Brady, 1995).

The consequences of this are that public officials are disproportionately more likely to hear from people with certain politically relevant characteristics – the higher an individual's family income, the more active in politics. Using eight participatory acts as criteria (voting, campaign work, campaign contributions, contact, protest, informal community activity, board membership, and affiliation with a political organisation), groups of American stratified by family income displayed the same patterns of "success" or "benefit" as is true for positive health outcomes – those with the greatest income (or education or occupational level) are most likely to be active in politics (and thereby most likely to ensure the protection or furtherance of their own interests) (Schlozman, 2004).

Examination of the actual content of the messages associated with participatory acts make it clear that the fact that public officials hear so disproportionately from citizens in different income (and educational and occupational) groups implies that they get a skewed set of messages about what the public wants and needs (Schlozman, 2004).

This impression is confirmed by an Australian study that found that "the higher a person's income the more likely they are to believe that politicians know what ordinary people think, excluding the lowest income bracket". Furthermore, people with university degrees and middle-class identifiers were more likely (than their less well educated counterparts) to believe that politicians know what ordinary people think (Brenton, 2005).

Schlozman (2004) found that, while both the advantaged and disadvantaged have wide-ranging policy concerns, they differ in the distribution of their concerns. Compared with the issue-based activity of the advantaged, that of the disadvantaged is more than twice as likely, and that of respondents in families receiving means-tested benefits four times as likely, to have been animated by concerns about basic human needs – poverty, jobs, housing, health, and the like. Moreover their activity is more likely to have been motivated by concern about drugs or crime. The activity of the advantaged, in contrast, is more likely to have been inspired by economic issues such as taxes, government spending, or the budget or by social issues such as abortion or pornography (Schlozman, 2004).

When discussing basic human needs policy issues, 15 percent of the disadvantaged – as opposed to 21 percent of the advantaged – indicated that the issue affects them as well as others. Taken together, of those who communicated to public officials about issues of basic human needs, 71 percent of the disadvantaged, but only 29 percent of the advantaged were discussing something with an immediate impact upon themselves or their families. It is axiomatic in the literature on lobbying that public officials listen more carefully to self-interested advocates who are affected by the policies they discuss (Schlozman, 2004).

But of course, precisely because the proportion of people acting as self-interested advocates from the most socially and economically disadvantaged groups in society is so much smaller than those from more advantaged groups, their voice is "lost" amidst those of the groups with greater numbers and greater access to the public officials. Conversely, because advantaged groups are so much more politically active than disadvantaged groups, public officials actually hear more from the advantaged urging reduced efforts to meet basic human needs than from the disadvantaged suggesting that more attention be given to issues such as jobs, housing, poverty and health care (Schlozman, 2004).

In sum, the same groups that have the greatest political voice are those who are likely to be healthiest – and, not coincidentally, to have the ability to amass the greatest proportion of societies' resources.

Indicators of the distribution of power include the extent to which the structures and processes of governance (of societies or of projects) demonstrate:

- representative range of citizens in elected or appointed positions
- mechanisms in place for civil society participation.

Reconceputalising Participation

Control of the structures and processes that enable participation (at any level of jurisdiction) – defining spaces, actors, agendas, procedures – is, largely, in the hands of governmental institutions and private companies. In some countries, the non-government sector and civil society have greater control of these structures and processes – often occupying a vacuum created by weak or disorganised governments.

Community or social participation refers to participation in the civil society sphere, in which citizens are the "beneficiaries" of government-resourced programs. Political participation, on the other hand, is the engagement of citizens in traditional forms of political involvement e.g. voting, political parties and lobbying (Gaventa & Valderrama, 1999).

Social and project participation has long been identified in health promotion as essential to sustain the relevance, quality and sustainability of projects and programs. This "type" of participation includes consultation or decision making in all phases of a project cycle, from needs assessment, to goal setting, implementation, monitoring and evaluation. Participation, in this sense, is seen not as related to broader issues of politics or governance, but as a way of encouraging action outside the sphere of formally constituted institutions. The focus is on direct participation of primary stakeholders, rather than indirect participation through elected representatives. The scale of such initiatives is, almost by definition, relatively small – local and project based. It has been viewed as impractical and difficult to engage large numbers citizens, in social decision-making (Gaventa & Valderrama, 1999).

Political participation involves the interactions of individuals or organised groups with the state, and involves indirect participation. Here the main focus is on action by citizens aimed at influencing decisions taken mainly by public representatives and officials. Political participation expresses itself in individual and collective actions that include, mainly, voting, campaigning, advocacy, group action and protest – all oriented towards influencing the representatives in government, rather than active and direct participation in the process of governance itself (Gaventa & Valderrama, 1999).

It is the contention of this chapter that if it is to be possible to influence equitable health outcomes it will be necessary to take steps to expand the meaning of participation in social decision making, from engagement of beneficiaries or people already marginalised or disenfranchised, to include the development of broad forms of engagement to enable all citizens to play an active part in policy formulation and decision making in key arenas which affect their lives (Gaventa & Valderrama, 1999). Table 16.1. presents their illustration of this shift.

Inevitably, the scaling up of participation leads those involved in development projects and programs to engage with the state, and with broader issues of governance, representation, transparency and accountability (Gaventa & Valderrama, 1999).

It also leads those involved to develop skills in facilitating participation – in working with the wide differences in perspective on goals, problems and solutions that inevitably arise when numbers of people, no matter how well intentioned, come together to make social decisions (Zakus & Lysack, 1998), and to identify processes to ensure that, having arrived at the table, each person has a voice. The methods of deliberative democracy are relevant, offering proven means of engaging multiple voices and perspectives in active debate and decision making on complex social issues.

TABLE 16.1. Redefining the concept of participation

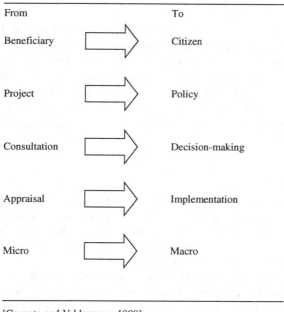

From		To
Beneficiary		Citizen
Project		Policy
Consultation		Decision-making
Appraisal		Implementation
Micro		Macro

[Gaventa and Valderrama, 1999]

Redefining participation in this way implies an expansion of its application in the field of health promotion, and takes up the challenge identified by Minkler (1998) through her work on the Tenderloin Project over many years. The evaluation found that, on the one hand, a theoretically-based and powerfully executed participatory approach did bring about significant shifts in social decision-making power that meant a socioeconomically disadvantaged community was able to improve its environment and health. On the other hand, the evaluation found that the power and sustainability of local actions were swamped by the lack of higher order and higher level political action (Minkler, 1998a). Exercising the rights of citizenship at all levels of governance in countries and communities is vital if health for all is to be achieved.

Indicators to use to evaluate participation as a component of good governance – at the level of a single project, or at different levels of government jurisdiction (local, state, national) might include:

- representativeness and proportion of citizen involvement in decision making – including, but not only, participatory planning, budgeting, implementation and evaluation;
- extent and range of participation in citizen education and awareness building;
- accessibility of and participation in training and sensitisation (to citizen participation) by local officials;
- number and accessibility of avenues through which citizens might participate in deliberating on problems, resources and solutions;

- legal requirements or public commitment by elected officials to account for progress (or at least action) to citizens.

In addition to assessing the "quantity" of participation, however, Laverack and Wallerstein (2001) pointed to the need to assess the extent to which such participation is empowering and developed a conceptual framework for the measurement of this.

Participation is the highest order criterion for good governance. But good governance cannot rest on participation, alone. Vital though it is, the criteria for good governance point to a range of other actions that are necessary if organisations and governments are to meet the standards of good governance.

Legitimacy

Good governance requires that the structures of governance have acknowledged legal and cultural capacity and authority to make and exercise laws, resolve disputes, and to carry on public administration. Among the means to ensure such legitimacy are the methods by which leaders are chosen, and the extent of constituents' confidence in and support of them.

Human societies and organisations have, across all time, developed structures and processes that have the power to decide on the distribution of social "goods and burdens" (Stanford Encyclopedia of Philosophy, 2001). Whether it is a local or at national or global levels, the mechanisms through which organisations are created and leaders chosen are indicative of the likelihood that the decisions made by that organisation will be effective in meeting the needs (including health needs) of their constituents.

For the World Bank and the International Monetary Fund there has been increasing discussion in the last decade of the poor representation, in terms of voting power, of their borrowing member countries compared to the non-borrowing industrialised countries.[*] They, too, are seeking means to better reflect the real changes in the relative weight of the developing countries in the global economy, and the potential to increase the institutions' legitimacy and effectiveness by giving countries most affected by their activities greater power in setting their agendas and policies (Birdsall, 2003).

Possible indicators to assess legitimacy would include:

- public mandate from "parent" organisation within the health sector
- opportunities to nominate for decision-making positions
- civil society representation on selection committees
- publication of the legal or contractual agreement upon which an organisation or project is based.

---

[*] Woods (2000) and Kapur (2002) discuss additional mechanisms besides voting for improving representation of developing countries, including staffing, location of the institutions, use of outside experts, etc.

Appropriate *Voice* Accorded to those whose Interests are Affected by Decisions

The idea of deliberative democracy is that decisions must derive from the collective will of its members based on transparent, inclusive processes of debate that enable all members to express their views and to participate in reaching collective decisions (Button & Ryffe, 2005).

The theory and practice of deliberative democracy offer insights into steps that can be taken to increase the range and extent of citizens' voices in social decision-making. The processes for effective civic engagement form the focal point for this field of scientific inquiry. They have the potential to add to the evidence of effective, empowering practice that has emerged from health promotion practice (and now, theory) and to increase the voices of populations and people previously unheard.

Indicators

Rowe, Marsh and Frewer (2004) developed a conceptual framework, including indicators and questions to evaluate a deliberative conference.
Evaluation criteria included:

- task definition
- representativeness
- resource accessibility
- structured decision making (including discussion)
- independence
- transparency
- influence (impacts)
- early involvement (timeliness)
- cost-effectiveness (cost benefit)

Accountability

Accountability is concerned with the extent to which those in power must justify, substantiate and make known their actions and decisions. Measures of performance need to identify the extent to which performance is responsive to the interests of citizens or stakeholders. This is far from simple – given the range of interests exhibited by different citizens and stakeholders, both across individuals' lifespans and circumstances, and among different groups – determined variously by language, race, culture, sexual preference, and by the consequences of oppression. This is one of the great challenges for the future – to build the capacity of heterogenous populations and communities to work together to make social decisions that are fair and just, as well as efficient.

Accountability is a combination of measuring progress toward goals or targets established through participatory planning and budgeting processes, and/or reporting routinely on this to stakeholders and citizens.

Accountability also rests on the *transparency and openness* in the conduct of the work being done, demanding that there be opportunities for scrutiny of and deliberation about decisions being made and actions being taken.

In many countries good governance is marred by corruption in all or most sectors, including health. Corruption presents a major barrier to action to promote health, particularly, although by no means only, in economically developing countries. It undermines human rights, prevents the application of effective policies or prevents them from achieving their intended outcomes, undermines citizens' confidence and trust in one another and in public officials and agencies, and can cause major health problems (as in, for example, illegal trading of blood or body parts; or selling spurious drugs), and reduce the quality of professional practice (by the use of bribes to obtain qualifications or marks).

Structures – Institutions and their Roles

The structures (or institutions) that make social decisions are critical to health promotion at every level of jurisdiction and practice. At global and national levels, the extent to which the structures enable the interests of a few or of many people or communities or countries to be represented has a critical role in the outcomes that are achieved. (Labonte et al, 2005). At project or program levels, too, the representation of residents or populations in decision making about every aspect of the work is critical to its later success – most particularly, success in reducing inequitable health outcomes.

Enabling Representation in Organisational Structures

Each of the institutions established by society (including those to promote health) needs to broadly represent the rights and interests of all its constituents, to enable them to achieve their collective (and individual) objectives, and to manage internal assets soundly if it is to retain its legitimacy and mandate. Jones (2000) describes the consequences of institutional discrimination for the health and well-being of, in this instance, African Americans.

Sound Corporate Governance

In a review of the literature on the characteristics of systems that have proven effective in ensuring that the governing bodies of organisations (including government, non-government and community organisations) are directed and managed Dodson and Smith (2003) identified the following:

- that the authority, roles and responsibilities of leaders, boards and managers are clearly set out in public policies, and given effect to;
- that decision-making is responsible and fair;
- that governing boards are of an effective composition, size and level of experience to adequately discharge their duties;
- that boards and management are able to understand their roles and responsibilities, evaluate risks, and to safeguard and facilitate the rights and interests of all their members;
- that these roles and responsibilities are periodically reviewed;
- that remuneration for leaders, managers and boards is transparently defined in terms of actual performance against these. (Australian Stock Exchange, 2003: p. 11; Sterritt, 2001).
- that managers and employees are trained, qualified and competent;
- that there are mechanisms for review of complaints and for redress of grievances;
- that civil society (represented by an organisation such as, for example, the People's Health Movement) establishes a strong mechanism to "watch and review" the decisions of organisations and projects; and
- that countries move to establish electoral systems that extend rights to vote to all citizens.

The Limitation and Separation of Powers

There is a need for systems and processes that prevent people who exercise legitimate powers from using that power for their personal (or class or race or gender) gain and from making or changing rules to suit their own interests. This, too, is self evident – but presents a major barrier to overcoming inequity.

Fundamental though the separation of powers is to the successful functioning of states, businesses, and communities, much work is still required to address this issue successfully. In all countries there is evidence of systematic discrimination against the interests of some people and groups or, conversely, of systematic privileging of the interests of some people and groups.

Privilege can be difficult to see for those who are, themselves, the beneficiaries. Power to shape and influence social decisions can be invisible to those who have it; or, if it is not invisible, people and our institutions find ways to codify difference in order to justify discrimination (on the grounds of sex or race or religion, for example) (Jones, 2000).

Explicit actions to limit and separate powers within organizations and government are necessary, combined with strict adherence to transparent decision-making and accountability mechanisms.

Effective Financial Management and Administrative Systems

Sound governance necessitates having access to, and control over, financial, social, economic and natural resources and technology, including information technology (Dodson & Smith, 2003).

Measuring the Effectiveness of Governance

Evaluating the effectiveness of governance for health promotion highlights the fact that the power to make many of the decisions that shape individuals' and populations' opportunities and health choices are often in the hands of relatively few people. Even where these people are highly trained and committed to the principles of justice and equity, there is the potential for the organisations and people committed to change unwittingly (or, perhaps deliberately) to limit the power of their "clients" or "target groups" or citizens to actively participate in decisions that affect their health (in particular).

Governance – the structures and processes through which power to make social decisions is harnessed – has a vital role to play in health promotion, particularly, if it is to be possible to close and ultimately, to eliminate the unjust inequalities in health that have proven so persistent into the 21st century.

The social contract between a government and its citizens is, essentially, a relationship based on trust. The same might be said about the contract (which is often implied) between any organisation and individual working to promote health at any level in society – that a high level of trust among the stakeholders is essential to achieving effective outcomes.

Corruption leads to high levels of distrust among citizens, between citizens and government and its agents, and between government and the private sector (particularly, investors). Transparency and accountability are the significant features of good governance. Corruption, although often linked with the misuse of financial resources, can also involve the misuse of power – unjustly and unfairly excluding people from decision-making and from the benefits of these decisions.

The chapter attempts to identify some implications of the introduction of the concepts and practice of good governance for health promotion theory and practice.

But what criteria might be used, therefore, to assess the quality of governance in general and in relation to health promotion in particular? In what ways can the concept, characteristics and practices be applied to health promotion, particularly, to assist in overcoming current weaknesses in the field and the growing evidence of the social determinants of health with particular emphasis on equity? Some of the key questions that follow are:

Representation

What "structures" or "organisations" play major roles in public decision making relevant to the health of populations?

Who is responsible for making public decisions within (or on behalf of) these organisations?

How are they selected and by whom? How "representative" are they of the diverse populations and perspectives of the citizenry of a given nation, region, or community?

Voice

How to ensure that a full range of citizens (particularly those who constitute minorities within larger dominant cultures) have a voice in social decision making?

What constituencies do the people participating in decision-making represent? How well organised are these constituencies? (e.g. formulating and endorsing policies and agenda items; briefing and supporting representatives)

What capacity (including financial resources) do they have to participate in the process?

What processes are used to set agendas? What processes are used to deliberate on agenda items? How respectful and inclusive are the processes?

What information, from what sources, is included in the debate? Is there an active exchange of social and technical knowledge among diverse citizens? Is learning promoted?

Influence

What methods are used to arrive at decisions – e.g. majority vote, consensus, secret ballot?

What methods are in place to ensure that equity is given priority over efficiency in social decisions?

Why, though, has there been such limited research to establish evidence of a relationship between governance and population health and well-being?

It is, perhaps, a function of the fact that the field of population health has evolved within the context of health systems that are dominated by a view that western bio-medical science (and its 'hierarchy of methods') can and will provide all the answers to improving the health of populations. It is the case that these scientific methods have contributed to significant gains in the health of populations. This "way of seeing" and "of thinking" has close links with contemporary economic theory based on the notion of the "rational man" making decisions based on analysis of "perfect" information.

For health promotion, however, it has never been the case that such rational, research-derived evidence has been sufficient (on its own) to drive the widespread changes in social policy and practice that are necessary to improve the health of populations. The need to engage in the politics of social change has always been obvious. However, the resources invested in health promotion have been limited for the most part so that much of the work has been carried out on a relatively small scale, as projects in local communities. This has resulted in a significant body of evidence of the role of community capacity and empowered citizenship in promoting health, and has resulted in the development of measures of these roles. The challenge of scaling up to national and global levels of action to prevent unjust inequalities in health – as well as to alleviate the consequences of existing inequalities – requires us to revisit the early roots of public health. The scale of change, the need to engage actively in the politics of social decision making, and to work from within governments and organisations, as well as from without, means that a focus on governance is of vital importance.

References

Arneson R. 2004. Democracy is not intrinsically just. In: Dowding K, Goodin R, Pateman C. eds. 2004. Justice and democracy: essays for Brian Barry. Cambridge: Cambridge University Press.

Australian Stock Exchange (ASX) 2003. Principles of good corporate governance and best practice recommendations. Sydney: ASX Corporate Governance Council.

Bachrach P & Baratz M. 1970. Power and Poverty. New York: Oxford University Press.

Bartels L. 2002. Economic inequality and political representation. Campbell Public Affairs Institute. New York: The Maxwell School of Syracuse University. www.campbellinstitute.org

Benn H. 2006. Political governance, corruption and the role of aid. 3rd White Paper speech, London: Royal African Society. www.dfid.gov.uk/news/files/Speeches/2p2006-speeches/gov Accessed on 17 July 2006.

Birdsall N. 2003. Why it matters who runs the IMF and the World Bank. Working Paper No. 22. Center for Global Development. www.cgdev.org/content/publications/detail/2768 Accessed on 2 August 2006.

Brenton S. 2005. Public confidence in Australian democracy. Democratic Audit of Australia. Canberra: The Australian National University. http://arts.anu.edu.au/democraticaudit/ retrieved 6 June 2006.

Button M & Ryffe D. 2005. What can we learn from the practice of deliberative democracy? In: Gastil J, Levine P. eds. The deliberative democracy handbook: strategies for effective civic engagements in the 21st century. San Francisco: Jossey-Bass.

Chandler M, & LaLonde C. 1998. Cultural continuity as a hedge against suicide in Canada's First Nations. Transcultural Psychiatry; 34(2): 191–219.

Crisp B, Swerissen H & Duckett S. 2000. Four approaches to capacity building in health: consequences for measurement and accountability. Health Promotion Internationals 15 (2): 99–107.

Dodson M & Smith D. 2003. Governance for sustainable development: strategic issues and principles for Indigenous Australian communities. Canberra: CAEPR Discussion Paper No. 250, CAEPR, Australian National University. Available: http://www.anu.edu.au/caepr/Publications/DP/2003DP250.pdf Accessed on 30 June 2006.

Frey B & Stutzer A. 2005. Beyond outcomes: measuring procedural utility. Oxford Economic Papers 57 (1): 90–111.

Gaventa, John. 1980. Power and Powerlessness: Quiescence and Rebellion in an Appalachian Valley. Urbana, IL: University of Illinois.

Gaventa J & Valderrama C. 1999. Participation, citizenship and local governance. Background note prepared for workshop on "Strengthening participation in local governance". Institute of Development Studies.

www.ids.ac.uk/ids/particip/research/citizen/gavval.pdf Accessed on 13 May 2006.

Graham J, et al. 2003. Principles for good governance in the 21st century. Ottawa: Institute On Governance.

Hawe P, King L, Noort M, Jordens C & Lloyd B. 1999. Indicators to help with capacity building in health promotion. Sydney: NSW Health Department.

Hess D. 1999. Community organizing, building and developing: their relationship to comprehensive community initiatives. Working Paper for COMM-ORG. the On-Line Conference on Community Organizing and Development. http://comm-org.utoledo.edu/papers/htm. Accessed on 27 June 2005.

Heywood A. 2000. Key concepts in politics. Hampshire and New York: Palgrave.

Institute On Governance. 1999. Understanding Governance in Strong Aboriginal Communities - Phase One: Principles and Best Practices form the Literature. Ottawa: Institute on Governance. http://www.iog.ca/about_us.asp Accessed on 15 May 2006.

Jackson S, Cleverly S, Poland B, Burman D, Edwards R & Robertson A. 2003. Working with Toronto neighbourhoods toward developing indicators of community capacity. Health Promotion International 18(4): 339–350.

Jones C. 2000. Levels of racism: a theoretic framework and a gardener's tale. American Journal of Public Health, 90: 1212–15.

Kaufmann D, Kraay A & Mastruzzi M. 2005. Governance Matters V: governance indicators for 1996–2005. Washington D.C.: The World Bank.

www.worldbank.org/wbi/governance/govmatters5 Accessed on 31 October 2006.

Labonte R, Schrecker T & Sen Gupta A. 2005. Health for some: death, disease and disparity in a globalising era. Toronto: Centre for Social Justice. Accessed on 22 May 2006.

Laverack G, Wallerstein N. 2001. Measuring community empowerment: a fresh look at organisational domains. Health Promotion International 16(2): 179–185.

Lukes, Steve. 1974. Power: A Radical View. New York: Macmillan.

Minkler M. ed. 1998. Community organizing and community building for health. New Brunswick, New Jersey, London: Rutgers University Press.

Minkler M. ed. 1998a. Organising among the elderly poor. Community organizing and community building for health. New Brunswick, New Jersey, London: Rutgers University Press.

Navarro V, Muntaner C, Borrell C, Benach J, Quiroga A, Rodriguyez-Sanz, Verges N & Pasarin M. 2006. Politics and health outcomes. The Lancet Early Online Publication DOI:10.1016/SO1040–6736(06)69341–0, 14 September, 2006.

Ober J. 2006. Learning from Athens: success by design. Boston Review (March/April)

O'Hara K. 2004. Trust: from Socrates to spin. Cambridge, UK: Icon Books.

Plumptre T. 2006. What is governance. Ottawa: Institute on Governance. www.iog.ca Accessed on 13 January 2006.

Plumptre T & Graham J. 1999. Governance and good governance: international and Aboriginal perspectives, unpublished report. Ottawa: IOG.

Putnam, R. D. 1993. Making democracy work: civic traditions in modern Italy. Princeton, NJ: Princeton University Press.

Rowe G, Marsh R & Frewer L. 2004. Evaluation of a deliberative conference. Science, Technology and Human Values 29 (1): Winter, 99–101.

Schattschneider E. 1960. The Semisovereign People: A Realist's View of Democracy in America. New York: Holt, Rinehart and Winston.

Schlozman K. 2004. What do we want? Political equality. When are we going to get it? Never. Inequality and American Democracy, Campbell Public Affairs Institute. New York: The Maxwell School of Syracuse University.

Schlozman K, Verba S & Brady H. 2004. Political equality: what do we know about it? In: Neckerman K. ed. Social Inequality. New York: Russell Sage Foundation.

Sen A. 1999. Development as freedom. New York: Knopf.

Stanford Encyclopedia of Philosophy (Stephen Gosepath). Oct 8, 2001. Equality. California: Stanford Encyclopedia of Philosophy, Metaphysics Research Laboratory, Centre for the Study of Language and Information, Stanford University. http://setis.library.usyd.edu.au/stanford/entries/equality/ Accessed on 1 June 2007.

Sterritt N. 2001. First Nations Governance Handbook: a resource guide for effective councils. Prepared for the Minister of Indian and Northern Affairs, Canada.

Szreter S. 2003. The population health approach in historical perspective. American Journal of Public Health 93(3): 421–432.

Tronto J. 1992. Moral Boundaries: A Political Argument for an Ethic of Care. New York: Routledge.

United Nations Development Programme. 1997. Good governance and sustainable human development. New York: UNDP.

Verba S, Schlozman K & Brady H. 1995. Voice and Equality: Civic Voluntarism in American Politics, Cambridge, Mass.: Harvard Univ. Press.

Wallerstein N. 2006. What is the evidence on effectiveness of empowerment to improve health? Copenhagen: WHO Regional Office for Europe (Health Evidence Network report). www.euro.who.int/Document/E88086.pdf Accessed on 1 February 2006.

Westbury N. 2002. The importance of Indigenous governance and its relationship to social and economic development. Unpublished Background Issues Paper produced for Reconciliation Australia, Indigenous Governance Conference 3–5 April, Canberra.

Zakus J & Lysack C. 1998. Revisiting community participation. Health Policy and Planning 13: 1–12.

Section 4
Global Debates about Effectiveness of Health Promotion

17
Evidence and Theory
Continuing Debates on Evidence and Effectiveness

DAVID V. MCQUEEN*

At the heart of the Global Programme on Health Promotion Effectiveness (GPHPE) is the notion of evidence. While most in health promotion desire to prove that there is evidence, even considerable evidence, that supports the work of those in the field of health promotion, one cannot escape the view that the notion of evidence rests uncomfortably with many of the concepts and principles of health promotion. That is one reason why the IUHPE, as the unique global professional organization for health promotion, took up the considerable task to address evidence effectiveness in a prolonged and ambitious project. The results of this project, which will continue at least through the decade, are a surprising and hopefully enlightening discussion of the debate around evidence in health promotion.

The field of health promotion is eclectic and multi-disciplinary. Many would argue that the great strength of the field is that it values pragmatism and eschews more narrow approaches. Indeed, part of the mantra of the field is to not work in silos, to value that which is cross-cutting and partnership enhancing. Similar to most fields of practice, analogous to medicine itself, there is both an art and a science base to the practice.

Multiple approaches to improve health, reorient health care systems, and empower people are welcomed (WHO EURO, 1984). Many of the principal activities of health promotion pertain to advocacy, partnerships and coalition building, areas considered more an art than a science. Furthermore health promotion is a field of action, highly applied, and having few characteristics of a discipline. Unlike medicine, health promotion is relatively new as a concerted field of action, still defining its terms. Many key concepts which health promotion hopes to embrace, including the word "evidence", do not appear in the WHO Health Promotion Glossary (WHO, 1998a).

Despite many definitional and conceptual challenges health promotion is quite well established in many dimensions. There are foundations, centers, institutes, schools, departments, buildings, professorships and programs named with the term "health promotion". Thus health promotion presents a dilemma with regard to the debates and discussions about evidence and effectiveness. The dilemma is

---

* The views and opinions in this chapter are those of the authors and do not necessarily reflect the views of the Centers for Disease Control and Prevention of the Department of Health and Human Services.

simply this: should health promotion look to classical scientific approaches for the assessment of evidence and effectiveness? Or is it more appropriate to take a very different approach? Because this is a true dilemma, the answer cannot be one position or the other. Recognizing this dilemma opens the possibility to explore the successful evaluation of health promotion practice on many different terms. Of particular note is the possibility to explore the dimensions of individual academic disciplines in contrast and their relationships to one another in an effort to lead to an approach that is acceptable to the multi-disciplinary field of health promotion practice.

The advantage of exploring the individual disciplinary approaches is that many people who work in health promotion, especially those who need to be convinced of its importance and effectiveness, are discipline trained. The very nature of our Western-based university system is to organize both the sciences and humanities around disciplinary bases that have been articulated over a considerable period of time. Thus there is a good rationale for respecting the "rules of evidence" put forward by scientists working in public health when making the case for the effectiveness of health promotion. At the same time, there is the need to respect and assist in the development of health promotion's own efforts to define the evidentiary field of health promotion.

The debate on evidence for health promotion centers on the fundamental problem of defining the field and the dimensions that belong to its practice. Part of the problem lies with the theoretical underpinning of the field, an issue that will be more elaborated elsewhere in this chapter. Health promotion is not alone in theoretical weakness; both public health and health promotion have been theory-weak and practice-strong. This is the product of their developments as fields of action. They share the constant challenges of whether they should focus on the individual or the social context or some combination of the two. They share the ongoing debate of how much they are rooted in the biomedical or in the social/behavioral sciences. The outstanding feature that would distinguish health promotion from public health is the stronger implied foundation of theory and practice based on the social sciences, whereas the biomedical model strongly underpins much of the practice of public health. Nevertheless, the development of health promotion is closely related to the historical and practical development of public health.

The Growth of Tradition and Ideology

Over the years different orientations towards health promotion have developed in the research and practice community, stemming from perspectives of public health. Roughly speaking, a dichotomy exists between two traditions which could be termed "medical public health" and "social public health". These two traditions are not necessarily in conflict, but they often give rise to differing interpretations of the underlying mission of public health which in turn affects the evidence debate. Essentially, medical public health regards epidemiology as the basic science of public health with a view of causation that is linear. This perspective relies heavily on "evidence" gathered by methodological approaches which feature experimental designs. In addition there is usually a stress on the individual as the focus of public health programs with the goal to influence changes in behavior. In contrast, a "social public health" considers many disciplines to be relevant and places emphasis on the human sciences such as sociology, politics and economics. Causation is not regarded as necessarily linear, with patterns of change and complexity as expected outcomes of interventions.

Health promotion fits historically with both of these public health traditions. However, in addition, health promotion has an underlying ideology that distinguishes it. Elsewhere I have argued for an ethos of health promotion, which helps define the nature of the field (McQueen, 1996). This ethos is manifested through a debate primarily on methodology, but seldom on theory. This ethos also helps to shape the evidence debate. This "ethos" in health promotion has research consequences: there is less emphasis on sophistication in quantitative analyses, and more on qualitative approaches. Further, the ethos was increasingly framed in post-modern terminology, for example one position is that sophistication in data analysis may have the effect of providing detail too elaborate or inscrutable for the general needs and use of community health workers and policy makers, introducing the paradox that some of the key notions such as dynamism, multi-disciplinarity, complexity and context might demand rather innovative and complex data collection procedures and analyses, whether quantitative or qualitative. This ethos helped reform the evidence debate.

Complicating the picture on assessing evidence and effectiveness for health promotion is the history of health promotion itself. As it developed in the last third of the 20th century health promotion took on different perspectives in different countries. Notable was the difference between the United States and the European Continent. In Europe, health promotion was largely framed by concerns with the social, economic and political roots of health and offered a strong focus on the sociopolitical environment as the place for health promotion action. This was also the primary experience of Canada as witnessed by the elements and importance of the Ottawa Charter. This focus remains a strong component in European health promotion. (The emphasis on the "social determinants" of health is an element of this way of thinking about public health and health promotion). In the USA, health promotion developed largely by extension of the traditional scope of health education, an area of work and academia that was quite well developed institutionally. Given its roots in education and educational psychology, it was logical that the primary focus of health promotion action should be on the individual and on changing attitudes, opinions, beliefs and behaviors. Whether or not modern health promotion, that is the health promotion practiced globally now, has fully integrated these two traditions remains the subject of historical analysis and not of this chapter. Nonetheless, these two traditions will and do influence the meaning and scope of evaluation, evidence and effectiveness in health promotion

A feature that unites these two different perspectives of the field of health promotion is the relationship to the established medical professions and the institutions of medical practice. In both perspectives there has generally been reliance upon the support of established medical care institutions for the appropriate part-nerships to guide the field. On both the continent and in the Americas it is rare to find an institutional base for health promotion outside of a primary medical care center. Health promotion as an academic area is found primarily in schools of public health, medical schools, and allied medical professional schools. Health promotion, as a field of study, is rarely found in disciplinary academic depart-ments such as sociology, psychology, biology, political science, et cetera. In fact, it is still rarely established as a first degree or undergraduate field.

Why is defining the field of health promotion such a critical issue for assess-ing evidence of effectiveness in health promotion? Partly the answer is that core disciplinary areas are generally ancient and have over many years defined their boundaries and the core concerns of their discipline. In addition, they have usu-ally developed a strong methodological approach that allows members of the discipline to recognize what the rules for evidence are in their discipline. There is not a remaining need to convince outsiders of the tenets and standards of the discipline; fundamental questions of theory and method have been addressed.

As a relatively recent field of practice, health promotion does not have the luxury of years of theoretical and historical development, thus the need for health promo-tion to prove its utility to both the sceptics and those who support the rhetoric of health promotion; thus the rise of what I have termed elsewhere the "evidence debate" (McQueen, 2002).

In the 1990's the evidence-based medicine discussion was extended to both health promotion and community-based public health interventions. The assump-tion is that this is a critical debate, and that it is necessary to demonstrate what constitutes evidence and proof that actions are effective. Although, the terms of the debate stem from clinical medicine rather than preventive medicine, the appli-cation of evidence criteria has taken evaluation down a path implying scientific rigor and justification.

Evidence, Effectiveness, Evaluation

These three words are commonly found in the health promotion literature. They have very different meanings, while at the same time sharing poor definitional clarification. Even in a chapter devoted to evidence, there is little hope to ade-quately define the words evidence, effectiveness, and evaluation. It is not because of a lack of definitions available, but rather that there are many definitions avail-able. In general, the definitions tell you more about the definers than the object being defined. To begin with, these are all highly conceptual terms, and as such, are all linked to areas of knowledge that are also conceptual. To the extent possi-ble these concepts will be defined here in terms of their usage in the development of the GPHPE program, and in addition the reader should rely upon the myriad definitions and uses of these terms as applied by the authors of the other chapters.

When one asserts that a causal relationship exists between one variable and another, the strength and validity of that assertion is evidence that the relationship is real. In another sense, evidence is the strength of the knowledge base for what works. In any case, evidence remains a highly conceptual word used when we have knowledge that something strongly relates to something else. In positivistic science this "evidence" can often be precisely stated, in many cases modeled, and in some cases even expressed in a deterministic mathematical formulation. In empirical science this "evidence" is often the end statement that results after observing in a large number of cases that two or more variables always (or in general) relate to each other in a highly probabilistic way. In more general usage "evidence" may be a statement based on judgment that when one entity is present another entity is generally present. An example of each of these will suffice. In the first case when one drops an object from a height, it will fall to the ground in a fashion that is almost entirely described by a deterministic mathematical formula; in the second case when one sees dark cumulus clouds in the sky there is a very high chance that there will be rain; in the third case, if we see a person discharging a pistol into a crowd, there is an expectation of harm. In each case there is a conceptualization of evidence and one would argue that in each case there is a reasonably high expectation of the outcome. Nonetheless, the reader will immediately recognize that these are simple, not complex, examples of the concept of evidence. By changing the context in any of the examples, the notion of evidence becomes more problematic. For example, if one "drops" an object while in orbit around the earth, the mathematical formula becomes unclear; if one sees dark clouds when the temperature is far below freezing, we may have no precipitation; if the pistol is a stage prop with blanks, we expect no harm.

Effectiveness is quite different from evidence. Unlike evidence, it does not arise from a strong epistemological base. Effectiveness is much more about translating evidence into application. Judgment plays a major role in the concept of effectiveness. Effectiveness is related to the understanding of change processes, as opposed to the description of causation itself. An underlying assumption in the GPHPE is that we are interested in how to intervene in the causal process in order to stop, retard, maintain, or accelerate the causal relationship. For example, if we show evidence that smoking can, with a definable probability, lead to lung disease, then we want, as health promoters, to intervene in that causal process. In the case of smoking we would strive for interventions that prevent or stop an individual from initiating the possible causal chain – a no smoking approach. Effectiveness is concerned with our intervention's ability to actually affect the causal pathway. Effectiveness, like evidence, is easier to assess and measure when the intervention is simple and the causal pathways are well described.

Evaluation is a very broad concept, much more open to interpretation than evidence or effectiveness. Nearly every field of human endeavor may be evaluated whether or not there is any relationship to science. However, in the second half of the 20th century evaluation took on a strong scientific-based dimension in the natural and social sciences. As a result there is a huge interest in evaluation, a large industry of consultants and specialists in many different forms of evaluation. Furthermore, there is almost an expectation that any program or human effort should be evaluated. From its beginnings health promotion has been concerned with evaluation. In the early 1990s a group of health promoters concerned with evaluation efforts in health promotion formed a working group that met for nearly a ten year period, producing a number of products, but chiefly resulting in a WHO publication on evaluation in health promotion (Rootman et al., 2001).

The working group consisted of some 18 people drawn from Europe and North America. Their task was to better define the principles and perspectives of evaluation in health promotion. Indeed, at an early stage the discussion centered on trying to carefully distinguish evaluation as it applied to health promotion and to develop those characteristics most salient to the field. As the discussion developed over the years, there was an effort to carefully define evaluation in terms of health promotion and set out a general model for evaluation. The subsequent main publication from this working group consisted of chapters by authors from the working group mixed with chapters that were invited by a core editorial team from the working group. The resulting publication was eclectic, but also critically defined evaluation in health promotion and examined the chief problems arising in carrying out evaluation.

What is remarkable about the work on evaluation in health promotion is how the themes that must be dealt with are so similar to the issues around evidence and effectiveness. In that sense, one can view the evidence debate as a drilling down into one particular aspect of evaluation. What is most pertinent in the 10 year study of evaluation in health promotion is the role of theory and methodology. These two areas remain highly pertinent to the evidence debate as well. Furthermore, many of the issues associated with theory and methodology bring in the same debates about complexity and contextualism. In brief, the related notions of evidence, effectiveness and evaluation share a commonality when it involves the world of health promotion.

Organized Efforts to Discover Evidence of Effectiveness

Throughout the globe, there have been many efforts to undertake comprehensive approaches to answer questions with regard to evidence and effectiveness in public health and medicine. It is not the purpose of this chapter to provide a guide or review all of these efforts. In any case it is clear that there is a huge literature available on the subject of evidence and effectiveness in public health and medicine, a literature that has been steadily accumulating during the past 15 years. The reader who wants further insight into all these efforts should consult the numerous websites, documents and the considerable literature that has accumulated. (e.g. www.keele.ac.uk/depts/li/hl/pdfs/ebhi4patients.pdf, www.cochrane.org/, www.thecommunityguide.org/, www.nice.org.uk/, www.health.vic.gov.au/healthpromotion/quality/evidence_index.htm).

Despite the accumulated literature, it would be incorrect to assume that there is anything nearing completeness to this effort to assess evidence and effectiveness. In addition, with specific regard to health promotion and its concerns, there is far less available than one expects. The efforts to work on evidence and effectiveness for health promotion are far more recent, far less developed and woefully under-funded in most instances. Furthermore, when we look to see the efforts on building evidence in interventions that focus on areas that are outside the medical context, for example interventions that focus is on changing social determinants or communities or that are complex in their number and variety of variables, then the efforts are few. That is why the GPHPE effort was undertaken by the IUHPE.

In the United States, there are the ongoing efforts of an independent Task Force to produce a *Guide to Community Preventive Services* (referred to as the *Guide*). The Guide defines, categorizes, summarizes, and rates the quality of evidence on the effectiveness of population-based interventions and their impact on specific outcomes. The Guide summarizes what is known about the effectiveness and cost-effectiveness of population-based interventions for prevention and control, provides recommendations on these interventions and methods for their delivery based on the evidence, and identifies a research agenda. This effort is an example of an approach that takes a strong biomedical/epidemiological definition of evidence (Zaza, Briss & Harris, 2005). Much of the Guide's work has gone into defining evidence in terms of how interventions are designed (SAJPM, 2000). What this effort has revealed is that finding evidence of health promotion effectiveness is not an easy task and that methodological decisions steer the type of results that emerge.

The scope and size of the task taken on by the Guide is huge, and this illustrates the potential breadth of studying interventions in a field like health promotion. In the case of the Guide there are some 20 members of the Task Force, chosen because of their broad knowledge of public health, preventive medicine, and health promotion. They are an independent body with representatives from local health departments, health care organizations, NGOs, and universities. In addition consultants are attached to the Task Force. The Task Force is supported at the HHS agency CDC by a staff of senior researchers, research assistants and administrative workers, federal agency liaison members, outside organization liaison members, and multiple liaison representatives of CDC offices, institutes and centers. The author of this chapter has served as a senior advisor since its inception.

The aim here is to illustrate the size and scope of effort that is necessary to take on a systematic, long term review and assessment of a large body of interventions in many fields that are pertinent to health promotion. In the evidentiary assessment of interventions, hundreds of studies are reviewed, evaluated and examined by a team of many abstractors using a rigorous evaluation protocol. Nonetheless, this search for evidence has been limited to published literature accessible to data retrieval systems such as MEDLINE, Embase, Psychlit, CAB Health, and Sociological Abstracts. Generally only publications written in English, published since 1979, and conducted in industrialized countries and studies that meet the evidence criteria laid out by the Guide team (SAJPM, 2000) are considered. This is not to criticize the effort, but rather to emphasize that even a large-scale project has necessary limitations and has to define its parameters. A large body of findings has been produced by the Guide and should be carefully considered by those working in the field of health promotion.

European Efforts: The IUHPE Report to the European Commission

An approach to evidence more rooted in health promotion was taken by the International Union for Health Promotion and Education (IUHPE). An advisory group, consisting of 13 senior persons in the health promotion field, 15 authors and a "witness group" of some 25 "political experts" produced a report for the European Commission (EC) on the evidence of health promotion effectiveness (IUHPE, 1999). The great value of this report, required reading for those in the field of health promotion, is that it identifies a considerable body of evidence pointing to the value of health promotion and attesting to its effectiveness. The report was also clear to recommend those areas where more research was needed, as well as those open to debate about effectiveness. Some areas of health promotion activity stand out as having unquestionably powerful value, for example the evidence of a strong inverse relationship between price and use of tobacco. Therefore, health promoting efforts that lead to price increases of tobacco, should lead to less use of tobacco. This finding mirrors those of the CDC group working on tobacco for the Guide. Thus there is an accumulating international evidence-base for global efforts to reduce tobacco consumption through pricing.

Health promoting efforts with regard to tobacco control appear as the "strong case" in the evidence debate. Other areas of health promotion activity noted by the IUHPE Report, however, require careful thought and further analysis to reveal effectiveness. For example, transportation policies impact health in many ways. However, demonstrating the efficacy of such policies is difficult. In this case complexity begins to play a major role. While many may believe that there is a highly probable association between transportation policy and the general health of a population, the evidence mechanisms to prove any scientific basis for this belief still need refinement. The derived standard is to develop as a first step a distinctive logic model or logic framework to demonstrate the causal links of each area of a health promotion intervention to an outcome. This logic model helps map out the links between social, environmental and biological determinants and related interventions. These models then serve as a guide for assessing where the evidence challenges are. The challenge is for the model to lead to an understanding of apparently true relationships, such as that between transport policy and health.

Despite all the difficulties with the notion of evidence, the writers of the EC report concluded that evidence clearly indicates that: 1) comprehensive approaches using all five Ottawa strategies are the most effective; 2) certain "settings" such as schools, workplaces, cities and local communities offer practical opportunities for effective health promotion; 3) people, including those most affected by health issues, need to be at the heart of health promotion action programmes and decision making processes to ensure real effectiveness; 4) real access to information and education, in appropriate language and styles, is vital; and 5) health promotion is a key "investment" – an essential element of social and economic development (IUHPE, 1999). These findings ultimately led to the development of the idea for a more comprehensive global approach that became the GPHPE.

Evidence and Conceptual Challenges for Health Promotion

During the past 30 years of the growth of health promotion we have witnessed a number of key theoretical ideas entering into the conceptual background of health promotion. Many of these ideas are discussed in detail in a recent publication on modernity and health (McQueen et al., 2007). However, in this chapter the emphasis is on three theoretically based ideas that impinge on the search for evidence in health promotion. Each idea presents a significant challenge to the field and merits the attention of anyone concerned with evidence and effectiveness in health promotion.

As mentioned earlier, health promotion prides itself on being multi-disciplinary, multi-sectoral, and embracing of many different perspectives in its practice. However, a major by-product of such openness is the introduction of complexity. Complexity as a concept has two general forms, in the simplest form it alludes to the general difficulty to understand something and in a broader sense the degree of complication of something, for example a system or a structure, in terms of the number of components, intricacy, and connectedness of the structure. Many now recognize the complexity of social structures, social change, and the complex infrastructure that derives from the context of health promotion practice. The idea of multivariate settings and situations is an idea that grew in part in response to the ability of modern day computers and statistics to handle multivariate problems. It is not that the world wasn't complex before, but that the computer has allowed scientists to address more complex problems. Health promotion picked up this profoundly different and emergent idea of complexity.

With regard to assessing evidence and effectiveness, complexity makes the effort extremely difficult. Several factors are pertinent. First, causal relationships that may indeed be operating in a complex situation cannot be "seen". That is, the methodological skills to analytically "pull out" the true relationships either do not exist or may be inaccessible to most practitioners in the field. Second, few practitioners can imagine and/or construct a complete model of the complexity. That is, when the system is very complex so many variables are operating that the researcher/practitioner cannot possibly anticipate all those that should be included in a relevant model. Third, measurement (discussed in Chapter 18 by Campostrini) of many important variables remains problematic. Often variables under consideration range from dichotomous to ratio and often possess non-linear characteristics. Despite these difficulties health promotion can hardly deny that it is a complex field of action.

Those forces that deny complexity are a challenge for health promotion. Simplicity is easier to argue than complexity because: a) cognitively, people want a single direct causal connection to an outcome; b) most causal models are conceived of as linear with discreet interconnecting causes; and c) traditionally science tends to be reductionist in its relationship between theory and proof, stripping away complexity to understand the "true cause". Further the placement of health promotion institutionally has generally been in places with more traditional approaches to science and public health. Complexity is a real problem because it masks what many would like to see as the real or main reason why something happens. Further, there seems to be an innate need in people to understand precisely why something succeeds or fails. In short, simple answers are preferable for many.

The second theoretically based idea that impinges on the search for evidence in health promotion is that of "contextualism". To begin with contextualism is an idea that is anathema to theory building because it goes against the grain of the search for standards, universality, comparability and best practice. Obviously all human activity takes place in contexts; exploring the idea more deeply only adds layers to that observation and reveals how social actions are related to the context. The challenge is trying to grasp the meaning of contextualism when we want to understand evidence.

Contextualism reveals the limitations of the science related to logical positivism, the view that reason alone may lead to an understanding of society. This view, of course, has been severely challenged by recent thinking in the philosophy of science that more or less parallels the modern thinking leading to health promotion. The philosophy of science has moved relatively seamlessly from the logical positivism of the Vienna school (Suppe, 1977) to embrace those of Kuhn and followers. Further, contextualism has allowed cynicism, skepticism, relativism and deconstructionism to be seen as appropriate approaches to understanding the human condition. For health promotion, a field of action steeped in practice that occurs in a context, contextualism provides an approach to excuse the idea that there is any easy way to link practice to observation or observed effects that can be generalized. Indeed the principal effect of contextualism as an idea is not skepticism or hopeless complexity, but its attack on the notion of generalizability. Further it argues that reality is directly in the context and not in a more abstract notion derived from theory. In turn this notion implies that it is the context itself in which consensus can be found. Many health promoters practicing "in the field" have this notion almost as a mantra. If one argues that a health promotion program that works in Chicago couldn't possibly work in Jakarta because of contextualism, then it is *ipso facto* difficult to come up with a common theory of a health promotion program for large cities. Thus so-called evidence of best practice and notions of "effectiveness" are seriously compromised.

The third theoretically based idea that impinges on the search for evidence in health promotion is the notion of reflexivity. In contrast to contextualism, which lies mainly in the social fabric outside the individual, reflexivity lies primarily within the individual. This is an elaboration of the concept as developed by Gouldner and others. Essentially the argument is that we frame or construct our theories based on our own biography. For example, if one develops a theory that is based on dynamism, accenting change over time, it is in response to a deep-seated inner need to understand why change occurs. Furthermore, and most pertinent for health promotion, deep-seated opinions and beliefs may be highly emotional and even based in moral consciousness. But Gouldner makes another linkage on reflexive sociology that is relevant to this evidence: " . . .those who supply the greatest resources for the institutional development of sociology are precisely those who most distort its quest for knowledge. And a Reflexive Sociology is aware that this is not the peculiarity of any one type of established social system, but is common to them all" (Gouldner, 1970, p 498). The parallel to the development of health promotion as a field and its institutions is clear. Health promotion, as a field of action, often fails to be reflexive and reveal the parameters of individual motivations for its work. For evidence this is a threat of prejudice and error.

Reduction Versus Complexity

In the real world of events, whether they are physical, biological, or social, complexity is the operating principal. Everything takes place in a context that is open to the impact and relationship of many variables. In the classical, notably positivist, approach to science experimentation often follows a methodology that calls for the reduction of complexity in a multivariate situation. This is the classical case where one tries to "control" for all variables other than those directly in the causal relationship you want to test. The RCT is a classical reductionist approach. However, most other experimental designs, including quasi-experimental designs are also reductionist. The underlying assertion is that, by holding constant all other variables that might interfere with the ability to see a causal relationship which does exist, but is masked by other causal variables, one can reveal the primary relationship that one desires to prove. Essentially, reductionism is a simplifying process.

The acceptance of complexity leads one away from reductionist methodologies. There are a number of reasons for this. First, the real world of events consists of phenomena that are made up of many elements (variables) that interact in a mixture of orderly and chaotic ways that are the parts of the whole phenomenon. Second, the whole is more than the sum of the parts; that is why simple reductionism, or deconstruction, does not always work as a methodology. Third, it is entirely possible that changes in parts of the whole are difficult because of the properties that bind all the different components of the whole. Fourth, the argument is also made that change can occur in complexity primarily because of forces within the whole and not due to any external forces or agents. Fifth, the relationships of component parts may not be simply deterministic, but in fact random or even chaotic, which leads to grave problems in assigning or seeing causal relationships. Finally, complexity makes the idea of knowledge very problematic, particularly how one creates knowledge. There are other important elements of complexity that go beyond these six issues, but are not considered in this brief chapter.

For the assessment of evidence as it relates to health promotion effectiveness, the position one takes on the continuum of absolute reductionism to total complexity determines not only an investigator's methodological approach, but also one's view of how evidence is created. Clearly evidence is easier to agree upon in situations where complexity is minimized; where very clear causal pathways operate and variation among very few variables is limited, linear and highly deterministic. As the health promotion interest or intervention becomes more multivariate, less metric and measurable, and highly contextual, that is as complexity increases, evidence of effectiveness becomes difficult to explain in positivistic terms and the more one turns to judgment as a form of evidence.

Building Evidence, Methodologies and Values

It can be argued that the type of methodology we use will determine the kind and nature of evidence that we will find. It is not the purpose of this chapter to go into the details of the debate on methodology ; that can be found elsewhere and it is well discussed in numerous publications. However it is important to see the methodological concerns as very broad. Too often, those seeking methods for evidence are mired in the intricate details of constructing abstracting forms, analyses of research designs and assessing whether an intervention has drawn an appropriate statistical sample. In reality, methodology begins with a careful conceptual consideration of how one is to develop the evidence in a particular area of intervention.

The concepts and principles of health promotion directly impact the methodological debate. As discussed in considerable detail in the book *Evaluation in Health Promotion* (Rootman et al., 2001) health promotion is an area of involvement that stems largely from some underlying values that relate public health actions to health. Evaluation efforts and their underlying methodological approaches are informed by and transformed by these values. Thus one cannot separate the concepts and principles of the field of health promotion from the methodologies that are appropriate to its evaluation. Indeed, it is a value that evaluation itself should, in the general case, be health promoting.

Similar arguments may be made for the methodological approach to evidence in health promotion. This raises a peculiar issue for health promotion and evidence, because in most of the "classic" literature on evidence, scientific-based methodology is at the forefront. Thus the literature in this "classic" approach debates issues such as random controlled trials versus comparison studies. The approach is clearly one of what is the appropriate "scientific" methodology. However, as will be seen in much of the discussion throughout this book, "scientific" methodology gives a secondary role to methodologies based on judgment. Operationalizing judgment is a key methodological problem in the health promotion literature.

As values enter into the debate around methodology and evidence the concept of harm rises in importance. As is often found, despite the best efforts to find evidence of the effectiveness of an intervention, we are often left with the conclusion that there is "insufficient evidence" to recommend the intervention. This does not mean that the intervention is not effective; it means that one cannot clearly show that it is. Finding insufficient evidence to recommend a health promoting intervention heightens the need for assessing that the intervention at least does not do any harm to the public's health. Despite the considerable importance of this idea of no harm, there is little in the way of methodological guidance as to how to assess it. Human judgment remains the key approach.

Why Theory?

Theory is vital to help set the parameters for a scientific discipline. Nonetheless theory serves a critical role in the conduct of most any interventionist activity and health promotion is no exception. Most critically, theory enters into the evidence debate because it helps avoid a narrow empiricism that concerns itself only with observation and the undirected collection of data. In addition, a sound theoretical base can help one avoid unanchored abstract thought. Health promotion practice has had a history of carrying out complex interventions that are not anchored in any systematic theoretical approach. At the same time large conceptual ideas that are discussed in health promotion are equally found wanting an underlying theory. Finally theory anchors explanations in a field in the rich contextual efforts of many others, particularly those from the basic academic disciplines, who have thought long and hard about why social life is the way it is.

A theoretical perspective forces one to take a certain distance from the object of study and to become skeptical and critical. It also challenges the practitioner to be more reflexive about their individual ideology. That is why a good theoretical approach is so practical for those in health promotion. Consider that many of the chapters in this book are concerned with issues of evidence and effectiveness related to broad conceptual notions such as settings, systems, urbanization, globalization, and peace. These types of topic areas of necessity lead to theoretical approaches from the more macro social sciences as well as the natural sciences. Theory thus becomes a guide to thinking about practice, interventions, and ultimately the evidence debate.

Most academic disciplines have an agreed upon theoretical framework. Health promotion as a non-disciplinary field of action or, in some instances, an ideological stance or "ethos" (McQueen, 1998) lacks a distinctive and consensual body of knowledge. There are numerous introductory textbooks to the field that are very dissimilar in content; this is in sharp contrast to the well-established disciplines in the natural sciences. In the established disciplines basic instructional texts for university are rarely different in content or underlying theoretical perspective. The texts are full of evidentiary illustrations of the practice in the field; underlying theory explains the observed practice.

The lack of theory is not unrelated to the lingering problem of defining health promotion. In essence, to define health promotion is to state a theory of health promotion. Efforts have been made to distinguish the concepts and principles of health promotion, and these efforts have been somewhat documented and at times addressed in a critical discussion (WHO EURO, 1984). The Ottawa Charter has served in many cases as an ideological and conceptual guideline for the field. There have been efforts to describe health promotion in terms of the new public health. Furthermore there have been other efforts to build a consciousness about health leading to a health promotion that goes beyond the medical model. However this effort has been guided to a great extent by force of argument and persuasion as opposed to a link to any theory. It is safe to say that there is not a clearly identifiable theoretical underpinning to the current concepts and principles of health promotion.

Opinion, Judgment, Expertism and Evidence

In a monograph on evidence and information, Robert Butcher (1998) defined evidence in a fashion that is most pertinent to health promotion. He wrote: "A piece of evidence is a fact or datum which is used, or could be used, in making a decision or judgment or in solving a problem. The evidence, when used with the canons of good reasoning and principles of valuation, answers the question why, when asked of a judgment, decision, or action." The challenge for the notion of evidence from a health promotion perspective is on the role of judgments in relation to assessing the effectiveness of action. However it is more than simply a matter of judgment. What is experienced in the quest for evidence of effectiveness is often confounded with issues of expert opinion and bias. In essence it is only once you frame what you are looking for, in terms of postulated effectiveness that one begins to define the criteria for gathering and collecting the evidence.

What becomes very clear in this monograph and in the evidence-effectiveness world outside this monograph is that some areas of health promotion cannot be discussed easily in terms of evidence. Many people, including world recognized experts in health promotion, fall into the trap of stating what would be effective rather than discussing how we could know effectiveness when we see it. Certainly this is not unique to the field of health promotion, but it is exacerbated in health promotion because so many of the topical areas in the field are complex and large in scope.

To illustrate, consider the area of health policy. There is a voluminous and rich literature on policy; it is an area that is addressed globally by many academics as well as those in the non-academic area that are concerned with policy. Yet as a content area it is full of assertions and opinions about what constitutes good policy; it is largely hortative literature. This in itself is not a negative criticism for it is difficult to imagine how else such literature might be. Nevertheless, such an approach rarely sets itself up in a way that can be considered for evaluation. For one thing, in the policy arena there are often many competing expert views on what policy should be as well as the methods to attain it. In the real world few policy decisions are realized in the terms that any single expert or policy advocates specify. In general, policies that do arise are a mixture of many different opinions and the result of complex political and administrative decisions. Thus to trace the evidence that a particular policy approach has been effectively undertaken becomes a monumental if not impossible task. And yet, we are still in need of knowing or estimating whether a particular or general policy has been effective. That is the conundrum that is faced by the search for evidence of effectiveness in some areas.

The above illustration is neither to discount the critical importance of judging effectiveness nor to criticize one particular area of work. Many of the same considerations apply to work on other large topic areas such as globalization, governance, urbanization, and peace-building, and other areas that appear in this monograph. It is simply that often the search for assessment of effectiveness must then turn to questions that assess who are the experts, or put in another way, who are those that have earned the right for their opinion to be so judged. Furthermore, once the experts have been identified, be they academics, lay leaders, practitioners, decision-makers, how can we assess whether their judgment is correct or adequate with regard to assessing effectiveness? A clear difficulty here is that models for assessing such judgmental ability either do not exist or are not as clearly specified and established as those for assessing evidence of effectiveness in "scientific" areas. It remains for future texts and volumes of the GPHPE to address these issues.

Issues Arising in the "Evidence Debate"

Above all, the evidence debate has served to illustrate the need for a stronger theoretical base for health promotion. The debate has made explicit theoretical notions such as contextualism. More than ever health promoters are aware of the social and cultural context in which they carry out their work. This awareness applies at all levels of society. At the local level they are sensitized to local needs and public understandings of health. At the global level they recognize the incredible diversity of nations in terms of development, cultural beliefs, and governance. Despite this accepted awareness of the great diversity in populations, some may still hold the belief that the evidence discussion is not affected by the contextual diversity.

Given the lack of a strong theoretical base, health promotion practice has been and remains difficult to define. The field of practice seems eclectic, encompassing many approaches from a wide range of research perspectives. Every approach seems relevant: policy research, evaluation research, survey research, action research, and social epidemiology. Many concerned with health promotion practice might disagree on the relative importance of the major areas for health promotion, but most would agree that there are critical issues with regard to the following areas: (1) theories and concepts in the field; (2) methodology and the whole issue of the style of research which is appropriate to practice; and (3) issues of application of findings, with an emphasis on translation of research and practice into something useful and oftentimes for the formation of policy.

Methodology remains a critical issue for research and practice in health promotion and directly relates to the evaluation of evidence. Even as the methods used in health promotion have ranged from the qualitative to the quantitative, there is still unease as to what is appropriate. Despite its apparent implausibility as a methodological approach suitable to health promotion, the RCT, or randomized control trial, remains for many who would term themselves health promoters as an ideal to which health promotion research should aspire because it is seen as the most powerful method to use in evaluating interventions. The lingering power of the RCT is witnessed in numerous debates at health promotion meetings for its application. Despite forceful arguments to the contrary by leaders in health promotion evaluation the RCT remains the bulwark for many public health practitioners that are either highly sympathetic to health promotion or would even classify themselves as health promoters. When control of the setting and population under study can be achieved for the time of the trial, and where there is a focus on a single intervention with an expected dichotomous outcome of success or failure, the RCT is indeed a powerful methodology, and there are those who argue fiercely that the RCT or a modified version thereof can be developed for health promotion. Thus the post-modern separation implied by the rejection of a model like the RCT has not impacted on these researchers and practitioners. Nevertheless, the strength of the RCT is directly related to rigidly meeting the restrictive assumptions of experimental design. When the severe restrictions of experimental design are not met, the utility, validity and power of the RCT diminish rapidly. The misapplication of the RCT in health promotion research is now legend (Rootman et al,. 2001). Even if one rejects the strictest classical RCT model, the notions of experimental and control groups remains in studies and projects which use quasi-experimental designs, controls, and all the trappings of the RCT. Unfortunately, for many at the so-called hard end of the hard to soft science spectrum, a softer health promotion methodology seems implausible. In health promotion interventions, control and experimental populations are often unlikely if not impossible. It is part of the very nature of health promotion interventions that they operate in everyday life situations, in a particular context, involving changing aspects of the intervention; outcomes are often decidedly different from expectations; unanticipated consequences of interventions are common and sometimes better than expected outcomes.

Evidence of Health Promotion Effectiveness: Issues for Consideration

The importance of evidence as a topic for health promotion practice should be seen in a larger context of discussions on evidence-based medicine taking place in much of the world, a debate which cannot be dismissed as pertinent only to medicine. Health promotion is also challenged by the debate (Adrian, 1994; Allison and Rootman; MacDonald et al. 1996; Nutbeam, 1998, Sackett, 1996).

Today, health promotion practitioners and researchers are urged to base their work on evidence. In May 1998, the 51st World Health Assembly urged all Member States to "adopt an evidence-based approach to health promotion policy and practice, using the full range of quantitative and qualitative methodologies" (WHO, 1998b).

Notions such as "Evidence", Effectiveness" and "Investment" are rightly viewed as Western derived, European-American, and in many ways European language concepts. Most of those who have written and write about evidence have Western approaches and Western training. These concepts and the biases inherent in them developed largely out of philosophical conjectures of the past two centuries, notably from debates around logical positivism (Bhaskar, 1997; Suppe, 1977). Logical positivism operates on the tenet that meaning is only verifiable through rigorous observation and experiment. In this context the word evidence has a very strict analytic meaning. Similarly, the RCT and the quasi-experimental approach are largely creations of a Western literature and reflect a reification of the positivist notion. Many social sciences, particularly anthropology and sociology, have alternative, but none the less Western-derived approaches to assessing evidence and the effectiveness of interventions.

If there are alternative approaches to the issues of evidence from developing countries, they are less readily accessible even on the global Internet. Yet, the Internet is a hope for the future once access to it becomes more readily available globally. Nevertheless there is another consideration; that is the urgency of emerging public health problems outside the West. We may not have the luxury or time to develop alternative approaches before the problems being faced significantly develop.

Should health promotion programs in the developing world simply proceed with the assumption that they will use approaches that have been shown to meet evidence criteria drawn up in the West? Should there be caution in accepting a Western-based evidence criterion for health promotion? Can developing countries in their search for best practice offer better guidance on how best to evaluate programs with minimal resources? Would other approaches be useful and/or transportable to those many Western countries with great inequities in population health? Addressing these questions is not easy, but they need to be recognized as legitimate concerns.

While the evidence debate in the West has been prolific, voices from developing countries are still missing from the debate. This lack of developing country participation is exacerbated by a debate that has been mainly conducted in the English language by those educated in a European-American context. Furthermore the debate has been largely by a privileged academic elite. The debate must find a way to uncover approaches used by developing nations that are meaningful and these must be incorporated into the existing body of the "evidence debate". However, the mechanism for this remains very unclear and one can even question the legitimacy of such an elite positing an appropriate mechanism for inclusion in the debate.

What the Field Needs

When looking at the state of the art of evidence for health promotion it may seem easy to be pessimistic. Even if we do possess some initial evidence that in some situations health promotion interventions are effective, it is only a small portion of the vast amount of work that is considered health promotion practice. Nonetheless, health promotion has come a long way since its inception and in particular its growing concern with good evaluation. Further, it is difficult to foresee a time when the funders and policy makers of health promotion will cease to be interested in the effectiveness of what they are supporting. Although, health promotion practitioners may not have been able to agree upon the nature of evidence, it is clear that evidence is expected by those who support the field. What can be done to improve the situation?

To begin with, it would be prudent to have a single source for obtaining information about evidence and effectiveness efforts around the world. There are, of course, numerous types of clearing houses, library reference websites and toolkits available to the practitioner. However, to date these always seem to have limitations, particularly in scope. They tend to work primarily with material that is already published, usually in English, and contain literature reviews of mixed standards. The reader of this chapter is invited to search the internet, using any of the powerful, readily available search engines using the words "evidence, effectiveness, and interventions." A wide and diverse inventory of databases and articles will result. Such information may, in fact, be extraordinarily helpful to the health promotion practitioner trying to design a particular intervention. The main difficulties are that the material found in this way is neither systematic nor particularly vetted, and that the literature is limited almost entirely to Western examples. These two difficulties could be surmounted with a dedicated, multilingual, multi-regional effort.

Secondly, we desperately need systematic monitoring or health related social and behavioral data on populations. This data has to be routinely collected as part of an ongoing and sustained information source. Over time, such data provides the baseline information about changes and trends of many of the social and behavioral determinants of health that health promoting interventions are trying to change in order to improve health. Because so many of the topics of interest to health promotion, topics such as urbanization, communities, etc. are population level phenomenon, one must have the background information as to how these phenomena are changing. This is particularly true if, as argued earlier, most health promotion takes place in a complex contextualism, which can only be understood accepting the wholeness. Fortunately we have some monitoring systems such as the US Behavioral Risk Factor Surveillance System (BRFSS) that have been collecting data over time for many years. The potential to use such systems as part of a broad approach to community interventions is worth exploring further.

Thirdly, we need to further develop both the methodological and theoretical bases for evaluation of effectiveness in health promotion. It seems clear that the borrowing or adapting theory and method from approaches to evidence by other fields has left health promotion without a clear vision of how to obtain evidence of effectiveness. In this book other chapters have addressed this in many ways. Sometimes there has been the outright rejection of the approaches of some of the sciences. For example, with few exceptions, there has been a rejection of the use of the RCT design for assessing evidence of effectiveness in health promotion. Nonetheless, it has been difficult to advance alternatives that provide the level of scientific confidence that strong experimental designs offer. The solution would appear to be in more explicit understanding of the theory base of the field. In principal it can be argued that health promotion should look to the sciences that deal with complexity, particularly social complexity, in order to discover the methodological requirements for explanation in these broad sciences.

Finally, and most important, we must realize that health promotion as a practice is in its early stages. We do not have a lot of interventions to evaluate. Further, because our interventions are contextual and complex, we need to have many more interventions to evaluate. The parallel to the broader sciences, e.g. geology or biology, is clear. In order to understand such sciences and develop a theory of explanation, one needs hundreds, if not thousands of observational examples. It is because each observation is so complex and so contextual that one cannot generalize beyond that given example. Imagine trying to derive a theory of evolution by studying a few birds non-systematically over time. What is needed is systematic, over time, careful observation of selected variables in selected contexts that can be consistently and accurately measured. It is this approach that will reveal the evidence that something has indeed changed.

What can we Conclude?

This book, along with the previous literature from IUHPE, CDC, NICE, Cochrane, among others, is proof that there is already available a large literature written about evidence and effectiveness in and of health promotion. Indeed it is certainly safe to say that we have a considerable amount of "evidence" that some health promotion interventions are effective. However it is also clear that systematic and/or comprehensive reviews have only been conducted on a relatively few interventions and these reviews are almost completely based on reviews of published materials appearing in Western journals and primarily in English. It is also clear that the field of health promotion does not possess an agreed upon methodological approach for assessing evidence of effectiveness.

To try and summarize the state of the art is too daunting a task. However, after more than a decade of being directly involved in systematic efforts to look at evaluation, evidence and effectiveness in health promotion it is possible to reflect on some general considerations that are shared by most all efforts to understand evidence. This understanding must be seen in the context of interventions.

When one looks at the many interventions that have been carried out in the name of health promotion, several themes appear. First and foremost, interventions vary

300 David V. McQueen

considerably within themselves. Rarely do interventions share the same variable mix. For example, one may be looking at community based interventions in poor communities in city neighborhoods; interventions that are designed with a participatory approach with the goal to improve the general dietary habits of the participants. In searching the scientific published literature you find that there are some 500+ such interventions that have been carried out and reported upon during the past five years. Seemingly this should be rich terrain for a systematic review. However, as one begins to read through the reported studies it soon becomes apparent that the quality is very mixed. But that is not the chief problem. The chief problem is the apparent lack of shared variables that are going into the interventions. In short, each intervention, as one places it under the microscope appears to be unique, sharing few common characteristics at the specific level. Thus comparability, an underlying assumption one has made about these 500+ interventions is only at the most general and often superficial level. This problem is a direct result of both contextualism and complexity and presents the biggest challenge to the search for evidence.

A second conundrum occurs on further examination of the scope and size of the 500+ interventions we are examining. That is, the scope and size may not be as broad as first appears. Those who practice in the field of health promotion rarely do so independently of one another. In the real world, most interventions are the product of group of like minded thinkers exploring a particular subject of personal interest. This is partly where reflexivity comes into play. Interventions are reported in the literature in patterns that are the product of the producers of the interventions. Typically a study will be analyzed and presented in a number of deconstructed ways in a number of publications. Thus, what may appear as ten articles on an intervention is in fact only the same intervention in ten different lights, often published in a diverse literature in order to spread the potential readership. Further, because research is often the product of a school of thought or tradition, one may simply be viewing the same or similar intervention carried out by students and former students of primary researchers. Thus these studies are not necessarily attempts to replicate findings from a scientific point of view, but rather a shared ideology of how such research should be verified. Thus, the conundrum is that while our 500+ studies are on the one hand difficult to compare, they may also share a common bias that arises from shared values about the intervention.

Third, there is another profound source of error that relates to assessing evidence of effectiveness. Secular trends at the population level occur naturally and may either mask any evidence of effectiveness or may be attributed as an effectiveness of an intervention. This is a profound problem, because health promotion interventions generally are attempts to change behaviors, communities, and systems over time. Yet all these variables change over time in any case. This is in essence the "background noise" of society as it changes over time. It may be seen as a powerful confounding variable in any intervention. The only way to "control" for such a powerful source of error is to understand it by having extremely good over time measures for changes in the population. This assumes that there are available data streams to account for such variables.

Finally, health promotion prides itself in taking an ethical stance that it is concerned with values such as equity, empowerment, participation, et cetera. Given that, it is remarkable how little attention the evidence debate as placed on the notion of "harm". Perhaps this is because, in the early days, it was not easily perceived that one might do harm by "doing good." However, it is easy to make the case that interventions may have negative side effects. Change, whether at the individual or social level, always implies that something else is given up. When change is made in a highly complex system it becomes much more difficult to see what exactly is exchanged. What is remarkable is that most groups that work with the question of evidence invariably turn to the problem of harm. In the most obvious case the notion of harm is a consequence of a common finding of evidentiary review groups. That finding is that, following extensive reviews of a particular intervention, the review group can only conclude that there is "insufficient evidence" to make a recommendation of whether or not the intervention is effective. Unfortunately this is a very common outcome. Why it is so is the core of an extensive discussion, but it remains a fact. The finding of "insufficient evidence" is particularly troubling because of the need to make a recommendation. Should one encourage the continuation of this type of intervention until we can conclusively say it is effective or not? Or, should one take up the question of potential harm done by the continuation of such interventions. In fact there are at least two highly credible harms to consider: 1. the harm to the individuals and/or community being intervened upon, and 2. resources that are taken away from other important intervention areas by the continuation of an intervention considered to lack evidence.

Conclusion

It would be unfortunate to end a chapter such as this on a non-optimistic note. It is very clear that health promotion has taken on the challenge to produce an evidence base for its actions. The "evidence debate" has resulted in all the costs and benefits implied by such a debate and the careful examination of the very premises of health promotion action that such a debate entails. At this point of time it is an assertion of this author that the benefits to the field of engaging in the debate have been highly positive. Some years ago, in the beginning of the last decade of the 20th century I argued that the field of health promotion was at a watershed. It had had its period of intense rhetoric, partly enshrined in the Ottawa Charter and all the hopes being put forward for the future that that document implied, but that it ultimately had to face its won accountability. The evidence debate was part and parcel of that accountability.

Obviously health promotion has not been capable of delivering on all its promises, nor has it been able to show hard evidence for all its work. But show us another area of medicine, public health or social justice that has delivered evidentially on all its promises. Unlike many other areas however, health promotion has taken the proof of practice mantra most seriously and the work on evaluation, evidence and effectiveness to date illustrate that fact. More than perhaps any other field health promotion needs to be careful with what it does. It is a field, unlike clinical medicine, that has limited resources. Therefore it has a mandate to do that which is most effective for the limited resources it has. The attention to issues of evidence and effectiveness will continue to guide the work of the field of health promotion.

References

Adrian, M. et al (1994). Can life expectancies be used to determine if health promotion works? *American Journal of Health Promotion*, 8(6): 449–461.

Allison, K. & Rootman, I. (1996). Scientific rigor and community participation in health promotion research: are they compatible? *Health Promotion International*, 11(4): 333–340.

Bhaskar, R. (1997). *A Realist Theory of Science*. 2nd ed. New York, Verso.

Butcher, R. B. (1998). "Foundations for Evidence-Based Decision Making," in *Volume 5: Evidence and Information, Canada Health Action: Building on the Legacy*, Editions MultiMondes, Quebec.

CDC (2007). *The Community Guide*. http://www.thecommunityguide.org/ Accessed on April 27, 2007.

Gouldner, A. W. (1970). *The Coming Crisis of Western Sociology*. New York, Basic Books.

IUHPE, (1999). *The Evidence of Health Promotion Effectiveness: Shaping Public Health in a New Europe.*A report for the European Commission by the International Union for Health Promotion and Education, ECSC-EC-EAEC, Brussels – Luxembourg. Paris: Jouve Composition & Impression.

MacDonald, G. et al. (1996). Evidence for success in health promotion: Suggestions for improvement. In: Leathar, D., ed. *Health Education Research: Theory and Practice*, 11(3): 367–376.

McQueen, D.V. (1996) "The Search for Theory in Health Behaviour and Health Promotion", *Health Promotion International*, 11:27–32.

McQueen D.V. (1998). Chapter 3, Theory or Cosmology: The Basis for Health Promotion Theory. In: Thurston W.E., ed. *Doing Health Promotion Research. The Science of Action* 29–40, University of Calgary Press, Calgary, Alberta, Canada.

McQueen, D.V. (2002). The evidence debate. Invited editorial in *Journal of Epidemiology and Community Health*. 56: 83–4.

McQueen, D.V. et al. (2007) *Health and Modernity: The Role of Theory in Health Promotion*. New York: Springer.

Nutbeam, D. (1998). Evaluating health promotion – progress, problems, and solutions. *Health Promotion International*, 13(1): 27–44.

Rootman, I. Goodstadt, M., McQueen, D., Potvin, L., Springett, J. & Ziglio, E. Eds. (2001). Chapter 24, There is a shortage of evidence regarding the effectiveness of health promotion. *Evaluation in health promotion: Principles and perspectives*. WHO (EURO), Copenhagen.

Sackett, D. et al. (1996). Evidence-based medicine: What it is and what it isn't. *British Medical Journal*, 150: 1249–1255.

SAJPM, Supplement to American Journal of Preventive Medicine, January (2000). Introducing the Guide to Community Preventive Services: Methods, first recommendations and expert commentary. *American Journal of Preventive Medicine*, 18(1).

Suppe, F., ed. (1977). *The Structure of Scientific Theories*, 2nd ed. Urbana, IL, University of Illinois Press.

WHO(1998a). *Health Promotion Glossary*, WHO: Geneva.

WHO(1998b). World Health Assembly resolution WHA51.12-Health Promotion. (Agenda item 20, 16 May 1998). Geneva: WHO.
http://www.who/int/healthpromotion/wha51-12/en/print.html. Accessed: February 19, 2007.

Zaza, S., Briss, P. & Harris. K. (2005). *The Guide to Community Preventive Services*. Oxford: Oxford University Press.

18
Measurement and Effectiveness
Methodological Considerations, Issues and Possible Solutions

STEFANO CAMPOSTRINI

Effectiveness of interventions in health promotion (HP) is often difficult to articulate, assess, and measure because the outcomes of any policy, program or intervention are often far distant in time from the intervention. Moreover, the observed outcomes may be further complicated by interactions (or effects) from other HP efforts or as a result of the "natural" evolution or "history" of the phenomena upon which a HP intervention takes place. Indeed, changes over time are difficult to detect measure and evaluate. This chapter concentrates on some of the measurement issues.

Given this, knowledge and evaluation of HP effectiveness is quite limited, and often, indirect. As in the Platonic shadows of the *Republic*, effectiveness can be captured by studying the *evidence* that can be produced by an intervention. Like in Plato's allegory of the cave ("To them . . .the truth would be literally nothing but the shadows of the images") it is quite often impossible to decide the absolute truth of the HP effectiveness but rather do one's best in observing (measuring) its shadow (the evidence) and analyze and interpret this to better understand the *noumena*, the realities. In few cases, researchers can organize their effectiveness studies like in many other disciplines, using standard research design (such as random trials) and standard measurement and analytical tools (e.g. standardized survey questionnaire and statistical tests). Often this is simply not possible for theoretical, methodological or feasibility (practical) reasons. So, researchers seeking information about effectiveness of a HP program or intervention should work on looking into which measure (which shadow in the Platonic metaphor) can be more suitable, how this can be properly analyzed and interpreted to gain useful information to evaluate HP effectiveness.

The aim of this chapter is that of offering a first methodological discussion on some of the issues that a researcher should or could afford in the evaluation or, more generally, in the study of HP effectiveness. Since the author acknowledges that to properly discuss many of the methodological issues presented here would require more space than this chapter provides, the goal is to offer an overview of the major issues of HP effectiveness and building the evidence based upon empirical research and evaluated practice from the scientific literature. After this "stroll," more in-depth discussions are provided in the cited literature.

This chapter begins with a fundamental discussion about the importance of time as an essential variable in measuring the evidence of effectiveness in HP: effectiveness often, if not always, is interested in changes or trends of *dynamic* processes. HP wants to offer to the target population knowledge, tools, etc. to allow them to make something to eventually increase their own level of health. This process that operates at individual level, from the HP perspective, is observed at aggregate level, observing changes, trends that show what the HP effort has produced over time. For this reason, e.g. prevalence measures are important in HP, but not as much as knowing their evolution over time: to know that in an interested area the prevalence of young female smokers is 15% could be interesting, but no one can say how much worrying, or how many resources for intervention requires a 15%. To know, instead, that the prevalence of smoking among the young female population in that area is increasing, stable or decreasing could be of dramatic importance, information that could drive HP efforts. HP is not particularly interested in the reality as it appears, as much as in the dynamic that is behind it. To embed time in the measurement and analysis process is the only way to understand these dynamic processes.

The Measurement Process: Measuring Effectiveness, Measuring Health Promotion

The Measurement Process

Before discussing the intricacies of measuring HP effectiveness, it is important to recall the fundamentals of any measurement process. Here I will briefly mention the basics steps (see Fig. 18.1) to help focus the discussion. In the following paragraphs I will look to HP effectiveness in context.

In the measurement process, it is often the case that we are not dealing with easily measurable concepts; i.e., attitude, behavior change, knowledge attainment are not objective outcomes, such as height, length, weight, that are more directly measured. For the latter the only challenge of measurement is that of finding a valid and reliable measurement tool. Rather, in HP we are trying to measure *abstract* concepts that first require a study of their conceptualization (Blalock, 1979) and definition in a more operative way, even to have a broad idea about the kind of measurements that can be applied.

Devising a clearer, more "usable" definition for the concepts in a hypothesis is called *operationalization* or *operationalizing concepts* – because it makes the hypothesis operational or ready to be used. Emphasizing the difficulty of doing this, Julie Ford (Ford, 1975) compares it to building a rope bridge across a chasm between the world of ideas and the world of observation (which she also calls "the world of appearances"). Once the process is established, one needs to define *measurement design*. Social science research offers several approaches

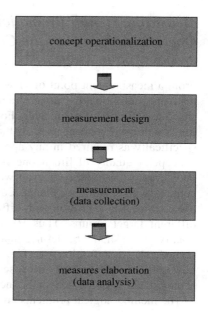

FIGURE 18.1. The fundamental steps of the measurement process

to obtaining "good" measures (valid, reliable, and usable). None can be considered better or always "superior" for it is dependent upon the context, the desired outcomes to measure, funding and time for the activities to be executed. For example, for many years randomized controlled trials (RCT) have been considered the gold standard for research however, other designs have shown improved or similar results, and not only due to reasons of practicability (Black, 1996; Victoria et al., 2004).

Once we have defined what we want to collect and how, the following step is the *data collection* (the third main step). At this point, there is only one worry: measurement error. In real life, errors are omnipresent, as in any process of measurement. Having said this, there are two fundamentals topics upon which we should elaborate: error control and error measurement. These are of major importance because:

• Errors cannot be avoided, but can be reduced;
• Errors *always* influence any estimates, but to know their magnitude can help in allowing for improved interpretation of what has been measured.

We cannot ignore that data collection does not complete the measurement process: data are not, generally, information that can be used, but require analyses and thoughtful reflection to provide insight to any policy and/or decision making process. We use data to create and provide information in many forms: from the construction of simple indicators (like computing simple ratio between two measures) to more sophisticated statistical analyses.

Measuring Health Promotion Effectiveness: Operationalization of the Concept – What do we Want to Measure?

From a measurement point of view one should accept the idea of having more than one definition for an abstract concept; for many abstract concepts an absolute definition it not tenable. For example the abstract concept of quality of life is a derived concept itself that should be defined and declined *hic et nunc*, specifically as required in any application. Thus there is a different notion or concept of quality of life if one is working on the elderly population, or on people with disabilities, or even with the same target population in a specific context, with specific problems. Consequently, it is widely recognized that the same concept is measured with different instruments when one is dealing with different target groups. Thus HP effectiveness related to a concept such as quality of life should be defined in an "operative" (measurable) way, with a contextual relative definition (see Fig. 18.2 for an example). This is perhaps obvious; still, it is rarely done, because of many reasons including a false sense of standardization of a contextual concept.

The methodological problems are related to the fact that the concept of effectiveness usually refers to the outcomes of an intervention, not to the process. As we know, in many HP interventions, outcomes are not observable, either for the time lag in which they can happen, or for the presence of so many other external effects that the practicability of isolating outcomes due to the intervention is substantially impossible. In practice, when outcomes could be reasonably defined, this is not done, or, more often than not, it is done in such a broad sense

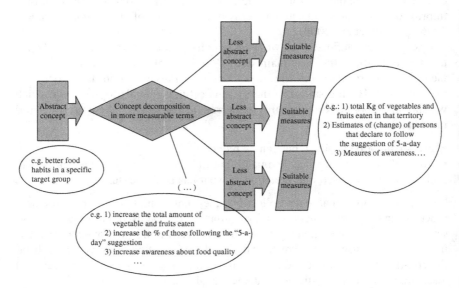

FIGURE 18.2. An example of operationalization of a concept

that the concept of effectiveness is, practically, declined as "any good change"; and outcomes are seen as any improvement in the health status (generally defined) of the targeted population. Because in HP, and generally in public health, often experts are convinced that any intervention is good, or more precisely will do some good to the target. And this is not only a belief; it is given by the simple practical observation that, as opposed to other health interventions or disease care, public health interventions do (generally) no harm to anyone.

If outcomes are too far in time to be measured or too difficult to be reasonably "isolated", one should work on the more proxy outputs, or even process of intervention. Proxy defined here in the sense that when these successful outputs or process elements are observed, a successful outcome is more likely to result. In any case it is of fundamental importance that what is effectiveness of any particular intervention is defined at the very beginning.

Measuring Health Promotion Effectiveness: How can we Measure? Measurement Design and Data Collection

Evidence requires good information and good data. While this is also true in health promotion, evidence in this area is a little different. Many health promotion interventions (programs, policies) across the globe are of limited scale, (e.g. smoking cessation efforts, sanitation and access to clean water, among others) and may also be considered "public health". Health promotion efforts are also generally concerned with looking at evidence from within the parameters of the intervention of interest. Therefore many of the variables one wants to assess are within the intervention study and easily obtainable. For example in a smoking cessation study one usually has a circumscribed setting, such as a workplace, clinic, etc. and a readily defined population, e.g., workers in a factory. Before the intervention, all the important variables regarding the target population can be easily assessed and, in this case, the necessary measurements are well understood: the number of smokers is assessed along with their potential confounding variables, such as demographics, gender and then the cessation program is introduced. The intervention group is followed and assessed at a later point in time with a new measurement to see if the smoking behavior has changed. This is a fairly straightforward as the "evidence data" has clear outcomes measures. And we can measure the "effectiveness" of the intervention quite easily. The measures of evidence are straightforward as the link between evidence and effectiveness: in these simple cases are essentially the same. The evidence of a change in the measures important for the interventions *is* (again, in this case) a measure of effectiveness. However many other concerns in health promotion globally fall into a category of very broad initiatives, such as efforts to address globalization, peace building, equity, urbanization. One provides relevant data for these types of "interventions" at the population level, involving complex variables assessed over time. Moreover, quite often it is difficult to attribute observed changes in the population to the initiatives of interest, provided that there are a myriad of other possibly interacting effects, or the "natural" evolution of the phenomena has affected the population, or the complexity of the effects often concern using more than one variable.

We must interject here that, in addition to these challenges, two other aspects should be considered in the study of effectiveness in these settings:

- time lag between the outcome of interest and a reasonable time for measurement;
- effect of the context on the outcome.

Classical examples for the first kind of challenge are preventive interventions, such as addiction prevention at school, of which effects are expected also a few years after the intervention. It is unreasonable and highly unlikely that one can wait to assess the program effectiveness, and so suitable design and (often proxy) measures should be found. For example, indicators of increase in knowledge among participants (in comparison with non-participants) and attitudinal changes prior to potential use of dependent substances, although output measures, can help in assessing the success of such a preventive intervention.

With regards to the second challenge mentioned above, it is common to assess the effectiveness of the intervention of interest in more than the specific setting in which these have been realized. Such is the case of pilot programs, founded just to observe their feasibility, etc., and then, eventually, their effectiveness. This is well known in the social science research literature as the problem of generalization: the observed (as effective) in a context may not be able to be considered, if not in some way proved, as potentially effective in a different context.

Randomized controlled trials (RCT) are certainly good and suitable approaches for the interventions that are discrete, have an incredibly defined population and outcomes easily measured. RCTs are essential to evaluate the effectiveness of clinical interventions in which the causal chain between intervention and outcomes is "measurably" short and simple. For the interventions that address larger and broader questions, such, for instance, those that affect general health, globalization, urbanization, et cetera, the utility and feasibility (this latter often questionable also for the first kind of interventions) of RCTs are difficult to demonstrate given their limitations, which may show them as unnecessary, inappropriate, impossible or inadequate (Black, 1996). It should be remembered that leaving the track of RCT does not mean abandoning a scientific approach or methodological rigorousness; scientific approaches are clearly found also in non-experimental designs (Des Jarlais et al., 2004).

What then are possible solutions to evaluate effectiveness, when the main so-called classical road is difficult or impossible to take? And, if evidence is a major indication to get some information about effectiveness, what is the better way to retrieve "evidence data"? Here, briefly, are a few possibilities. When generalization of results is the major challenge, one can obtain the information from specific settings through the use of meta-analysis; much literature has shown that this can be an effective approach. A meta-analysis pools together single "small" (in terms of being statistically representative) results to infer a more generalizable or "good enough" data and information on the effectiveness of similar interventions and programs. Although meta-analysis is an already well-developed social research method (Glass et al., 1981), it cannot be considered as the best panacea for many effectiveness analyses and, as with all methods and approaches, it is not free from biases (van Driel & Keijsers, 1997).

Recently meta-analysis has been embedded (and so systematized) into a larger category: the so-called *systematic review*, which proposes a general methodology to perform an overview of primary studies that used explicit and reproducible methods on the subject the researcher is interested (Murlow, 1994; Greeenhalgh, 1997). The idea of systematically assembling information from published material, that at the beginning occurred independent from the meta-analysis movement, has been applied successfully also in public health (Jackson et al., 2004) and specifically in assessing effectiveness (Bridle et al., 2005). Systematic reviews begin from the need to efficiently integrate existing information in order to provide reliable and sufficiently generalized information for rational decision-making. The purpose of introducing a method in the reviewing process is that of performing integration among different studies dealing with the same, or similar, subject, enhancing efficiency, and at the same time providing more generalizable outcomes, assessing the consistency of relationships among different studies (and/or explaining the inconsistencies). Systematic reviews are discussed in more detail elsewhere in this monograph.

Another important approach is that of *surveillance* (McQueen & Puska, 2003) or of *surveillance systems*: Public health (PH) systems in which data on several variables are routinely collected and analyzed, offering a suitable evidence based upon data concerning the evolution and changes in many variables of interest for PH and HP. These systems can offer also evidence for effectiveness when HP interventions deal with variables already routinely collected (along with information on contextual variables). The flexibility of surveillance allows, in other cases, to include in the data collection process new variables, just to offer information on specific subjects that are part of (usually major) new interventions / policies. Surveillance is an important tool for public health as it provides researchers, practitioners and decision-makers the information to measure and understand the dynamic evolution of behaviors and attitudes, a feasible way to collect necessary data. Its relative novelty makes this approach so unique and important for HP effectiveness, to deserve a specific discussion, that we will propose in the following paragraphs.

In the search for measures of effectiveness in health promotion, in the context of the theoretical and practical challenges and complex methodological issues previously discussed, one is often left with that of a "practical wisdom" which involves a broader concept of rationality (Sanderson, 2004). This does not mean to forget the scientific approach. Since the moment of deciding what data or information should be gathered and how, when the complexity is really high, the need is that of going behind the standard quantitative, solid, classic research approach.

This could be done, for example, integrating more sources, both quantitative (different surveys, social indicators, context indicators, etc.) and qualitative, such as experts' opinion (Thurston et al., 2003) or policy-makers' experience (Rütten, 2003). Indeed, particularly when one is dealing with complexity, (and this is quite often the case in evaluating HP effectiveness, from the definition, to the measurement, and to the analysis process) building evidence is often a matter of using multiple methods and multiple sources of data (Nutbeam, 1998). Specifically, the integration between qualitative and quantitative data/information (Steckler et al., 1992; De Vries et al., 1992; Baum, 1995) is promising, given the limits and potentialities of both, and particularly the advantages from a merge in which each can bring its specific strengths: the flexibility and consequent ability of an in-depth comprehension and interpretation of the qualitative approach, and the solidity and the ability to quantify, showing the size of what we are observing that only the quantitative approach can offer.

Whatever the intervention, and the design adopted to measure its effects, attention should be paid to the ("natural") evolution of what we are measuring in respect to the design. In the following figure, one can find a simplified example of this.

Let's observe Fig. 18.3a; there is a target variable, say prevalence of sedentary people in a particular setting observed before and after a specific intervention (I). Observing Fig. 18.3a, one would conclude that the intervention has not been effective since there is no observed change in prevalence? Let's look at Fig. 18.3b. Here we have added only some additional information: two observations before the intervention. Well, the assessment about the effectiveness of the intervention now changes: would you say that there was an increasing trend in the prevalence of, keeping the example, sedentary people, that, after the intervention has been modified? So, now, one would say that the intervention has been effective. Now let's pass to Fig. 18.3c, which provides new observations (please note, *not* modifying the ones given in the previous figures). Here the assessment changes again. We note that what we have first interpreted as an increase was only perhaps a seasonal variation of a phenomenon that, if we take out seasonality, is fairly stable over time, and that has not been modified by the intervention, so again, the intervention seems to be not effective. This helps us to visualize the importance of the "time component" in the study of effectiveness and in understanding the potential risk of too simple approaches, such as the observational design pre-post intervention.

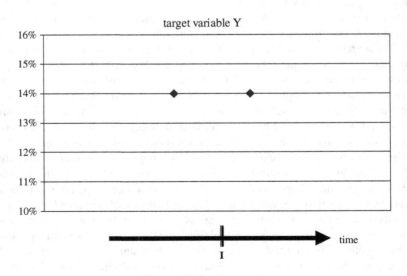

FIGURE 18.3a. (pre-post)

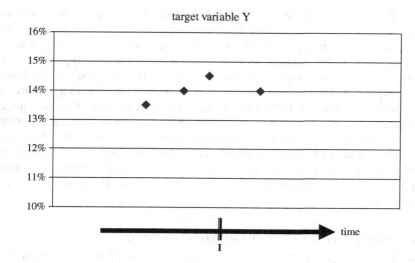

FIGURE 18.3b. (few observations)

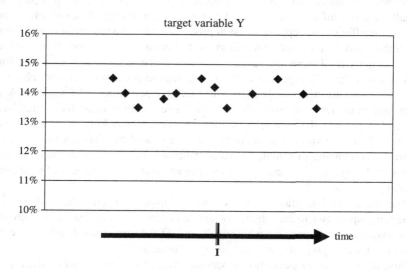

FIGURE 18.3c. (continuous observation)

So, if there is no single perfect design to collect data and/or evidences to assess the effectiveness of an HP intervention/program/policy, it is fair to say that in many cases it is possible to judge if an approach is suitable or not for a certain situation. For instance, as we have seen in the example reported in the previous figures, a pre-post design can be really dangerous to evaluate effectiveness for intervention on the general population. Another important consideration at this point should be made concerning the risk of single source of information. Evidence, in fact, can be gathered also combining different sources, and this is particularly recommendable when one lack of strong assumption and/or of optimal data collection designs. Conversely, as we have seen in the example presented above, the threat of drawing wrong conclusions can be high, when interpreting the results from a single, weak, source of information.

Measuring Health Promotion Effectiveness: The Transformation of Data to Information Through Analysis

It is not all in design and in data collection. Once data are gathered, the most important step is yet to come. Any data must be elaborated, and transformed to become information. Information can be defined as "everything capable in decreasing the uncertainty linked to a decision process"; data, given this purpose, usually, are not information: "raw" data (as they come from data collection) are usually insufficient to support decision processes, they are not capable of removing uncertainty. Data must be transformed to become informative. To know that in the target school there are, say, 225 female smokers is not useful information, to know that this 225 represents 25% of the female population of that school in certainly more informative. Then, to know that the percentage of female smokers decreased in the last year from 30% to 25% is even more informative, particularly if this has happened just after you have run an anti-smoking program in that school. Finally, to know that in another similar school that has not run any program the percentage of female smokers remained more or less the same in that period, helps you to elaborate some evidence about the effectiveness of your anti-smoking program.

The "data transformation" process typically involves several steps, which can, depending upon case to case, be fairly simple or terribly complicated. It is impossible to describe this process exhaustively and, at the same time, briefly. Here we will only try to highlight some typical "transformation".

First of all, measurement should become "readable"; this could be done (following the kind of measurement and the purpose of the transformation) selecting suitable indicators or performing suitable statistical analyses. Given the relevance of indicators of HP effectiveness we will discuss this subject separately in the following paragraph.

A discussion of statistical analysis for the study of HP effectiveness is far from the purpose of this chapter. What is emphasized here is the strong relationship between data analysis and its interpretation. Too often data collection, data analysis, and interpretation have been kept independent, often performed by different persons, who have little contact with another. This is a bad mistake. Data collection, analysis, interpretation are part of the same process, and are highly interrelated and therefore the quality of this interrelation is, often, what can assure the quality of the final results, of the information that results from this process.

In dealing with evidence one typical challenge is that of going behind the "statistically significant": often times, it is not enough to find, say a difference, in the statistical test significant enough to say that the observed effect is "evidence" of effectiveness. In medicine, progress has been made in defining the level of effectiveness for any intervention that is (also) "clinically significant". Only a combined consideration about statistically and clinically significant allows one to evaluate the real evidence of effectiveness.

In many HP interventions data analyses do not lack statistical evidence (given by power of tests, good samples, limited measurement errors, etc.), rather they lack "clinical evidence", that is it is not clearly defined what change can be considered significant from a theoretical point of view. For example, statistical tests show that there is a significant decrease in the number of smokers of 1.1% among the general population. Is this decrease significant also from a public health ("clinical") point of view? Quite often the answer is "it depends". For instance if, after several years of increase in the number of smokers in the particular population we are dealing with, we observe this 1.1% decrease, well, we can be happy about it, think that our programs have been effective and say that, yes, this is a significant change. Instead if, for example, the 1% decrease is the "natural" evolution of smoking and this is observed after some billion dollar interventions on our target population, we can easily say that the 1% decrease is *not* significant for our purposes.

As we have already pointed out, in some cases assessing effectiveness is not necessarily assessing evidence. In programs in which expected results are clearly defined, easily isolated from other possible interactive effects, there is no need to look for "some sort of evidence": evidence is what we observe, evidence is not "a shadow of effectiveness", it is effectiveness itself. In these cases the analysis itself could be different. For instance, specific statistical tools can be applied when experimental designs are possible (different from those applicable in non-experimental designs), and recent literature has shown that this is possible even in the presence of weaknesses in the application of the "experiment", as, in the case of non-random selection of participants (see the works of the Nobel-prize winner Heckman in Heckman et al., 1999).

Effectiveness Indicators: Reliability and Validity Issues

Indicators play an important role in informing any social and health action. Indicators represent substantial informative support for any policy, offering useful information for directing, monitoring and evaluating any sort of intervention. In health promotion they may play a specific role in the process of HP programming, from the very first step of need analysis to the final evaluation (see Noack in the editorial intervention, Noack, (1988), in an issue of the journal *Health Promotion International*, entirely devoted to health promotion indicators). It has been noted that HP should have specific indicators, usually different from those applied in measuring aspects, such as health status, that can be important also for HP, but which are specific for HP purposes (Dean, 1988). From a methodological point of view, indicators constitute a form of translation from an unobservable, abstract concept to a proxy measure, usually done through (simple or complex) transformation of suitable data.

From a practical point of view, indicators help the decision making process with regard to policy or program intervention, to better direct, monitor, or, eventually, evaluate the outcomes and/or allocation of resources. We may like indicators or not, but certainly decision makers, public health practitioners, and stakeholders expect and require information from which indicators are derived (McQueen & Anderson, 2001). In order to best choose indicators, the importance of the link with the policies cannot be overemphasized: policies generate the information needed, and consequently, the indicators then will help, with a sort of circularity, the policies themselves.

It is from this double nature of the indicators (methodological and practical, theoretical) that the choice and the construction of indicators call upon both methodological and substantial aspects, seeking an answer to the question "What research will lead to appropriate indicators?" (McQueen & Noack, 1998).

From a methodological point of view, the indicator construction follows what is illustrated in Fig. 18.2, after operazionalizing the concept, and selecting suitable measures, following data collection, the step is that of combining together data in order to give sense and readability. In so doing, the researcher finds several options (among different measures and different way of combining them). The choice of suitable indicators is driven by considerations both concerning methodological aspects and substantial ones. The methodological aspects with which we are concerned revolve around reliability, validity and sensitivity. Here are briefly noted the meaning of these terms without going into the detail found in the vast literature for a broader presentation (see Miller, 1991). *Reliability* is the ability of the indicator to render the same result over repeated trials. *Validity* is referred to the capability of the indicator to measure what it is supposed to measure. *Sensitivity* is the ability to catch and measure differences, even small but that are significant in the phenomenon that the indicator wants to measure. The ability to respond relatively quickly and noticeably to real changes is also referred as *responsiveness*.

Beside these important methodological characteristics, there are others that can help in providing the most appropriate choice in the construction of an indicator. These apply differently, with different relative importance that is specific to the challenges being addressed. To name only a few: *Readability*, how easy is an indicator understood by interested stakeholders; *Pertinence*, how closely it is related to the subject; *Relevance*, relative importance of a change in that indicator for a change in the subject; *Sharing*, how much the value/use will be/is shared among stakeholders;

TABLE 18.1. Contrasts and trade-offs between
positive characteristics of indicators

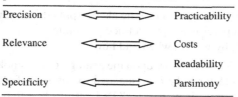

Precision	⟸⟹	Practicability
Relevance	⟸⟹	Costs
		Readability
Specificity	⟸⟹	Parsimony

Comparability, how much it helps in comparing and benchmarking (to other context); *Practicability*; how easily it is to compute. It should be noted that the choice among indicators sometimes is difficult because one has to consider trade-offs between potential good characteristics that could be compared to one another. In Table 18.1 we summarize possible contrasts (trade-offs).

Surveillance as a Tool for Measuring Health Promotion Effectiveness

In the search for suitable tools to study HP effectiveness, we have seen that quite often "classical" approaches can be limited, inappropriate or simply impossible to realize. In all these cases, the availability of surveillance concerning people's risk behavior and attitudes can be of great importance. In some case this can even offer a fertile ground to evaluate HP effectiveness (see Campostrini et al., 2006). In many ways, surveillance can provide a broad view of the general results of many interventions, thus providing insight into the interplay among them, as well as observations of the "natural" evolution of the phenomena of interest. And this, as we know, it is not only "better than nothing", but it is, when well studied and properly interpreted, invaluable information for HP future policies and programming. For these reasons, a more detailed description of behavioral risk factor surveillance and the related methodological topics is presented here, partly because surveillance has so rarely been seen as a primary way of assessing evidence and effectiveness in health promotion.

A Definition of Surveillance

The use of the word *surveillance* with regard to human behavior is fairly recent phenomenon. That is, surveillance that monitors health-related behaviors in a general population over time (McQueen, 1996). Although the origin of this word is straightforward in the health system (in chronic diseases it has been "borrowed" in the 90s from the non-communicable diseases), it is worthwhile to outline the main characteristics that the use of this word evocate.

1) *Time flow of observation*: surveillance cannot be a random activity, carried out once in a while, with long time lags between observations (no one would like a smoke detector that is switched on only two hours a week!). Surveillance requires

continuity in the measurement process (the meaning of continuity in a survey system will be discussed below).

2) *Systematic approach*: surveillance needs be applied in a suitable, institutionalized, context with precise and pre-defined procedures, which will outline what, should be surveyed, by whom, when and how.

3) *Link to interventions:* to follow upon the analogy of the smoke detector, would you like a smoke detector to be disassociated to any sort of alarm that indicates when the level of smoking is worrisome? Perhaps it is best to be linked to an efficient alarm system and, able to contact the fire department, or others capable to assess the emergency and act on it!

Behavioral Risk Factor Surveillance (BRFS) is all this. It is a systematic system of data collection, analysis, interpretation and reporting, of behavior of the general population, which is useful in informing public health interventions and services.

The availability of such a continuous stream of information has been shown to be highly important to address, monitor and evaluate issues in public health, as well as effectiveness of HP intervention.

– *Address*: any HP effort moves from the theoretical rationale (why one would promote something) *and* from an understanding of the level of knowledge, attitudes and behaviors of the target population. Surveillance systems can offer invaluable information about these latter aspects.
– *Monitoring/evaluate:* once HP objectives have been established (in a measurable way) and the program / policy has been implemented, surveillance can offer unique information about its effectiveness, offering always the information in "context", often valuable "evidence" for evaluating its effectiveness, and in some cases (as will be shown further on), also a perfect set for specific, solid, quantitative evaluation.

Methodological Aspects of Surveillance

BRFS has been around for some twenty to thirty years, beginning in the US and the UK with some pilot testing in the '80s. These efforts have produced a fully implemented surveillance system, such the US's BRFSS (Gentry et al., 1985; Nelson et al., 1998), as well as the Scottish LAH (Lifestyle and Health Survey, McQueen et al., 1992) that is not running any more as a system, although it remains a complete research and study experience that can be seen as a model for other applications). Over the past two decades, several countries have also developed BRF surveillance systems (US, UK, Canada, Australia, to name a few) and others are in various stages of full implementation (many South American countries, Italy, Singapore, among others). It is fair to say that most of the methodological aspects linked to surveillance have been addressed, discussed, experimented and resolved. Many methodological topics are, in the surveillance scientific and practitioners' community, fully researched. Still, many other topics require

TABLE 18.2. Synopsis of methodological issues related to BRF surveillance

Surveillance Topics Widely Accepted	Accepted but still problematic	Challenging (need further studies)
Surveillance approach (time perspective, etc.)	How to measure Social determinants Diet and physical activities Urban sprawl, etc. . . .	Data analysis: small area statistics
Questionnaire development	Data collection - Is the telephone the best way of collecting data on BRF?	Data analysis: analysis of interactions and complexity
'System' and empowerment issues	Survey errors Is it all in weighting? errors measurement and control	Integration Data linkage, but also Information linkage

attention, either because of new technologies (e.g., the increased use of cell phones, which fewer home lines, creating practical and methodological problems for those systems relying on CATI – computer assisted telephone interviewing – data collection), or brought about by new policy needs (e.g., local data/information are more and more expected), or simply because many topic areas are yet to be appropriately addressed (e.g., how best to measure physical activity). In Table 18.2 we summarize the most important methodological topics linked to BRFS, categorized by how these have been already discussed and acquired in the surveillance community.

This information is based upon the work in which we have been involved and the colleagues from whom we have learned over the past decade; in addition this is collaborative work that has been carried out in more than ten countries and reinforced by face to face scientific meetings every two years.

Surveillance Topics Widely Accepted

Over twenty years of study and practice of BRFS has brought at least a clear definition of the approach, as already pointed out, with *time* as the main variable, and continuity in data collection, at least as a theoretical rationale to follow. Continuity in data collection, as has been already pointed out (Campostrini, 1996), can be defined in a relative way as "observations sufficiently near one another to catch significant changes in the variables of interest". This could, practically range from yearly observation for some stable variable (phenomenon) to weekly for some unsteady ones. As previously stated, the more observations the researcher has, the more precise will be the time trend / time change analysis. This latter consideration argues that one should collect observations as often as possible, practically translated into monthly sampling by many BRFS systems now running.

The other pillar of BRF surveillance is that it is a systematic approach that integrates into the wider system of public health information and dissemination of analyzed data. Although several systems are still in various stages of progress, years of experience from other countries and a robust and shared literature (Campostrini & McQueen, 2005) has resulted in a global view of the importance of a systematic approach to surveillance.

Thus, many years of discussion and study (inside and, perhaps even more, outside the surveillance community) on questionnaire development have yielded reliable and valid ways of measuring attitudes, opinions, beliefs, behaviors, and some social-cultural variables that offer international comparisons and benchmarking.

Surveillance Topics Accepted but Still Problematic

In health prevention and promotion nothing is static; new knowledge and novel problems demand new information, more specific or, simply, different. So, the *learning system* (Campostrini, 2003) of surveillance addresses new challenges in "how to measure" variables. Keeping the core of the questionnaire as stable as possible is critical, thus offering the possibility of time comparison, the use of new modules to better measure new "hot topics" such as social determinants or old ones such as physical activity and diet that, for the actual level of knowledge about their relation with health, need to be better or differently measured from past work. As the discussion about how other factors can influence health is learned, surveillance systems should be able to adapt these new findings and learn how to best measure these phenomena or establish collaborative links to what is collected through surveillance. Let's take as example the case of urban sprawl; some now consider this social phenomenon a new and potential risk factor for health. When and if urban sprawl is proven (by other studies: the mission of surveillance is not that of doing research, but that of providing information) to be an actual risk factor, it is important to provide the methods by which this can be measured through addenda to questionnaires or by linking surveillance to other sources of routinely collected information (such as census data).

Many behavioral monitoring systems rely on the proven methodology of telephone interviewing. After two decades, now the question rises again: is the telephone the best way of collecting data on risk factors and social determinants? Much research has shown in the past how telephone surveys, and particularly computer aided telephone surveys (CATI) are not only an efficient way of data collection, but also a valid and reliable one, even for sensitive questions (Nelson, et al., 2001). There are various aspects to consider when addressing this very basic and important methodological issue. Firstly, in economically developed countries, in which telephone coverage is almost 100%, technology has changed the way in which we communicate. Many residents have opted for cell phones in place of secured landlines. In addition, in particular in many economically developing countries in which surveillance is desired, (landline) telephone coverage is low, while cell phone coverage is incredibly increasing. Solutions are available; we know that if we adopt a divergent method for data collection different results will be reported. Mixed methods to data collection, meaning face-to-face interviews coupled with telephone surveys, can be explored. This must be understood and adapted.

Every researcher wishes to provide error-free measurement, but is cognizant of the fact that indeed there is no such thing as error-free measurement. This is a topic that has been discussed, studied and written about in the literature extensively, (see Groves, 1989); however, there still remain challenges. While statistical methods for "correcting" errors are quite established, these methods cannot be seen as a perfect panacea. For example, often data weighting (post-stratification) is considered adequate, that is if we have weighted the data it must be okay. We weight data using few known, variables such as gender and age, and adjust our estimates by these characteristics, and, hopefully, this would lead to unbiased (or better less biased) estimates for those variables that are highly correlated with these characteristics. But what about the many other variables that are independent from the variables used in the weighting? It is worthwhile, then, to remember that weighted data can lead to unbiased estimates, but generally gives biased (non consistent) estimates of the standard errors. Because of this, specific procedures (now available in much statistical software) should be adopted to compute confidence intervals or to run statistical testing.

Challenging Topics about Surveillance, Measurement and Effectiveness

Think globally, but act locally. This well-known motto is so shared around the world that the request for reliable data at the local level is constantly increasing. Good data and reliable information provide the basis on which we can not only think, but more importantly also act based upon needs and priorities. Since many health promotion activities are at the local level, surveillance systems must face the challenge to offer *reliable information at the local level*. In this regard, two points must be considered. First, information "to act" is generally not the same as the information required "to think". For example, often at the local level information are needed for comparison, benchmarking, goal-setting and evaluating; the information at the local level is not used to understand the mechanisms of behaviors and behavioral changes: this task is usually performed by people working at national level, and the results of these studies are, generally, applicable at any level. To examine the relationship among several risk factors, something that requires "big samples", much data, generally has to be done by national agencies using national data; but when a relationship is proven, often this is valid for many different geographical areas, although the level of prevalence of the risk factors may be different in different locations. So, if the study of relationship among variables, or the study of patterns of behavioral change and attitudes require much data, this is usually not done at local level, where usually are sufficient "simple" measures that require smaller sample sizes. So, the need to reproduce at local level the same sampling size as a national surveillance system is not necessary. Nevertheless, quite often the "local" level is corresponding to such a small geographical entity (province, defined region, even county) that in any case the sample size of each observation is, in a "normal" surveillance system, so small that it is hard to say that it can be informative. Here, luckily, comes an important point about surveillance. To have a continuous data stream, to have time embedded in the system, helps, a great deal in offering reasonable estimates at the local level. This for two reasons: the first is that an aggregation of observation over time is always possible, so if for a reasonable estimate of the prevalence at national level we put together monthly observations, for estimates at county level we have possibly to aggregate observation over two or three years to have reasonably comparable estimates. The second reason comes from the Statistics: in doing this, techniques belonging to the so-called "small area statistics" can be applied to perform more efficiently a comparative analysis among small area. Usually, this is done "borrowing" information on a local area from the nearer ones, and in this way improving the accuracy of the estimates based on small samples. In surveillance this can be done "borrowing" information also from observations, nearer in time, made on the same local area.

The second challenging topic we think germane to briefly discuss here is concerned with data analysis. Researchers, and also HP practitioners, often have to deal with complexity: behaviors are complex and behavioral change is even more complex. Indeed, it is challenging to understand why people act in a particular way, and at times appears to be even more difficult to understand what the influences are that can change behaviors. With the exception of a few success stories in HP, we find many challenging, never-ending stories. An example of this is the effort to control the "obesity epidemic". Many interventions have been implemented, many resources allocated to address the determinants of the risk factors and behaviors related to obesity and yet, the percentage of persons overweight or obese is steadily increasing across the globe. Indeed, this public health issue is complex. Obesity is a good example, because, thus far, surveillance systems have been limited in measuring the increases in rates of obesity; little has been done to measure the reasons why and how. If this has been done, little information has been produced. There is no single risk factor linked to obesity. It is complex: people are less sedentary (BRFSS, 2006) and still obesity increases; more attention is paid to diet, and yet rates of obesity increase. Why? Well, perhaps we should have *complex tools to deal with this complexity*. Surveillance offers a perfect response in order to address this challenge. There remain many variables related to obesity but there is also the time aspect and its evolution over time. This is a challenging and relevant topic: to study the evolution of several variables over time, and the evolution of the relationship among them.

Data Analysis of Surveillance Data: The Last Step for Measuring Effectiveness

Data analysis and data interpretation is a fundamental step in producing useful information, and surveillance is no exception. Perhaps the need for linking data analysis with the other fundamentals of the information process is even more relevant, given the need for surveillance to become an (information) system (Campostrini & McQueen, 2005). Several are the issues that are necessary to address specifically in surveillance, where data analysis is linked to the availability of continuous data stream of which the researcher would likely to take advantage (Campostrini, 2003).

In a chapter as brief as this we are not able to cover all possible methods and techniques of analysis useful in measuring effectiveness, but only to position analysis in the framework of the study of HP. Concerning specifically the issue of evidence and effectiveness, analysis of surveillance data can provide a lot of information. Using standard statistical techniques such as the so-called interrupted time series approach (Box & Tiao, 1975; Orwin, 1997) one can look into the surveillance data for possible effects of interventions on behavioral and attitudinal trends (Campostrini et al., 2006).

Given the availability of several attitudinal and behavioral variables collected over time, surveillance data can be analyzed not only to show trends and detect change, but also to link these one with the others. To conclude, measurement remains an essential area of concern for assessing effectiveness, but it must go hand in hand with careful analysis of the data that have been measured.

Acknowledgments. To write a chapter on this subject is certainly not an easy task. In summarizing many years of diverse research, studies, and approaches, one has to deal with many contrasting viewpoints. At the same time one must be brief, clear and not too technical. If at the end of this effort what is written can be useful, this is due only partially to the author. One has to acknowledge the many persons that in the last decades worked both on the methodological and the practice side of issues related to how to measure effectiveness in health promotion. The acknowledgment for some of these is already given with the citations recommended for a better understanding. Many of the issues discussed here are more extensively and better explored in the references. Many others who have done excellent work on this broad and difficult subject are not even cited and to these my humble apologies. Among several colleagues that helped me in better focusing on the methodological issues related to health promotion, notably effectiveness, measurement problems and surveillance, I acknowledge the major contribution of David McQueen. Most of what is written here has been discussed, in one way or another, with him; his suggestions have been very helpful in the study, in the practice, as well as in writing about this area.

References

Baum, F. (1995). Researching public health: beyond the qualitative-quantitative method debate. *Social Science and Medicine, 55*, 459–468.

Black, N. (1996). Why we need observational studies to evaluate the effectiveness of health care. *British Medical Journal, 312*, 1215–1218.

Blalock, H. (1979). Measurement and Conceptualization Problems: the major obstacle to integrating theory and research. *American Sociological Review, 44*, 881–894.

Box G. & Tiao G. (1975). Intervention Analysis with Applications to Economic and Environmental Problems, *Journal of the American Statistical Association, 70*, 70–92.

BRFSS (2006). www.cdc.gov/brfss

Bridle, C., Riemsma, R.P., Pattenden, J., Sowden, A.J., Mather, L, Watt, I.S. & Walker, A. (2005). Systematic review of the effectiveness of health behaviour interventions based on the transtheoretical model. *Psychology and Health, 20*, 283–301.

Campostrini, S. (2003). Surveillance systems and data analysis, in D.V.McQueen & P.Puska (eds.) *Global Behavioral Risk Factor Surveillance*, 47–55, New York: Kluwer.

Campostrini, S. (1996). Dynamic approaches to the study of behaviour. The continuous collection of data in comparison with panel surveys, *Statistica Applicata, 8*, 695–708.

Campostrini, S., Holtzman, D., McQueen, D. V. & Boaretto, E. (2006). Evaluating the Effectiveness of Health Promotion Policy: Changes in the Law on Drinking and Driving in California. *Health Promotion International, 21*, 130–135.

Campostrini, S. & McQueen, D.V. (2005). Institutionalization of social and behavioral risk factor surveillance as a learning system. *Social and Preventive Medicine, 50 Suppl 1*, S9–S15.

Dean, K. (1988). Issues in the development of health promotion indicators. *Health Promotion International, 3*, 13–21.

Des Jarlais, D.C., Lyles, C., Crepaz, N. and the TREND Group (2004). Improving the Reporting Quality of Nonrandomized Evaluations of Behavioral and Public Health Interventions: The TREND Statement. *American Journal of Public Health, 94*, 361–366.

De Vries, H., Weijts, W., Dijkstra, M. & Kok, G. (1992). The utilization of qualitative and quantitative data for health education program planning, implementation, and evaluation: a spiral approach. *Health Education Quarterly, 19*, 101–115.

Ford, J. (1975). *Paradigms and Fairy Tales. An Introduction to the Science of Meanings.* London: Routledge Kegan Paul.

Gentry, E.M., Kalsbeek, W.D. & Hogelin, G.C., et al. (1985). The behavioral risk factor surveys. II design, methods, and estimates from combined state data. *American Journal of Preventive Medicine*, 1(6), 9–14.

Glass, G. V., McGaw, B. & Smith, M.L. (1981). *Meta-analysis in social research.* Newbury Park, CA: Sage.

Greeenhalgh, T. (1997). Papers that summerise other papers (systematic reviews and meta-analysis). *British Medical Journal, 315*, 672–675.

Groves, R. M. (1989). *Survey errors and survey costs.* Jon Wiley & Sons.

Heckman J., LaLonde R. & Smith J. (1999). "The economics and econometrics of active labor market programs", in O. Ashenfeltere D. Card (eds.), *Hanbook of Labor Economics* – Vol. 3A, Amsterdam: North-Holland.

Jackson, N. & Waters, E. (2004), and the Guidelines for Systematic Reviews of Health Promotion and Public Health Interventions Taskforce. The challenges of systematically reviewing public health interventions. *Journal of Public Health, 26*, 303–307.

McQueen, D.V. (1996). Surveillance of health behavior. *Current Issues of Public Health*, *2*, 51–55.

McQueen, D.V. & Anderson, L.M. (2001). What counts as evidence: issues and debates, in *Evaluation in health promotion*, WHO Regional Publications, European Series, No. 92.

McQueen D. V. & Noack, H. (1998). Health promotion indicators. *Health Promotion International*, *3*, 73–78.

McQueen, D.V. & Puska, P. (Eds.) (2003). *Global Behavioral Risk Factor Surveillance*, New York: Kluwer.

McQueen, D.V., Uitenbroek, D. & Campostrini, S. (1992). Design, Implementation and Maintenance of a Continuous Population Survey by CATI, Bureau of Census, *Annual Research Conference proceedings*,.

Miller, D. (1991). Handbook of Research Design and Social Measurement. CA: Sage.

Murlow, C. D. (1994). Rationales for systematic review. *British Medical Journal*, *309*, 597–599.

Noack, H. (1988). Measuring health behaviour and health: towards new health promotion indicators. *Health Promotion International*, *3*, 5–12.

Nelson, DE., Holtzman, D., Waller, M., Leutzinger, C. & Condon K. (1998). Objectives and design of the Behavioral Risk Factor Surveillance System. Dallas, TX: *proceedings of the American Statistical Association Annual Conference, Section on Survey Methods*, 214–218.

Nelson, D. E., Holtzman, D., Bolen, J., Stanwyck, C. & Mack, K. (2001). Reliability and validity of measures from the Behavioral Risk Factor Surveillance System (BRFSS). *Social and Preventive Medicine, 46*, 1–42.

Nutbeam, D. (1998). Evaluating health promotion – progress, problems and solutions. *Health Promotion International, 13–1*, 27–44.

Orwin, R.G. (1997). Twenty-one years old and counting: the Interrupted Time Series comes of age, in Chelimsky E., Shadish W.R. (eds.) *Evaluation for the 21st Century*, Sage, Thousand Oaks, 443–466.

Rütten, A., Luschen, G., von Lengerke, T., Abel, T., Kannas, L., Diaz, J. A. R., Vinck, J. & van der Zee, J. (2003.). Determinants of health policy impact: comparative results of a European policymaker study. *Social and Preventive Medicine, 48(6)*, 379–391.

Sanderson, I. (2004). Getting evidence into practice. Perspective on rationality. *Evaluation, 10(3)*, 366–379.

Steckler, A., McLeroy, K. R. & Goodman, R. M. (1992). Towards integrating qualitative and quantitative methods: an introduction. *Health Education Quarterly, 19*, 1–8.

Thurston, W. E., Vollmann, A.R., Wilson, D. R., MacKean G., Felix, R. & Wright M.F. (2003). Development and testing of a framework for assessing the effectiveness of health promotion. *Social and Preventive Medicine, 48(5)*, 301–316.

van Driel, W.G. & Keijsers, J. (1997). An instrument for reviewing the effectiveness of health education and health promotion. *Patient Education and Counseling, 30*, 7–17.

Victoria, C.G., Habicht, J. & Bryce j. (2004). Evidence-Based Public Health: Moving Beyond Randomized Trials. *American Journal of Public Health, 94*, 400–405.

19
Healthy Settings
Building Evidence for the Effectiveness
of Whole System Health Promotion – Challenges
and Future Directions

MARK DOORIS, BLAKE POLAND, LLOYD KOLBE, EVELYNE DE LEEUW,
DOUGLAS S. MCCALL AND JOAN WHARF-HIGGINS

In this chapter, we focus on the settings approach to health promotion. We start with a brief review of its origins and development in relation to international policy; provide an overview of theory and concepts relevant to current practice; focus on the challenges faced in building evidence of effectiveness for the approach; and conclude by discussing several recent theoretical and methodological innovations that we believe offer potential ways forward.

While touching on the current state of the evidence base, the main purpose of the chapter is not to summarize past research but to illuminate clear theoretical underpinnings for the settings approach; examine the challenges to evaluating and demonstrating effectiveness and efficiency of such an ecological, whole system approach; and highlight implications and directions for future research.

The Settings Approach: Origins,
Development, and Policy Context

The settings approach to health promotion has developed during the past 20 years. Green, Poland, & Rootman (2000) note that health education and health promotion have a long history of being organized around settings such as health-care, workplaces, and schools – which provide "major social structures that provide channels and mechanisms of influence for reaching defined populations" (Mullen, Evans, Forster, Gottlieb, Kreuter, Moon, O'Rourke, & Stretcher, 1995, p.330). In this way, settings, alongside population groups and health topics, make up the traditional three-dimensional matrix used to organize programmes aimed at individual behaviour change (Dooris, 2004).

However, we would contend that "the settings approach"[*] represents an important development beyond this focus on carrying out interventions *within* a setting,

---

[*] A range of terminology has been used in relation to settings, as discussed by Whitelaw, Baxendale, Bryce, Machardy, Young, & Witney (2001) and Tones & Green (2004). This includes "settings for health", "the settings approach", "the settings-based approach",

recognising that place and context are themselves important and modifiable determinants of health and wellbeing, both directly and indirectly. Understood thus, the approach is acknowledged to have its roots in the *Ottawa Charter*, which highlighted "supportive environments for health" (a focus further developed in the *Sundsvall Statement* [WHO, 1991]) and stated that "health is created and lived by people within the settings of their everyday life; where they learn, work, play and love (WHO, 1986, p.2).

The Ottawa Charter stimulated WHO to prioritize the settings approach in its health promotion programmes, thereby "shifting the focus from the deficit model of disease to the health potentials inherent in the social and institutional settings of everyday life" and pioneering strategies that "strengthened both sense of place and sense of self" (Kickbusch, 1996, p.5).

Under WHO's leadership, the settings approach developed rapidly. Building on the 1984 Toronto "Beyond Health Care" meeting, Healthy Cities was launched in 1987 as a small European project (Ashton, 1988), quickly expanding to become a global movement for the "new" public health (Tsouros, 1991). In the European Region, developments subsequently took place within smaller settings such as schools, prisons, hospitals and universities (Barnekow Rasmussen & Rivett, 2000; Groene & Garcia-Barbero, 2005; Squires & Strobl, 1996; Tsouros, Dowding, Thompson, & Dooris, 1998). In the Region of the Americas, Canada initiated a Healthy Communities movement in 1986 (O'Neill, 2000; Wharf Higgins, 1992), both the United States and Canada developed comprehensive school health models in 1987 and 1988 respectively, and PAHO supported the development of the Healthy Municipalities and Communities movement in Latin America (Restrepo, Llanos, Contrera, Rocabado, Gross, Suárez, & González, 1996). The South-East Asia Region advocated a Healthy District programme as an umbrella for smaller settings projects (WHO, 2002a) and the Western Pacific Region supported Healthy Islands and Healthy Marketplaces initiatives (Galea, Powis, & Tamplin, 2000; WHO, 2004). And in Africa, Healthy Cities programmes have incorporated the settings approach, emphasizing the importance of action within and across a range of settings (WHO, 2002b), with a particular focus on creating healthy settings and environments for children – an emphasis echoed in the Eastern Mediterranean and other regions involved in the Healthy Environments for Children Alliance (WHO, 2006a).

The approach was strengthened by a number of further publications – most notably the *Jakarta Declaration* (WHO, 1997a), which suggested that settings "represent the organisational base of the infrastructure required for health promotion" (p.4) and "offer practical opportunities for the implementation of comprehensive strategies" (p.2). Whilst focusing strongly on "macro" issues as determinants of health in a

---

"health promoting settings" and "healthy settings". Whilst it is possible to identify semantic differences between terms such as "health promoting settings" and "healthy settings" – the former more clearly suggesting a focus on people and a commitment to ensuring that the setting takes account of its external health impacts (Dooris, 2006b) – they have increasingly been used interchangeably, with a dual focus on both context and methods.

globalized world, the *Bangkok Charter* (WHO, 2005) follows on from Ottawa, Sundsvall and Jakarta in further highlighting the role of settings.

Healthy Settings: Theory and Practice

The Rationale for the Settings Approach: The Importance of Context

A "setting for health" has been defined as: "The place or social context in which people engage in daily activities in which environmental, organisational and personal factors interact to affect health and wellbeing . . .where people actively use and shape the environment and thus create or solve problems relating to health . . .normally . . . having physical boundaries, a range of people with defined roles, and an organisational structure" (WHO, 1998a, p.19).

Thus, a settings approach not only recognises that contexts influence both health and the achievement of the core goals of a setting, but also contends that health improvement requires investment in the social systems in which people spend their daily lives (see Figure 19.1). Health is, then, both a critical asset for and an outcome of the effective functioning of settings (Dooris, Dowding, Thompson, & Wynne, 1998; Grossman & Scala, 1993). This system-level investment is mirrored in parallel developments: for example, educators have developed "effective schools" strategies, business has adopted Total Quality Management programs, and many sectors have used the "the learning organization" concept (Senge, 1990).

The value of such investment has been acknowledged not only internationally (e.g. through the inclusion of a specific target on settings within the European Health for All Policy Framework [WHO, 1998b]), but also at national level. For example, the Northern Ireland public health strategy states that "many risk factors are interrelated

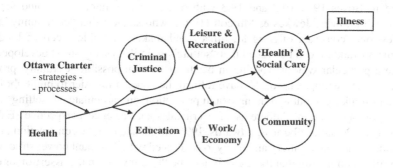

Figure 19.1. Putting 'health' into settings

Source: Dooris (2004) produced with permission from Critical Public Health http://www.tandf.co.uk/journals (adapted from Grossman & Scala, 1993, with permission from WHO)

and can be best tackled through comprehensive, integrated programmes in appropriate settings where people live, work and interact" (Department of Health, Social Services, & Public Safety, 2002, p.134).

Contemporary health promotion programs consist of complex *social* interventions slotting intentional change efforts into pre-existing contexts. Yet, "whilst programs are initiated in prisons, hospitals, schools, neighbourhoods, and car parks, it is the prior set of social rules, norms, values and interrelationships gathered in these places which sets limits on the efficacy of program mechanisms" (Pawson & Tilley, 1997, p.70). Context, is therefore fundamental to health promotion.

Although context receives attention in health promotion texts (e.g. Bartholemew, Parcel, Kok, & Gottlieb, 2006; Green & Kreuter, 2005), it is typically neglected during planning, implementation, and evaluation. Indeed, the dominant post-positivist paradigm sees context as a source of potential confounders to be "factored in" (as variables that apply across cases) or "factored out" (controlled for statistically or through study design such as randomization). While some authors (e.g. Kahan & Goodstadt, 2001) emphasize the importance of context to understanding and applying "best practices" in health promotion, the overwhelming tendency is to see context as a nuisance to be overcome.

In summary, although the inherent "messiness", unpredictability and uniqueness of context is anathema to an administrative (if not scientific) rationality intent on procedural standardization (Malpas, 2003), the settings approach asserts the importance of physical and social contexts to programme design, implementation, and evaluation.

Conceptualizing Settings

The theory and practice of the settings approach have been discussed by several authors (e. g. Barić, 1993; Dooris, 2004; Dooris et al, 1998; Green et al, 2000; Kickbusch, 1995; 2003; Paton, Sengupta, & Hassan, 2005; Poland, Green, & Rootman, 2000; St Leger, 1997; Wenzel, 1997; Whitelaw et al, 2001) and are illustrated in Boxes 19.1, 19.2 and 19.3 with reference to schools, cities and virtual settings. Following Jewkes & Murcott (1998), who suggest that "community" is a professional construct offering legitimacy and making possible a certain kind of modus operandi, it can be argued that "setting" is similarly a construct developed to make a particular way of working in health promotion possible. Certainly, proponents of the "settings approach" have refined the concept in order to highlight new ways of thinking about and doing health promotion, and articulate the setting as an object of intervention. Adherents of a critical social science perspective (Eakin, Robertson, Poland, Coburn, & Edwards, 1996) might add that the construction of the concept is far from arbitrary and likely to be aligned with dominant power structures.

Whilst recognising that there can indeed be "tyranny . . . in the assertion or creation of consensus" (Green et al, 2000, p.26), it remains that increased clarity of conceptualization can strengthen future practice, policy, research and evaluation. To this end, we would suggest that the settings approach is rooted in values such

as participation, equity, and partnership – and characterized by three interconnected dimensions (Dooris, 2006a; Dooris & Hunter, 2007).

Ecological Model of Health Promotion

Firstly, reflecting multi-disciplinary influences, the approach is based on an ecological model of health promotion in which health is determined by a complex
interaction of environmental, organisational, and personal factors. The approach
reflects a shift of focus from individuals to populations, from illness to salutoge-
nesis (Antonovsky, 1996), and from a reductionist focus on single issues, risk factors, and linear causality towards an holistic concern to develop supportive
contexts in the places that people live their lives.

This ecological perspective ensures that "settings" are conceptualized not
merely as culturally and socially defined locations in space and time, but also as
"arenas of sustained interaction, with preexisting structures, policies, characteristics, institutional values, and both formal and informal sanctions on behavior"
(Green et al, 2000, p.23).

Systems Perspective

Secondly, reflecting this ecological viewpoint and drawing on organisational theory, the approach views settings as complex dynamic systems with inputs,
throughputs and outputs (Paton et al, 2005). This systems perspective acknowledges interconnectedness and synergy between different components (Capra,
1983; French & Bell, 1999) and suggests that: "the healthfulness of particular settings and the well-being of their participants are jointly influenced by multiple
aspects of the physical environment . . .and the social environment" (Best,
Stokols, Green, Leischow, Holmes, & Buchholz, 2003, p.170). It also recognizes
that settings do not function as "trivial machines" (Grossman & Scala, 1993), but
are both *complex* systems (unpredictable) and *open* systems (interacting with the
other settings and the wider environment).

This latter point is important for a number of reasons (Dooris, 2001, 2004;
Poland et al, 2000):

- health issues do not "respect" boundaries and an issue made manifest in one
  setting may have its roots in a different setting (e.g. bullying in schools);
- people's lives cross different settings, concurrently and consecutively (e.g.
  someone's time might be divided between work, leisure and home; or a period
  of detention in prison might precede resettlement into the community);
- there are micro-environments within each setting that offer different experiences, to different people on different days;
- and settings function at multiple levels with shared and separate domains, and,
  as "elemental" or "contextual" settings (Galea et al, 2000), may, like "Russian
  dolls" be located within the context of another (e.g. a school may be located

within a neighbourhood, within a city, within a region) – constituting nested settings within interconnected spatial and temporal layers (Bronfenbrenner, 1979; 1994).

Whole System Organisation Development and Change Focus

Thirdly, the approach uses organisation development to introduce and manage change within the setting in its entirety (Grossman & Scala, 1993; Paton et al, 2005) – applying "whole system thinking" (Pratt, Gordon, & Plampling, 1999). Drawing on the work of Barić (1993, 1994), it is important that the approach uses multiple, interconnected interventions and programmes to embed health within the culture, routine life and mainstream business of a specific setting; ensure living and working environments that promote greater health and productivity; and engage with and promote the health of the wider community.

A number of models have been developed to help move from conceptualization to operationalization: Paton et al (2005) have proposed the Healthy Living and Working Model, which highlights the use of organization development and systems theory in creating change; and Dooris (2004) has highlighted the need for a values-based approach that balances organization development with high visibility projects, top-down commitment with bottom-up engagement, and the health promotion agenda with core business concerns (see Figure 19.2).

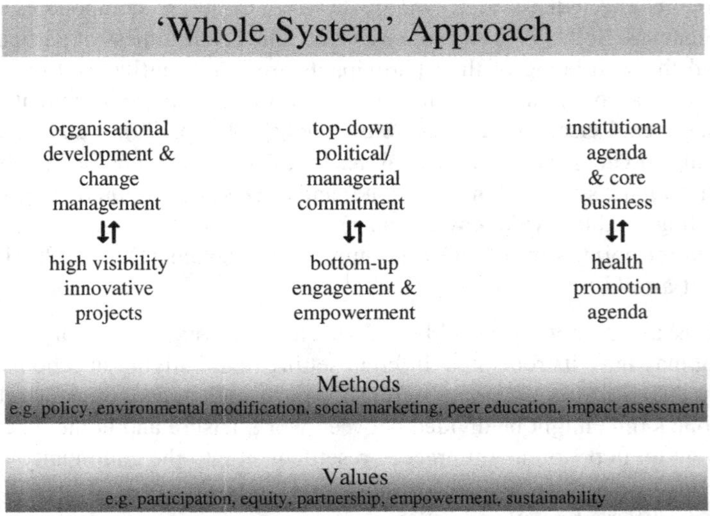

'Whole System' Approach

organisational development & change management	top-down political/ managerial commitment	institutional agenda & core business
↕	↕	↕
high visibility innovative projects	bottom-up engagement & empowerment	health promotion agenda

Methods
e.g. policy, environmental modification, social marketing, peer education, impact assessment

Values
e.g. participation, equity, partnership, empowerment, sustainability

FIGURE 19.2. A model for conceptualizing and operationalizing the healthy settings approach

Source: adapted from Dooris (2004), produced with permission from Critical Public Health http://www.tandf.co.uk/journals

Box 19.1. Theory and practice – schools

Schools could become one of the most effective settings in which to improve health, education, and other social outcomes among large populations (Kolbe, Jones, Birdthistle, & Vince-Whitman, 2000; Scottish Health Promoting Schools Unit, 2006; U.S. Centers for Disease Control, 2006a; WHO, 1997b, 2006b). In theory, schools could improve these varied outcomes (Kolbe, 2002) for students, employees (Kolbe, Tirozzi, Marx, Bobbitt-Cooke, Riedel, Jones, & Schmoyer, 2005), families and the wider community by simultaneously implementing action in a number of interrelated areas (Kolbe, 2005):

- safe, healthy and supportive physical and psychosocial environments
- health, counselling, and social services
- healthy nutrition
- enjoyable, lifelong physical activity
- education that informs, motivates, and empowers students and employees to work for sustainable health at individual, family, community, national, and global levels.

To do this effectively requires the integrated efforts of students, families, staff, and public, not-for-profit, and private-sector agencies in and out of school hours. Whilst such an approach is being advanced by the Health Promoting Schools movement, relatively few schools integratively plan, implement, and evaluate such actions. Rather, they usually offer fragmented efforts to meet urgent health *problems* and fail to build mutual trust, enjoyment, commitment, and collaboration. Furthermore, schools infrequently help young people to build *assets* such as caring for others, connectedness, or civic engagement (Institute of Medicine, 2002; Moore & Lippman, 2004).

Thus, whilst we have extensive data about the impact of fragmented risk-specific interventions implemented within schools, we have much less about the effects of school health interventions on education outcomes or social assets, or about the effectiveness of whole school approaches that strategically integrate multiple interventions.

Box 19.2. Theory and practice – cities

The WHO Healthy Cities project aims "to put health on the agenda of decision-makers" (Tsouros, 1995, p.133). The logic of this aim is that, with increased social and political status, more appropriate action for health can be taken in the urban context.

Cities were therefore encouraged to embark on innovative approaches to strengthen the presence of health in the social and political discourse. Some cities (e.g. Bologna, Horsens, Copenhagen) took a community perspective, opening 'health shops' – which used community development and self-help approaches to engage the public. Others (e.g. Kuressaare, Noarlunga, Bangkok) built on existing political debates, utilising community action, advocacy, and research to address issues such as tourism, sustainable economic development, environmental concerns, and transportation. A number (e.g., Krakow, Kuching, Accra) generated data demonstrating the epidemiological evidence for doing things differently: air pollution monitoring systems were established, communities were engaged in producing health information, and environmental aspects of sanitation were highlighted. Finally, a range of cities (e.g. Tainan, Torun, Johannesburg) were enabled, through the international prominence of the programme, to engage in interventions that were before considered unrealistic or unfounded: community empowerment programmes, a city-wide tobacco control strategy, or the use of televised health-oriented soap operas.

Whilst all found inspiration in the rich framework provided by Healthy Cities and grounding in the unique environmental, social and political contexts of their administrations' work, the sheer diversity illustrates just how challenging it is to establish 'across-the-board' evidence of effectiveness for Healthy City programmes.

Box 19.3. Theory and practice – virtual settings

Information technology provides countless settings (e.g. internet, telemedicine, health portals, online support groups) – where people can conveniently access and retrieve information, and be supported in their behaviour change efforts (Evers, 2006). However, technology may fail to address the broader determinants of health, further widening health inequalities, as health literacy issues compounded by the digital divide disenfranchise access for those with few resources (Hirji, 2004; Lorence & Greenberg, 2006; Nguyen, Carrieri-Kholman, Rankin, Slaugher, & Sulbarg, 2004; Norman & Skinner, 2006; Skinner, Biscope, & Poland, 2003). Furthermore, the growth of e-learning may well undermine the social connections that healthy settings facilitate (St Leger, 2006), changing as it does both the ethos of education settings and people's experience of education and professional development.

Calls for building social capital, networks and bonds virtually (Bolam, McLean, Pennington, & Gillies, 2006) cite examples from politics where online activity has influenced off-line activism (Wellman, Haase, Witte, & Hampton, 2002). For example, TeenNet (http://www.teennetproject.org/) encourages behaviour change as well as online activism, social support, and mutual aid, reflecting a 'virtual' community development approach (Lombardo & Skinner, 2003–2004; Lombardo, Zakus, & Skinner, 2002; Skinner, Biscope, Poland, & Goldberg, 2003).

Although descriptive research suggests that virtual settings are valuable channels for distributing health information or counselling support (Suggs, 2006), the challenges of conducting high quality research online have limited rigorous and wide-ranging evaluation (Bessell, McDonald, Silagy, Anderson, Hiller, & Sansom, 2002; Eng, 2002; Nguyen et al, 2004). Moreover with few exceptions, virtual settings – rooted in communication, behaviour change and psychological theories – have assumed an interventionist stance, perpetuating "traditional individually-focused intervention(s)" (Wenzel, 1997 cited in Dooris, 2006b, p.4).

Evidence of Effectiveness

Introduction

We have argued that the settings approach is essentially characterized by an ecological whole system perspective – and would further contend that this contributes a richness and coherence that can make health promotion more relevant, appropriate, and effective than "traditional" narrowly focused topic-based and disease-specific interventions. However, in asserting these benefits, we acknowledge the implications for building evidence of effectiveness – and make explicit the "evaluation paradox" that emerges.

In this section, we will briefly outline the current situation and consider the challenges presented. Rather than attempting a comprehensive review of the existing evidence base, we highlight key points and provide examples.

The Current Situation

In terms of effectiveness, the settings approach is perceived to have a number of benefits (Dooris, 2004). It encourages connections between people, environments and behaviours to be explored within everyday places; it allows relationships between different groups of people to be recognized; it enables interactions between different issues to be taken into account; it looks outward as well as inward, facilitating intra- and inter-organisational awareness of wider impacts on health and sustainability at local, national and global levels; and it provides opportunities to harness the contribution of a range of settings to "joined-up" public health.

Despite these perceived benefits and significant advances in evaluation, it would seem that the approach has an uneven and under-developed evidence base (see Boxes 19.4 and 19.5). Settings seem to provide a framework for planning, implementing, and evaluating comprehensive behaviour and environmental change interventions, and documenting health outcomes (Goodstadt, 2001; Nutbeam, 2000), yet significant challenges remain. As St Leger (1997, p.100) argues: "The settings

Box 19.4. Evidence – Schools

In relation to schools, the value of the 'whole school approach' is widely recognized. However, the belief that comprehensive programmes are most likely to achieve and sustain benefits (National Health and Medical Research Council, 1996; St Leger and Nutbeam, 2000) has not generally been translated into appropriate research – and the vast majority of studies concern the effectiveness of individual health interventions implemented *in* the school setting (see Chapter 8).

Thus, there is scant data on such comprehensive programmes, and there are ongoing difficulties with both evaluation and implementation (Deschesnes, 2003; Lister-Sharp, Chapman, Stewart-Brown, & Soden, 1999; McIntyre, Belzer, Manchester, Blanchard, Officer, & Simpson, 1996; Mũkhoma & Flisher, 2004). This is partly because of the variation between different schools (Honig, 2006), but also because the approach is relatively new and instruments are still being developed and tested (Australian Health Promoting Schools Association, 2002; Lee, Cheng, & St Leger, 2005; Lohrmann, 2006; Rowling & Jeffreys, 2006; US Centers for Disease Control, 2005, 2006b; WHO, 1996). Furthermore, there has been a tendency to "define out, simplify, or edit out 'complex variables', relationships, structures and processes in an attempt to gain insight into the complex organisations that are schools" (Colquhoun, 2006, pp.41–42).

More optimistically, in a recent synthesis, Stewart-Brown (2006, p.17) has concluded that effective school health promotion programmes are likely to be intensive and of long duration, and "complex, multifactorial and involve activity in more than one domain (curriculum, school environment and community). These are features of the health promoting schools approach, and to this extent these finding endorse such approaches."

Box 19.5. Evidence – Cities

In relation to Healthy Cities, de Leeuw & Skovgaard (2005) conclude that the general evidence that the programme works does not translate to a problem-solving perspective that can inform decision-making.

As stated in Box 2, although the general ambition of Healthy Cities is clear ('to put health high on social and political agendas'), evidence-related demands are extremely diverse:

Funders, often health agencies, want to know whether activities yield more health. When related to particular programmes in unique cities, there is ample evidence that programmes such as community empowerment (Wallerstein, 2006), adapted to specific urban environments and with appropriate developmental perspectives, are effective.

Politicians want to know additionally whether policies provide an appropriate return on investment – whether they advance political agendas. Whilst evidence on oral health in the Brazilian city of Curitiba shows that broad-based healthy public policies inspired by Healthy Cities are effective (Moysés, Moysés, McCarthy, & Sheiham, 2006), this is not to say that such evidence furthers a city's political agenda.

Academics have yet to accept fully that appropriate evidence cannot come from randomized controlled trials (RCTs) or quasi-experimentation alone – despite well-articulated arguments that evidence is multi-factorial, can be generated through multiple-method research designs, should involve health producers, and has to be weighed in an almost judicial approach (Tones, 1997).

Nevertheless, it is this approach that would do ultimate justice to the diversity of Healthy City characteristics. Kegler, Twiss, & Look (2000) have highlighted the centrality of systems thinking in Healthy City evaluation and Poland (1996) has argued that "the complex multifaceted causal web surrounding the sorts of long-term impacts the . . .[healthy communities] movement is seeking to make is a sobering reminder of the limitations of conventional evaluation science." The solution advocated by de Leeuw & Skovgaard (2005) is that 'real' evidence should be useful to those who need it – and that such 'utility-driven evidence' can only be generated through extensive collaboration between partners.

approach has been legitimated more through an act of faith than through rigorous research and evaluation studies . . .much more attention needs to be given to building the evidence and learning from it."

Challenges Faced in Evaluating the Settings Approach and Building Evidence of Effectiveness

Health promotion has experienced a number of general difficulties in responding to the demand for evidence of effectivenesss. Nutbeam (1999, p.99) has commented: "It is a challenge to assemble 'evidence' in ways which are relevant to the complexities of contemporary health promotion, and to avoid the possibility that this may lead action down a narrow, reductionist route." The response to this challenge has seen a call for the use of both quantitative and qualitative data, for a greater breadth of evidence, for an "evidence into practice into evidence" cycle, and for a consideration not only of what works, but also of how and under what conditions.

However, as discussed in detail by Dooris (2006a), it can be argued that for those using the settings approach, a number of specific challenges have made it problematic to undertake consistent, rigorous evaluation and have added to the general difficulties of building evidence of effectiveness.

Diversity of Conceptual Understandings and Real-Life Practice

Firstly, the settings "banner" embraces a diversity of both conceptual understandings and real-life practice (Green et al, 2000; Poland et al, 2000; Whitelaw et al, 2001), making it difficult to build a substantive body of research that allows comparability and transferability. A number of issues are of relevance:

Conceptual variation: Despite a growing literature prioritising an ecological systems perspective, there remains a tendency to conflate "health promotion in settings" with the settings approach (Wenzel, 1997). Recognising this conceptual variation and the confusion it can cause, Whitelaw et al (2001) have formulated a typology that distinguishes different forms of of settings-based practice, reflecting different analyses of the problem and solution in terms of whether the focus is more on the individual or the setting/system. The challenge to evaluation is evident – and constitutes "a political as well as scientific process" (Connell & Kubisch, 1998 cited in Mackenzie & Blamey, 2005, p.153).

Practical considerations: Whitelaw et al (2001) also discuss the influence of practical considerations on practice, highlighting real life constraints and opportunities within different settings, and the challenges of translating theory into action. As Dooris (2004, p.44) has noted, "whilst the theoretical framework guiding the work may be rooted in systems thinking and organisational development, the practice is often constrained to smaller-scale project-focused work around particular issues." In terms of evaluation and subsequent dissemination, this highlights again the centrality of context and of "exploring what works better for whom in what circumstances, and why" (Pawson & Tilley, 1997 cited in Stame, 2004, p.58).

Size and type of settings: As previously highlighted, the approach has expanded to include a wide range of settings, diverse in size and form. This suggests a need for clarification of similarity and difference within and across categories of settings (Dooris, 2004; Poland et al, 2000). Methods used within "total institutions" such as prisons or hospitals will differ from those used in less formal settings; and in terms of effectiveness, it may be easier to demonstrate whole system change within a small setting such as a primary school than in a large multi-layered setting such as a university, or indeed, a city.

Standards and accreditation: An additional distinction must be drawn between programmes with agreed accreditation criteria or standards (e.g. schools and hospitals) and those without a widely recognized programme (e.g. universities). Although subject to criticism (Jones & Douglas, 2002) in terms of their failure to take account of cultural, economic and social variations, accredited programmes clearly facilitate evaluation.

Focus on Diseases and Single Risk Factors

Secondly, the established evidence "system" for health promotion retains a primary focus on single risk factor interventions and specific diseases/problems rather than on multiple interventions and settings. A few reviews have looked specifically at programmes such as Health Promoting Schools (e.g. Lister-Sharp et al, 1999; Stewart-Brown, 2006) and drawn promising conclusions regarding the value of a whole system approach. However, most reviews that consider a particular setting are only concerned to assess the value of discrete interventions designed to impact on one specific risk factor.

It would, then, appear that the evidence base has continued to be structured following a medical model – despite discussion of a "paradigm shift" in health promotion (Barić, 1994). This reflects the continuing priority given to disease and behaviour based targets in health policy (Ziglio, Hagard, & Griffiths, 2000), leading to more funding being available for evaluation of issue-based than settings-based initiatives; and the fact that most research designed to evaluate complex, ecological programmes does not qualify for inclusion within systematic reviews and meta-analyses – although there is optimism that this will change with the general broadening of approaches (Nutbeam, 1999; Jackson & Waters, 2005).

Complexity of Evaluating Ecological Whole System Approaches

Thirdly, it *is* very complex to evaluate the settings approach as conceptualized above – characterized by an ecological model, a systems perspective and whole system thinking. Such an approach involves multiple interconnected interventions tailored to the culture and needs of a specific setting, and the prioritisation of organisation development, participation and empowerment to ensure that these interventions are owned and modified by local actors, and become embedded in routine life. Two points can be usefully highlighted:

Ecological complexity: An ecological perspective focuses on the interactions and interdependence between different elements within ecosystems, highlighting the relationships between people and settings (McLaren & Hawe, 2005). In applying systems thinking to health promotion, we are encouraged to focus not only on the individual components but on the spaces in between, on the arrows that join up the bubbles in addition to the bubbles themselves (Barić & Barić, 1995). As Senge (1990, p.68) has argued: "Systems thinking is a discipline for seeing wholes. It is a framework for seeing interrelationships rather than things, for seeing patterns of change rather than static "snapshots".

In relation to health-promoting schools, Rowling and Jeffreys (2006, p.708) have noted that: "Researchers fail to recognize and monitor the synergy created by integrating components, give it minor status in reporting or omit "process" completely. This ignores an essential quality in a settings approach – the interaction of components in a specific context." The need to acknowledge and take account of synergy *between* settings adds further complexity to the evaluation challenge, and highlights the value of networks operating "horizontally" as well as "vertically" (Dooris, 2004).

Integration and visibility: It can, paradoxically, be argued that the more successful a settings-based initiative is, the harder it will be to isolate its unique contribution to organisational and personal change. Effective mainstreaming is likely to make health promotion less visible as a tangible entity and a key challenge is to allow the language of health (as an enterprise somehow separate from the core business of the setting) to recede. This is illustrated in a review of workplace health promotion, which reflects that many organisation-level interventions are "performed without any direct link to health and thus have an unspecified effect on ill health and well-being" (Breuker & Schröer, 2000, pp.103–104).

Implications for Future Research

Whilst there has been a convergent recognition of the importance of ecology and systems thinking in fields such as health promotion (Best et al, 2003; Green, Richard, & Potvin, 1996; Stokols, 1996), education (Fullan, 2003; Senge, Cambron-McCabe, Lucas, Smith, Dutton, & Kleiner, 2000), and business (Gharajedaghi, 1999; Senge, 1990), this has not been translated into clear guidelines to inform research and evaluation. It would seem to us that, for the most part, those evaluating health promoting settings initiatives have struggled to apply such a perspective.

If we are to capture the added value of ecological, whole system working, and build convincing evidence of effectiveness for the settings approach, we cannot merely focus in isolation on individual interventions operating as part of a settings initiative. Instead, we must design evaluation studies that adopt non-linear approaches, looking at the whole and mapping and elucidating the interrelationships, interactions and synergies within and between settings – with regard to different groups of the people, components of the system and "health" issues. It is also important for researchers to utilize multi-method approaches (Pan American Health Organisation, 2005), acknowledge the synergistic effects of combining a variety of methods to answer different evaluation questions (Baum, 1995; Steckler et al, 1992), and integrate "health" measures with measures that relate to the core business of the setting (Lee et al., 2005).

With a particular focus on the third challenge outlined above, we will now highlight some key implications for future research, discussing key theoretical and methodological innovations in two related areas: critical realism and complexity theory. Critical realism emphasizes discovery of underlying logic, using theory to discern generative mechanisms that endure across space-time, but whose expression is highly variable, contingent, and context-bound. In contrast, complexity theory places more emphasis on the organic, emergent nature of innovation and adaptation, and suggests different principles for the management of organizational and social change initiatives.

We believe that harnessing and applying thinking from these two fields offers enormous potential for overcoming the limitations of traditional evaluation models and helping generate evidence of effectiveness for ecological, whole system settings-based health promotion.

Critical Realism and Critical Realist Evaluation

Critical realist evaluation represents a promising, but underutilized, approach to understanding how interventions work or fail in particular contexts – i.e. which elements of context matter, and why (Poland, Frohlich, & Cargo, 2007). Critical realism is a logic of inquiry, drawing on the work of Bhaskar (1979), whose central premise is that constant conjunction (empirical co-occurrence) is an insufficient basis for inferring causality, and that what is required is the identification of generative mechanisms whose causal properties may or may not be activated, depending on circumstance (Connelly, 2001; Julnes, Mark & Henry, 1998; Stame, 2004; Williams, 2003). It is a theory-driven approach whose starting point is the distinction between the *empirical* (what is observed), the *actual* (events and experiences that may or may not be observed/observable), and the *real* (the domain of underlying causal mechanisms) (Williams, 2003). Further, mechanisms can coincide under real world conditions to produce *emergent properties* contingent in time and space (Sayer, 2000).

Thus, from a critical realist perspective, context is not an undifferentiated social ether in which programmes and phenomena "float", but a series of generative mechanisms in constant interaction with complex and contingent combinations of events and actors. The notion of contingency contrasts with positivist notions of universal logical necessity (natural laws, generalizable truths) by highlighting the uncertain nature of phenomena (i.e. that propositions may hold true only under certain circumstances).

As these generative mechanisms may only be discernible because of their effects (contingent in space-time), critical realist program evaluations must be grounded in theories that specify what generative mechanisms are triggered (or suppressed) by which intervention elements, under which conditions. Generative mechanisms refer to program mediators that interventions seek to modify. Weiss (1997) argues for developing sound program theory, specifying the interrelated sequence of events expected to occur and how they relate to each other in space and time, thereby making transparent the underlying logic and assumptions of a given intervention.

From this perspective, the central evaluative question is not so much *whether* certain programmes (or parts of programmes) work – what Stame (2004) refers to as "black box" evaluation – but "to 'unpack the mechanism' of *how* complex programmes work (or *why* they fail) in particular contexts and settings" (Pawson, Greenhalgh, Harvey & Walshe, 2004, p.1). These "how" and "why" questions are critical to decision-making regarding which programmatic components are worth replicating in which circumstances.

Thus it is possible to (re)define context as: "The (local) mix of conditions and events (social agents, objects and interactions) which characterize open systems . . .whose unique confluence in time and space selectively activates (triggers, blocks or modifies) causal powers (mechanisms) in a chain of reactions that may result in very different outcomes depending on the dynamic interplay of conditions and mechanisms over time and space" (Poland, Frohlich, & Cargo, 2007). This gives us a more workable and concrete definition of social context that offers a way to transcend the "evaluation paradox" described above (i.e. that successful embedding of interventions in settings and systems makes their impacts harder to observe and measure). Moreover, a critical realist approach – with its emphasis on theory-based evaluation – provides a further motivation to address the first challenge highlighted, by clarifying the conceptual basis of settings-based health promotion and articulating the inter-related web of hypotheses, assumptions, processes and anticipated outcomes that constitute a complex initiative (Dooris, 2006a).

Complexity Theory

Complexity theory is the second theoretical perspective that we would suggest holds promise for those seeking to build evidence for the settings approach to health promotion. Its central object of inquiry is the complex adaptive system (CAS) – "a collection of individual agents with freedom to act in ways that are not always totally predictable, and whose actions are interconnected so that one agent's actions change the context for other agents" (Plsek & Greenhalgh, 2001, p.625). A CAS is thus a complex, non-linear and interactive system, within which "semi-autonomous agents . . .adapt by changing their rules and, hence, behaviour, as they gain experience" (Zimmerman, Lindberg, & Plsek, 2001, p.263).

Complexity theory is of particular interest because it shines a spotlight on those aspects of reality that traditional organization development theory sees as irrele-vant or troublesome, or doesn't see at all. It draws on new discoveries in the bio-logical and social/organizational sciences; empirical examples of the failure of central planning (e.g. strategic planning exercises that produce little change); and the power of groundswell, organic innovation from the margins (e.g. the emer-gence of the internet). It is a perspective that emphasizes the power of distributed (as opposed to centralized) control, relationships between relatively self-organiz-ing individuals, the co-evolution of systems in embedded environments, and the relationship of micro and macro.

Applied in the field of organization development, complexity theory differs from traditional management theories that emphasize planned change through better (more) specification and hierarchical control of players, processes, and outcomes that are inherently slippery, potentially resistant, and ultimately not always open to influence using traditional techniques. It suggests that the key to the kind of adaptive innovation required in a changing and fast-paced world is the identification of new ways to harness the creativity and knowledge of frontline staff, by stimulating and supporting "communities of practice" (Brown & Duguid, 1991; Wenger & Snyder, 2000; Westley, Zimmerman & Patton, 2006) and by drawing on the kinds of principles outlined in Table 19.1 (Zimmerman et al, 2001).

The result is a very practical, but very different, basis for initiating, supporting, and harnessing adaptive change that seems much more attuned to the realities of late-modern (organizational) settings. The many examples described by Zimmerman et al (2001) of how these ideas are operationalized in health care set-tings suggests what might be possible within the field of health promotion if those seeking to implement and evaluate settings-based initiatives and programmes were to harness and apply perspectives from complexity theory.

TABLE 19.1. Nine organizational and leadership principles from the study of complex adaptive systems

Principle	Full statement of principle	Further explanation or contrast to the traditional approach
1. Complexity lens	View your system through the lens of complexity . . .	. . . in addition to the metaphor of a machine or a military organization.
2. Good-enough vision	Build a good-enough vision and provide minimum specifications . . .	. . .rather than trying to plan out every detail.
3. Clockware/ swarmware	When life is far from certain, lead from the edge, with clockware and swarmware in tandem . . .	. . .that is, balance data and intuition, planning and acting, safety and risk, giving due honor to each.
4. Tune to the edge	Tune your place to the edge by fostering the 'right' degree of: information flow, diversity and difference, connections inside and outside the organization, power differential and anxiety . . .	. . .instead of controlling information, forcing agreement, dealing separately with contentious groups, working systematically down all the layers of the hierarchy in sequence, and seeking comfort.
5. Paradox	Uncover and work with paradox and tension . . .	. . .rather than shying away from them as if they were unnatural.
6. Multiple actions	Go for multiple actions at the fringes, let direction arise . . .	. . .rather than believing that you must be sure before you can proceed with anything.
7. Shadow system	Listen to the shadow system . . .	. . .realizing that informal relationships, gossip, rumour, and hallway conversations contribute significantly to agents' mental models and subsequent actions.
8. Chunking	Grow complex systems by chunking . . .	. . .by allowing complex systems to emerge, out of the links among simple systems that work well and are capable of operating independently.
9. Competition/ cooperation	Mix cooperation and competition	. . .it's not one or the other.

Source: Zimmerman et al (2001)

Conclusion

In this chapter, we have proposed a rationale for the settings approach to health promotion based on the importance of context and the need to invest in the places where people live their lives. We have also suggested that the approach reflects an ecological model of health promotion, is informed by systems thinking, and focuses on whole organization change through multiple interconnected interventions concerned to improve health and enhance productivity.

However, despite a widespread perception that the approach is both appropriate and effective, those engaged in evaluation and evidence generation face important challenges – including the diversity of both theory and practice that is presented as settings-based health promotion; the evidence system's continuing focus on diseases and single risk factors; and the very real difficulties of evaluating ecological, whole system health promotion characterized by synergy and integration. In addressing these challenges and considering implications for future research, we have suggested that the two related areas of critical realism and complexity theory offer potentially exciting and valuable opportunities to overcome the restrictions of traditional evaluation and help build evidence of effectiveness for settings-based health promotion.

Before concluding, it is useful to return to the values that underpin the settings approach – because evaluation and evidence are essentially value-based (Raphael, 2000). We want to highlight three key values – participation, equity, and partnership.

As the logic of the settings approach is a non-medical one, it may be more easily understood by community members and political decision-makers than by "health" professionals (Kickbusch, 1996). Participatory action research is entirely compatible with a systems perspective and ecological model, encouraging a shift away from a disease and risk factor mindset (Leung, Yen, & Minkler, 2004) and allowing a better understanding of the context and reality of life (Satterfield, Volansky, Caspersen, Engelgau, Bowman, Gregg, Geiss, Hosey, May, & Vinicor, 2003). As a method of inquiry, it is built on trust and equity, and characterized by working *with* community partners and citizens in all aspects of research from community assessment to evaluation (Kelly, 2005). It blends collaborative investigation, education, and action, and provides a mechanism to help make epidemiological findings locally relevant, setting specific, and provide apposite answers to community health issues (Kelly; Leung et al., 2004). It crosses disciplinary boundaries and is concerned with social justice and equity, drawing as it does on the settlement house tradition (in many ways a forerunner to the healthy communities movement), which in the late 19th and early 20th centuries responded to the problems of rapid industrialization and urbanization (Koerin, 2003).

In terms of equity, health promotion must grapple not only with the health-related impacts of inequality, but also with the way that social relations (economic and political systems, institutional and cultural practices) create, maintain, and reproduce inequalities in health (Eakin, et al, 1996). Such power relations play a central role in the marginalization and disempowerment of people locally and globally. Settings-based health promotion must therefore seek to address issues of equity and power relations – within, outside and across settings. Green et al. (2000, p.24) suggest that health promotion may have inadvertently "played into existing power relations and alliances" within settings by aligning itself with management, thereby marginalising or alienating less powerful groups (e.g. workers, students). A further concern is the need for health promotion policy, practice, and research to extend its focus to less traditional settings – recognizing that, with a few exceptions such as prisons, "the settings in which one is to find the unemployed, the homeless, the disenfranchised youth, the illegal immigrants, and so forth are not as well defined" (Green et al, 2000, p.25). The effectiveness of healthy settings initiatives must also be judged in terms of their focus on organisational structures, policies, and practices that redress inequalities, and their successful advocacy for macro-level social, economic and political change.

Issues of equity and power relations become even more evident within complex settings such as cities, which involve forming partnerships between a diversity of stakeholders from multiple sectors (Costongs & Springett, 1997), and when connecting between and working across settings. However, if we are to build credible evidence of effectiveness for the settings approach, we need to prioritize such collaboration and utilize networks (both setting-specific and cross-setting) to understand and capture the synergy and "added value" of whole system health promotion. This will require a dual focus, evaluating how the approach impacts on health and how it influences the achievement of "core business" goals. It will also require a broadening of the evidence base across sectors and disciplines to reflect the intersectoral nature of settings programs (Rowling & Jeffreys, 2006).

Looking to the future, we face considerable challenges in articulating with simplicity and clarity the theory and practice of the settings approach, and in building evidence of effectiveness for this ecological, whole system health promotion, in ways that reflect the underpinning values of participation, equity, and partnership. By harnessing innovations from critical realism and complexity theory, we have the opportunity to move beyond traditional evaluation – paying increased attention to "the social context of interventions that are evaluated" (McQueen, 2002, p.83) and understanding settings "in a way that celebrates complexity rather than trying to control for it" (Colquhoun, 2006, p.42).

References

Antonovsky, A. (1996). The salutogenic model as a theory to guide health promotion. *Health Promotion International, 11*, 11–18.

Ashton, J. (1988). Rising to the challenge. *Health Service Journal, 20 October*, 1232–1234.

Australian Health Promoting Schools Association (2002). *National framework for health promoting schools, 2002–2003.*
(http://www.ahpsa.org.au/files/framework.pdf accessed 06 October 2006).

Barić, L. (1993). The settings approach – implications for policy and strategy. *Journal of the Institute of Health Education, 31*, 17–24.

Barić, L. (1994). *Health promotion and health education in practice. Module 2: The organisational model.* Altrincham: Barns Publications.

Barić, L. & Barić, L. (1995) *Health promotion and health education. Module 3: Evaluation, quality, audit.* Altrincham: Barns Publications.

Barnekow Rasmussen, V. & Rivett, D. (2000). The European network of health promoting schools – an alliance of health, education and democracy. *Health Education, 100*, 61–67.

Bartholemew, L. K., Parcel, G. S., Kok, G., & Gottlieb, N. H. (2006). *Planning health promotion programs: an intervention mapping approach* (2nd Ed.). San Francisco CA: Jossey-Boss.

Baum, F. (1995). Researching public health: beyond the qualitative and quantitative method debate. *Social Science and Medicine, 55*, 459–468.

Bessel, T., McDonald, S., Silagy, C., Anderson, J., Hiller, J., & Sansom, L. (2002). Do internet interventions for consumers cause more harm than good? A systematic review. *Health Expectations, 5*, 28–37.

Best, A., Stokols, D., Green, L. W., Leischow, S., Holmes, B., & Buchholz, K. (2003). An integrative framework for community partnering to translate theory into effective health promotion strategy. *American Journal of Health Promotion, 18*, 168–176.

Bhaskar, R. (1979). *The possibility of naturalism.* Atlantic Heights, NJ: Humanities Press.

Bolam, B., McLean, C., Pennington, A., & Gillies, P. (2006). Using new media to build social capital for health. *Journal of Health Psychology, 11*, 297–308.

Breuker, G. & Schroer, A. (2000). Settings 1 – health promotion in the workplace. In International Union for Health Promotion and Education *The evidence of health promotion effectiveness. Shaping public health in a new Europe. Part two: Evidence book* (pp. 98–109). Brussels – Luxembourg: ECSC-EC-EAEC. 2nd edition. Paris: Jouve Composition & Impression.

Bronfenbrenner, U. (1979). *The ecology of human development. Experiments by nature and design.* Cambridge MA: Harvard University Press.

Bronfenbrenner, U. (1994). Ecological models of human development. In T. Husen & T. Postlethwaite (Eds.), *International encyclopedia of education*, Vol. 3, 2nd Ed., (pp. 1643–1647). Oxford: Pergamon Press/Elseiver Science.

Brown, J. S. & Duguid, P. (1991). Organizational learning and communities of practice: Towards a unified view of working, learning, and innovation. *Organization Science, 2*, 40–57.

Capra, F. (1983). *The turning point: Science, society and the rising culture.* London: Flamingo.

Colquhoun, D. (2006). Complexity and the health promoting school. In S. Clift & B. Bruun Jensen (Eds.), *The health promoting school: International advances in theory, evaluation and practice* (pp. 41–53). Copenhagen, Denmark: Danish University of Education Press.

Connell, J. P. & Kubisch, A. C. (1998). Applying a theory of change approach to the evaluation of comprehensive community initiatives: Progress, prospects, and problems. In K. Fulbright-Anderson, A. C. Kubisch, & J. P. Connell (Eds.), *New approaches to evaluating community initiatives. Volume 2: Theory, measurement, and analysis*, (pp. 15–44). Washington, DC: The Aspen Institute.

Connelly, J. (2001). Critical realism and health promotion: Effective practice needs an effective theory. *Health Education Research, 16*, 115–120.

Costongs, C. & Springett, J. (1997). Joint working and the production of a city health plan: The Liverpool experience. *Health Promotion International, 12*, 9–19.

Department of Health, Social Services & Public Safety (2002). *Investing for health.* Belfast: DHSSPS.

Deschesnes, M., Martin, C., & Jomphe Hill, A. (2003). Comprehensive approaches to school health promotion: How to achieve broader implementation? *Health Promotion International, 18*, 387–396.

Dooris, M (2001). The "health promoting university": A critical exploration of theory and practice. *Health Education, 101*, 51–60.

Dooris, M. (2004). Joining up settings for health: a valuable investment for strategic partnerships? *Critical Public Health, 14*, 37–49.

Dooris, M. (2006a). Healthy settings: challenges to generating evidence of effectiveness. *Health Promotion International, 21*, 55–65.

Dooris, M. (2006b). Health promoting settings: future directions. *Promotion & Education, 13*, 4–6.

Dooris, M. & Hunter, D. (2007). Organisations and settings for public health. In S. Handsley, C. Lloyd, J. Douglas, S. Earle & S. Spurr (Eds.), *Policy and practice in promoting public health*. London: Sage/Milton Keynes: Open University.

Dooris, M., Dowding, G., Thompson, J., & Wynne, C. (1998). The settings-based approach to health promotion. In A. Tsouros, G. Dowding, J. Thompson, & M. Dooris (Eds.), *Health promoting universities: Concept, experience and framework for action* (pp. 18–28). Copenhagen: WHO Regional Office for Europe.

Eakin, J., Robertson, A., Poland, B., Coburn, D. & Edwards, R. (1996). Towards a critical social science perspective on health promotion research. *Health Promotion International 11*, 157–165.

Eng, T. (2002). eHealth research and evaluation: challenges and opportunities. *Journal of Health Communication, 7*, 267–272.

Evers, K. (2006). eHealth promotion: the use of the internet for health promotion. *American Journal of Health Promotion, 20*, 1–7.

French, W. & Bell, C. (1999). *Organisation development: Behavioural science interventions for organisation improvement*. New Jersey: Prentice Hall.

Fullan, M. (2003). Change forces with a vengeance. London: RoutledgeFalmer.

Galea, G., Powis, B., & Tamplin, S. (2000). Healthy islands in the Western Pacific – international settings development. *Health Promotion International, 15*, 169–178.

Gharajedaghi, J. (1999). *Systems thinking: Managing chaos and complexity – A platform for designing business architecture*. Burlington, MA: Butterworth-Heinemann.

Goodstadt, M. (2001). Part 3: Settings – introduction. In I. Rootman, M. Goodstadt, B. Hyndman, D. McQueen, L. Potvin, J. Springett, & E. Ziglio (Eds.), *Evaluation in health promotion: principles and perspectives* (pp. 209–211). Copenhagen: WHO Regional Office for Europe.

Green, L. W. & Kreuter, M. (2005). *Health promotion planning: An educational and ecological approach*, 4th Ed. New York: McGraw-Hill.

Green, L. W., Poland, B. D., & Rootman, I. (2000). The settings approach to health promotion. In B. D. Poland, L. W. Green, & I. Rootman (Eds.), *Settings for health promotion: Linking theory and practice* (pp. 1–43). London: Sage.

Green, L. W., Richard, L. & Potvin, L. (1996). Ecological foundations of health promotion. *American Journal of Health Promotion, 10*, 270–281.

Groene, O. & Garcia-Barbero, M. (Eds.) (2005). *Health promotion in hospitals: Evidence and quality management*. Copenhagen: WHO Regional Office for Europe.

Grossman, R. & Scala, K. (1993). *Health promotion and organisational development: Developing settings for health*. Copenhagen: WHO Regional Office for Europe.

Hirji, F. (2004). Freedom or folly? Canadians and the consumption of online health information. *Information, Communication and Society, 7*, 445–465.

Honig, M. (2006). *New directions in education policy implementation: confronting complexity*. Albany, New York: State University of New York Press.

Institute of Medicine (2002). *Community programs to promote youth development*. Washington, DC: National Academy of Sciences.

Jackson, N. & Waters, E. (2005) *Guidelines: Systematic reviews of health promotion and public health interventions*. Melbourne: Cochrane Collaboration – Cochrane Health Promotion and Public Health Field.

Jewkes, R. & Murcott, A. (1998). Community representativeness: Representing the "community"? *Social Science and Medicine, 46*, 843–858.

Jones, L. & Douglas, J. from 1st draft by Adams, L. (2002). The politics of health promotion. In L. Jones, M. Sidell, & J. Douglas (Eds.). *The challenge of promoting health: Exploration and action* (pp.143–171). Basingstoke: Palgrave MacMillan.

Julnes, G., Mark, M., & Henry, G. (1998). Promoting realism in evaluation: Realistic evaluation and the broader context. *Evaluation, 4*, 483–504.

Kahan, B. & Goodstadt, M. (2001). The interactive domain model of best practices in health promotion: Developing and implementing a best practices approach to health promotion. *Health Promotion Practice, 2*, 43–67.

Kegler, M. C., Twiss, J. M., & Look, V. (2000). Assessing community change at multiple levels: The genesis of an evaluation framework for the California Healthy Cities Project. *Health Education and Behavior, 27*, 760–779.

Kelly, P. (2005). Practical suggestions for community interventions using participatory action research. *Public Health Nursing, 22*(1), 65–73.

Koerin, B. (2003). The settlement house tradition: current trends and future concerns. *Journal of Sociology and Social Welfare, XXX*(2), 53–68.

Kickbusch, I. (1995). An overview to the settings-based approach to health promotion. In T. Theaker & J. Thompson (Eds.), *The Settings-based approach to health promotion: Report of an international working conference, 17–20 November 1993* (pp. 3–9). Welwyn Garden City: Hertfordshire Health Promotion.

Kickbusch, I. (1996). Tribute to Aaron Antonovsky – "what creates health"? *Health Promotion International, 11*, 5–6.

Kickbusch, I. (2003). The contribution of the World Health Organization to a new public health and health promotion. *American Journal of Public Health, 93*, 383–388.

Kolbe, L. (2002). Education reform and the goals of modern school health programs. *The State Education Standard: The Quarterly Journal of the National Association of State Boards of Education, 3*, 4–11.

Kolbe, L. (2005). A framework for school health programs in the 21st Century. *Journal of School Health, 75*, 226–228.

Kolbe, L., Jones, J., Birdthistle, I., & Vince-Whitman, C. (2000). Building the capacity of schools to improve the health of nations. In C. E. Koop, C. E. Pearson, & M. R. Schwarz (Eds.), *Critical Issues in Global Health* (pp. 212–220). San Francisco: Jossey-Bass.

Kolbe, L., Tirozzi, G., Marx, E., Bobbitt-Cooke, M., Riedel, S., Jones, J., & Schmoyer, M. (2005). Health programs for school employees: Improving quality of life, health & productivity. *Promotion & Education, 12*, 157–161.

Lee, A., Cheng, F., & St Leger, L (2005). Evaluating health promoting schools in Hong Kong: the development of a framework. *Health Promotion International, 20*, 177–186.

Leeuw, E. de & Skovgaard, T. (2005). Utility-driven evidence for healthy cities: problems with evidence generation and application. *Social Science and Medicine, 61*, 1331–1341.

Leung, M., Yen, I., & Minkler, M. (2004). Community based participatory research: A promising approach for increasing epidemiology's relevance in the 21st century. *International Journal of Epidemiology, 33*, 499–506.

Lister-Sharp, D., Chapman, S., Stewart-Brown, S., & Soden, A. (1999). Health promoting schools and health promotion in school: Two systematic reviews. *Health Technology Assessment, 3*(22).

Lohrmann, D. (2006). *Creating a healthy school using the healthy school report card.* Alexandria, Virginia: Association for Supervision and Curriculum Development.

Lombardo, C. & Skinner, H. (2003–2004). "A virtual hug": Prospects for self-help online. *International Journal of Self Help and Self Care, 2*, 205–218.

Lombardo, C., Zakus, D., & Skinner, H. (2002). Youth social action: Building a global latticework through informtion and communication technologies. *Health Promotion International, 17*, 363–371.

Lorence, D.P. & Greenberg, L. (2006). The zeitgeist of online health search: Implications for a consumer-centric health system. *Journal of General Internal Medicine, 21*, 134–139.

Mackenzie, M. & Blamey, A. (2005). The practice and the theory: Lessons from the applications of a Theories of Change approach. *Evaluation, 11*, 151–168.

Malpas, J. (2003). Bio-medical Topoi – the dominance of space, the recalcitrance of place, and the making of persons. *Social Science and Medicine, 56*, 2343–2351.

McIntyre, L., Belzer, E. G., Manchester, L., Blanchard, W., Officer, S., & Simpson, A. C. (1996) The Dartmouth health promotion study: A failed quest for synergy in school health promotion. *Journal of School Health, 66*, 132–137.

McLaren, L. & Hawe, P. (2005). Ecological perspectives in health research. *Journal of Epidemiology and Community Health, 59*, 6–14.

McQueen, D. (2002). The evidence debate. *Journal of Epidemiology and Community Health, 56*, 83–84.

Moore, K. & Lippman, L. (2004). *What do children need to flourish? Conceptualizing and measuring indicators of positive development.* New York: Springer.

Moysés, S.J., Moysés, S.T., McCarthy, M., & Sheiham, A. (2006). Intra-urban differentials in child dental trauma in relation to Healthy Cities policies in Cūritiba, Brazil. *Health and Place, 12*, 48–64.

Mükhoma, W. & Flisher, A. (2004). Evaluations of health promoting schools: A review of nine studies. *Health Promotion International, 19*, 357–368.

Mullen, P., Evans, D., Forster, J., Gottlieb, N., Kreuter, M., Moon, R., O'Rourke, T., & Stretcher, V. (1995). Settings as an important dimension in health education/promotion policy, programs, and research. *Health Education Quarterly, 22*, 329–345.

National Health & Medical Research Council (1996). *Effective school health promotion: towards health promoting schools.* Canberra: Australian Government Publishing Service.

Nguyen, H., Carrieri-Kholman, V., Rankin, S., Slaugher, R., & Sulbarg, M. (2004). Supporting cardiac recovery through eHealth technology. *Journal of Cardiovascular Nursing, 19*, 200–208.

Norman, C. & Skinner, H. (2006). eHealth literacy: Essential skills for consumer health in a networked world. *Journal of Medical Internet Research, 8*, e9.

Nutbeam, D. (1999). The challenge to provide "evidence" in health promotion. *Health Promotion International, 14*, 99–101.

Nutbeam, D. (2000). Health promotion effectiveness – the questions to be answered. In International Union for Health Promotion and Education *The evidence of health promotion effectiveness. Shaping public health in a new Europe. Part two: Evidence book* (pp. 1–11). Brussels – Luxembourg: ECSC-EC-EAEC. 2nd edition. Paris: Jouve Composition & Impression.

O'Neill, M., Pederson, A., & Rootman, I. (2000). Health promotion in Canada: declining or transforming? *Health Promotion International, 15*, 135–141.

Pan American Health Organisation (PAHO) (2005). *Healthy municipalities, cities and communities: Evaluation recommendations for policymakers in the Americas.* Washington: PAHO.

Paton, K., Sengupta, S., & Hassan, L. (2005). Settings, systems and organisation development: the Healthy Living and Working Model. *Health Promotion International, 20*, 81–89.

Pawson, R. & Tilley, N. (1997). *Realistic evaluation.* London: Sage.

Pawson, R., Greenhalgh, T., Harvey, G., & Walshe, K. (2004). *Realist synthesis: An introduction. RMP Methods Paper 2/2004.* Manchester: ESRC Research Methods Programme, University of Manchester.

Plsek, P.E. & Greenhalgh, T. (2001). The challenge of complexity in healthcare. *British Medical Journal, 323*, 625–628.

Poland, B., Frohlich, K., & Cargo, M. (2007). Context as a fundamental dimension of health promotion program evaluation. In L. Potvin, D. McQueen, L. Anderson, Z. Hartz, & L. de Salazar (Eds.), *Health Promotion Effectiveness in Context: Issues and Perspectives from the Americas.*

Poland, B.D., Green, L.W., & Rootman, I. (2000). Reflections on settings for health promotion. In B.D. Poland, L.W. Green, & I. Rootman (Eds.), *Settings for health promotion: linking theory and practice* (pp. 341–351). London: Sage.

Poland, B. (1996). Knowledge development and evaluation in, of, and for healthy community initiatives. Part I: Guiding principles. *Health Promotion International, 11*, 237–247.

Pratt, J., Gordon, P., & Plamping, D. (1999). *Working whole systems: Putting theory into practice in organisations.* London: King's Fund.

Raphael, D. (2000) The question of evidence in health promotion. *Health Promotion International, 15*, 355–367.

Restrepo, H.E., Llanos, G., Contrera, A., Rocabado, F., Gross, S., Suárez, J., & González, J. (1996). The PAHO/WHO experience: Healthy municipalities in Latin America. In C. Price & A. Tsouros (Eds.) *Our cities, our future: Policies and action plans for health and sustainable development.* Copenhagen: WHO Regional Office for Europe.

Rowling, L. & Jeffreys, V. (2006). Capturing complexity: Integrating health and education research to inform health-promoting schools policy and practice. *Health Education Research, 21*, 705–718.

Satterfield, D., Volansky, M., Caspersen, C., Engelgau, M., Bowman, B., Gregg, E., Geiss, L.S., Hosey, G.M., May, J., & Vinicor, F. (2003). Community-based lifestyle interventions to prevent type 2 diabetes. *Diabetes Care, 26*, 2643–2652.

Sayer, A. (2000). *Realism and social science.* London: Sage.

Scottish Health Promoting Schools Unit. (2006). *Health promoting schools.* (http://www.healthpromotingschools.co.uk/index.asp accessed 06 October 2006).

Senge P. (1990). *The Fifth Discipline: The Art and Practice of the Learning Organization.* London: Random House

Senge, P., Cambron-McCabe, N., Lucas, T., Smith, B., Dutton, J., & Kleiner, A. (2000). *Schools that learn.* New York: Doubleday Press.

Skinner, H., Biscope, S., & Poland, B. (2003). Quality of internet access: Barrier behind internet use statistics. *Social Science and Medicine, 57*, 875–880.

Skinner, H., Biscope, S., Poland, B., & Goldberg, E. (2003). How adolescents use technology for health information: Implications for health professionals from focus group studies. *Journal of Medical Internet Research, 5*, e32.

Squires, N & Strobl, J. (Eds.) (1996). *Healthy prisons – a vision for the future. Report of the first international conference on healthy prisons, Liverpool, 24–27 March 1996.* Liverpool: University of Liverpool.

St Leger, L. (1997). Health promoting settings: From Ottawa to Jakarta. *Health Promotion International 12*, 99–101.

St Leger, L. (2006). Communication technologies and health promotion: Opportunities and challenges. *Health Promotion International 21*, 169–171.

St Leger, L. & Nutbeam, D. (2000). Settings 2 – effective health promotion in schools. In International Union for Health Promotion and Education *The evidence of health promotion effectiveness. Shaping public health in a new Europe. Part two: Evidence book* (pp. 110–122). Brussels – Luxembourg: ECSC-EC-EAEC. 2nd edition. Paris: Jouve Composition & Impression.

Stame, N. (2004). Theory-based evaluation and types of complexity. *Evaluation, 10*, 58–76.

Steckler, A., McLeray, K., & Goodman R. (1992). Towards integrating qualitative and quantitative methods: an introduction. *Health Education Quarterly, 19*, 1–8.

Stewart-Brown, S. (2006). *What is the evidence on school health promotion in improving health or preventing disease and, specifically, what is the effectiveness of the health promoting schools approach?* Copenhagen: WHO Regional Office for Europe. (Health Evidence Network Report http://www.who.dk/Document/E88185.pdf accessed 06 October 2006).

Stokols, D. (1996). Translating social ecological theory into guidelines for community health promotion. *American Journal of Health Promotion, 10*, 282–293.

Suggs, L.S. (2006). A 10-year retrospective of research in new technologies for health communication. *Journal of Health Communication, 11*, 61–74.

Tones, K. (1997). Beyond the randomized controlled trial: a case for "judicial review". *Health Education Research, 12*, 1–4.

Tones, K. & Green, J. (2004). *Health promotion: planning and strategies.* London: Sage.

Tsouros, A. (Ed.) (1991). *World Health Organization healthy cities project: A project becomes a movement. Review of progress 1987–1990.* Copenhagen: FADL Publishers/Milan: SOGESS.

Tsouros, A.D. (1995). *The WHO healthy cities project: State of the art and future plans. Health Promotion International, 10*, 133–141.

Tsouros, A.D., Dowding, G., Thompson, J., & Dooris, M. (Eds.) (1998). *Health promoting universities: Concept, experience and framework for action.* Copenhagen: WHO Regional Office for Europe.

U.S. Centers for Disease Control. (2005). *School health index: a self-assessment and planning guide.* (http://www.cdc.gov/HealthyYouth/SHI/paper.htm accessed 06 October 2006).

U.S. Centers for Disease Control. (2006a). *Healthy schools, healthy youth.* (http://www.cdc.gov/healthyyouth/index.htm accessed 06 October 2006).

U.S. Centers for Disease Control. (2006b). *The school health policies and programs study.* (http://www.cdc.gov/healthyyouth/shpps/index.htm (accessed 06 October 2006).

Wallerstein, N. (2006). *What is the evidence on effectiveness of empowerment to improve health?* Copenhagen: WHO Regional Office for Europe.

Weiss, C. H. (1997). Theory-based evaluation: Past, present, and future. *New Directions for Evaluation, 76*, 41–56.

Wellman, B., Haase, A., Witte, J., & Hampton, K. (2002). Does the internet increase, decrease, or supplement social capital? Social networks, participation and community commitment. *American Behavioral Scientist, 45*, 436–455.

Wenger, E. & Snyder, W. (2000). Communities of practice: The organizational frontier. *Harvard Business Review (Jan–Feb)*, 139–145.

Wenzel, E. (1997). A comment on settings in health promotion. *Internet Journal of Health Promotion.* (http://www.ldb.org/setting.htm accessed 06 October 2006).

Westley, F., Zimmerman, B., & Patton, M. (2006). *Getting to maybe: How the world is changed.* Toronto, Canada: Random House.

Wharf Higgins, J. (1992). The healthy community movement in Canada. In B. Wharf (Ed.), *Communities and social policy in Canada* (pp. 151–189). Toronto: McClelland & Stewart.

Whitelaw, S., Baxendale, A., Bryce, C., Machardy, L., Young, I., & Witney, E. (2001). Settings based health promotion: A review. *Health Promotion International, 16*, 339–353.

Williams, G. H. (2003). The determinants of health: Structure, context and agency. *Sociology of Health & Illness 25(3)*, 131–154.

World Health Organization. (WHO) (1986). *Ottawa charter for health promotion*. Adopted at an International Conference on Health Promotion – The Move Towards a New Public Health (co-sponsored by the Canadian Public Health Association, Health and Welfare Canada, and the World Health Organization), Nov 17–21, Ottawa, Canada. (http://www.who.int/hpr/NPH/docs/ottawa_charter_hp.pdf accessed 06 October 2006).

World Health Organization (WHO) (1991). *Sundsvall statement on supportive environments for health*. Copenhagen: WHO Regional Office for Europe.

World Health Organization (WHO) (1996). *Health-promoting schools series 5: Regional guidelines. Development of health-promoting schools – A framework for action*. Manila: WHO Regional Office for the Western Pacific.

World Health Organization (WHO) (1997a). *Jakarta declaration on health promotion into the 21st century*. Geneva: WHO.

World Health Organization (WHO) (1997b). Promoting health through schools. Report of a WHO Expert Committee on Comprehensive School Health Education and Promotion. *World Health Organization Technical Report Series, 870(i–vi)*, 1–93.

World Health Organization (WHO) (1998a). *Health promotion glossary*. Geneva: WHO.

World Health Organization (WHO) (1998b). *Health21: The health for all policy for the WHO European region – 21 targets for the 21st century*. Copenhagen: WHO Regional Office for Europe.

World Health Organization (WHO) (2002a). *Integrated management of healthy settings at the district level. Report of an intercountry consultation. Gurgaon, India, 7–11 May 2001*. New Delhi: WHO Regional Office for South-East Asia.

World Health Organization (WHO) (2002b). *Healthy cities initiative: Approaches and experience in the African region*. Brazzaville: WHO Regional Office for Africa.

World Health Organization (WHO) (2004). *Healthy marketplaces in the Western Pacific: Guiding future action. Applying a settings approach to the promotion of health in marketplaces*. Manila: WHO Regional Office for the Western Pacific.

World Health Organization (WHO) (2005). *Bangkok charter for health promotion in a globalized world*. Geneva: World Health Organization.

World Health Organization (WHO) (2006a). *Healthy environments for children alliance inter-regional consultation: Improving children's environmental health in settings – experiences and lessons for policies and action. Report of meeting held in Entebbe, Uganda from 29 November to 2 December 2005*. Geneva: WHO (Healthy Environments for Children Alliance Secretariat).

World Health Organization (WHO) (2006b) *School health and youth health promotion*. (http://www.who.int/school_youth_health/en/ accessed 06 October 2006).

Ziglio, E., Hagard, S., & Griffiths, J. (2000). Health promotion development in Europe: Achievements and challenges. *Health Promotion International, 15*, 143–153.

Zimmerman, B., Lindberg, C., & Plsek, P. (2001). *Edgeware: Insights from complexity science for health care leaders*, 2nd Ed. Irving, Texas: VHA Inc.

20
Feasibility for Health Promotion Under Various Decision-Making Contexts

LIGIA DE SALAZAR

This chapter addresses three issues regarding effectiveness evaluation in health promotion and its theoretical and practical applicability considering different decision making contexts. The first part deals with the question, what does health promotion mean in practice and how does this practical definition influence its evaluation of effectiveness? The second issue taken up is the socio-political context as a risk factor for the implementation of the intervention and effect modifier of the outcomes. And finally, the third issue focuses on aspects related to the search for evidence, to demonstrate that health promotion is a function of a complicated equation combining the country's wealth, political conditions, political will and the degree of influence, vulnerability and dependence of the territories in terms of factors that modify the population's living conditions.

What does Health Promotion Imply in Practice and What does this Practice Imply in Effectiveness Evaluation?

The answer to this question necessitates an analysis of the historical and political context in which the practice of health promotion takes place, looking at its feasibility in different socio-political scenarios, and as a result of this analysis, the identification of factors that condition its practice as well as its evaluation.

Therefore, before addressing effectiveness evaluation in health promotion it is obligatory to define, in operational and practical terms, what health promotion really means. Rychetnik, Hawe, Waters, Barratt and Frommer (2004) state that the way a problem is framed determines the research questions to be answered, and consequently, the type of evidence that becomes available; they recognize that frames are often tied to disciplinary perspectives, ideologies, or particular historical – political contexts. This definition also orients the evaluation question, as well as the standards and parameters for comparison.

Health promotion has been acknowledged as a strategy that inspires policies, actions, programs, and initiatives through the design of multi-focal interventions aimed at broad and sustainable social changes (Carvalho, Bodstein, Hartz & Matida, 2004) and as a social movement defending health agendas and strategies in all their dimensions, as a means to update and expand the debate on the social, cultural, political, and economic determinants of the health-disease process, reassuring health as an ethical imperative and a citizen's right (Carvalho et al., 2004). The World Health Organization, on the other hand, defines health promotion as "a process of enabling people to increase control over, and to improve, their health" (World Health Organization [WHO], 1998).

The above definitions not only highlight health promotion as both a political mean and a social end, but also demand evaluation questions and the inclusion of new and broader indicators to measure its effectiveness. These indicators must go beyond health outcomes, and beyond achievement and static indicators, to include indicators that account for the appropriateness, feasibility and sustainability of the political process that produce these changes, as well as collective, institutional and territorial (local) capacity to intervene. They also should include indicators of risk factors and social determinants of health; equity issues; intermediate outcomes associated with inter-sectoral and multilevel actions; balance of power relationships and social participation to negotiate decisions that affect population health; and governance, among others.

The Socio-Political Context as a Risk Factor for the Success of the Implementation and Effect Modifier of the Outcomes

Social practices are developed within complex systems-contexts, which are adaptive and unpredictable. The analysis of these contexts includes, among others, the socio-economic history of the territory, the demographic and cultural characteristics of the target population; the decision-maker's needs and interests; the political momentum; and the local and macro structural conditions influencing interventions aimed to improve health conditions and well-being.

The context could be a risk factor for the implementation of the intervention, as well as an effect modifier of the efforts to demonstrate effectiveness. Thus, an evaluation that excludes these variables from the analysis would not only be useless but also counterproductive. Although there is a universal conceptual definition of health promotion, its operational definition (the way it is implemented), differs according to the sociopolitical-context in which it is developed, the availability of certain conditions that make the implementation feasible, and the will of those responsible for it, as well as the political and cultural conditions.

Samaja (2004) and Max Neef suggest that context analysis be done by means of the paradigm of adaptable and complex systems with a history, considering that behind every historical process there is a dominant language and philosophy.

The study of the context and history involves the analysis of aspects that behave in a different manner for each territory, reaffirming the idea that health promotion and its evaluation are influenced by: the people and their socio-economic and cultural characteristics, the setting, the local infrastructure and institutional capacity to act; the availability of professional skills; information about the decision makers, who they are, what their objectives are; their time frame; the degree of independence and governability of territories, and how global phenomena such as globalization, urbanism and decentralization influence them.

The abovementioned aspects can act separately and in conjunction by the interaction among them, and manifest themselves in different ways. Different thinkers, politicians, and Latin American social movements have acknowledged that although there has been a European and North American influence in the theory and practice of public health in the Latin American region, there has also been a long history of struggle and contributions that have been represented in political proposals and methodological approaches. There have also been critical analyses of imported models that decontextualized and distort the Latin American reality, which do not acknowledge the fact that social phenomena, just as science, are not permanent, but transform themselves, according to Stern cited by Tetelboin, (2005).

Moreover, diverse and repeated problems have been the subject of analysis and debate. Among them are: 1) the static versus the dynamic nature of health-illness, looking at it as a dichotomous category rather than a dialectic process; the tendency to focus on the biological rather than on the social components, reducing the unit of analysis to the individual and obscuring social causes amenable to interventions at the societal-level; 2) the positive focus with which health phenomena and sickness have been analyzed and interventions have been evaluated, not acknowledging particular contexts and modes of attention in each place; 3) the growing demand for performance results that decontextualize and reduce the complexity of the phenomena in health to simplistic expressions that fit in existing investigative designs; 4) the need to investigate and apply new targets in order to value practice (Samaja, 2004); by establishing the dichotomy between the objectivity demand of positive science and the values and considerations related to the subject and population health, answering the question, "is scientific knowledge of health value possible?".

The need to conduct more research on health inequalities has been a recurring priority. This aspect has been at the heart of the Latin American health debate, with a long standing tradition of research, (Almeida-Filho, Kawachi, Pellegrini & Dachs, 2003) however, lack of information on trends and causes of health inequities in the region are still present. There is a need to include position and conceptual studies and analyses of macro contexts to show the situation of one of the regions with the highest degree of social inequity of the world (Almeida-Filho et al., 2003).

Many authors have made important contributions to the Latin American thinking and practice in order to promote population health (Almeida-Filho et al., 2003; Guba & Lincoln, 1989; Stake, 1975; Stake & Abma, 2005). Almeida–Filho (2000) sustains that building the new health object appears not only as a demand for scientists, but as the result of a changing conjuncture due to the consequences of the production processes and the social dynamics.

Waitzkin, Iriart, Estrada and Lamadrid (2001) cite different movements in the region that have made important contributions to the conception and practice of public health through adult literacy campaigns that encouraged people in poor communities to approach education as a process of empowerment; new approaches for medical education; health outcomes including social class as determinants of health; an ideological basis for discrimination against Latinos; poverty, inadequate housing and sanitation, and insufficient nutrition fostered epidemics; social changes oriented to income redistribution, state regulation of food and clothing supplies, national housing programs, and industrial reforms to address occupational health problems, among others.

The study of social determinants of health and their distribution is one of the priority areas of focus on the international scene and constitutes an opportunity to cultivate actions oriented towards the resolution of health problems and improve quality of life. The context in which these actions are developed is important for conducting this analysis and evaluating its achievements, and therefore, an evaluation that doesn't acknowledge this fact would be either unfruitful or unethical.

Most recent Latin American thinkers advocate for more holistic approaches to explain and understand complex social phenomena, instead of simplified causality chains that show incomplete realities, and to understand our inability to account for such complex realities. In their critique of the positivist character of the epidemiologists whose latest aim is to measure facts, Samaja (2004) and Almeida-Filho (2002) are explicitly clear about the risks that we face when we try to reduce health to objective terms, overlooking the fact that the health-sickness object and the modes of adapting them result from the social construction of valuing always performed in a culture, in a society and in a determined time, and responding to complex adaptable systems.

International Context and its Influence on Determining What is Local: "Tell Me About the Context and I'll Let You Know What Health Promotion is in Practice"

Each population has its own history, culture, organization, and socio-economic conditions that influence how and why people are exposed to and affected by these influences. International policies and movements such as globalization, decentralization, urbanization, and liberalization of the economy directly and indirectly influence health and well-being of populations as well as the programs and interventions to face their problems.

The level of governableness and grade of economic and technological dependency of developing countries are seen as seriously affected by these policies, manifesting themselves in free trade treaties, the burden of foreign debt, which demands regulatory policies, fiscal cuts, expenditure decrease in social sectors, and reduction of the state, among other changes.

Globalization and urbanization have been considered as societal determinants of health. Mehta (2005) identified some problems of the globalization and urbanization processes and their impact on health in developing countries, despite the recognition of some advantages. These policies have influences on: migration of health professionals; work patterns; physical infrastructure; pollution; inequity trends; marginalization; poverty; gaps in health of poor and non-poor populations; violence, crime and war; changes in social capital; international trade participation without protection; privatization of public institutions; power accumulation and impoverishment; state reduction; social exclusion and what he called the "urban health paradox," which states that despite "better health services and programmes, urban poor have lower health status than rural population".

It is worthy to highlight the negative tendency of the social indicators in Latin America. If you consider the realistic figure of US$ 5.00 per day as the poverty level guideline, more than 70% of Latin Americans live in poverty, and almost 40% are indigent – living with less than US$ 2.00 per day. In Argentina, the richest country in production of beef and cereals per capita, almost 60% of the population lives in poverty and one-third is destitute. Brazil has been undergoing a recession for over three years and has paid more than 60 billion of its foreign debt, while other governments have reduced public financing for housing, health, education and agricultural reforms. In Mexico, Uruguay, Bolivia, Colombia and Venezuela the economies are in a deep crisis as the neo-liberal model based on exports transfers abroad the resulting revenues in the form of benefit drafts, payments on debts and fiscal evasion. Inequalities have rapidly spread throughout Latin America over the past five years. Under the austerity programs introduced by Brazil, Argentina and Mexico, the upper classes increase their earnings thanks to lower taxes, lower salaries paid, and more reduced social security contributions – at the expense of workers.

Anyone unaware of these conditions and faced with the threat of not being able to show achievements on the conditions of health of the population could ask if the values and principles that drive the promotion of health should continue. I would say that today, more than ever, we should base our practice on obtaining the same. But also, today, even more, an articulated, local, regional, and national effort to do so is required, one that should be expressed on a political agenda that takes into consideration our particular context and includes the actions to improve our capability to intervene and motivate social change. The evaluation of effectiveness on promoting health should concentrate on analyzing and valuing coherence, sustainability and capability of this political action of the different territories.

A couple of questions to be broached are: What are the agreements, policies and legislation to make globalization an opportunity instead of a threat for development? Is the country in a position to control the negative consequences already mentioned? The economic tendencies have influenced in a differential manner the sectoral reforms. In the health sector, the values and principles that for a couple of decades had guided the health system were inverted, giving way to other values and principles tightly related to the actual market economy such as: high productivity; high coverage – although with low quality service; privatizing of services; segmentation of medical care and differentiated health services according to affordability. Fidler (2001) argues that globalization jeopardizes disease control nationally by eroding sovereignty, while the assertion of national sovereignty can frustrate disease control internationally.

Equally existing are the local conditions that worsen the problems already mentioned. The relationships of political actors in civil society and in governmental institutions, their discourse, the structures they represent, the networks they participate in, and their potential to produce social changes; territorial governability and institutional development are all conditions that impact the problem.

How are governability and the institutional development of territories affected by global phenomena such as drug trafficking and civil wars? Are state modernization processes conducted by the state's own people or by outsiders? Has the path for this quasi-autonomy been prepared? Does an institutional strengthening process exist in order to meet the demands that imply decentralization? Or, are we promoting the return of the centralist model due to the low institutional capability of official institutions?

Search for Evidence of Health Promotion Effectiveness – More than a Technical Endeavor

Effective health promotion is a function of a complicated equation consisting of a country's wealth, political conditions, – political will, – and the degree of influence, vulnerability and dependence of the territories in terms of factors that modify the populations' living conditions. On the other hand, behind what we define as successful, and the technical tools to measure success, to compare and to evaluate, there hides a system of principles and values that have ethical, philosophical, political and pragmatic aspects.

Evidence of health promotion effectiveness must be interpreted under two analytical dimensions: First, by its achievements in changing social determinants of health, equity and health status of the targeted population, and second, by its influence, as a political strategy, which is exerted upon the structural conditions that force the changes in order to make them happen. In the first dimension, there is a political and social expense that has to be considered when evaluating health promotion – changes in health determinants and health status – ignoring that these depend, in large part, on the capabilities of the government and of the population to change the true causes of the problems- the structural conditions in each geographic context.

In this sense, the evidence of health promotion effectiveness in Latin America must address the particular situation of this region. Therefore, we call attention to some indicators that, although inconclusive, taken into context become key elements to judge effectiveness of health promotion under the two dimensions given. The purpose is not to make a profound analysis of economic policies and their influence on social policies, a subject that has already been well documented, but rather to enhance the differential effect that these policies have on the health and quality of life of the population, as well as their influence on implementing social interventions and its results.

In many Latin American countries a contradiction has been present, which is the recognition of social causality of the disease and its negation in practice. Would it be just to ask oneself why this is? Is it because we adjust our actions to what can be done? Could it be that dependence and pressures from international entities do not give us enough room to adjust the politics according to our own real conditions of each region, country, or town? Could it be that the level of our countries' vulnerability does not give room for change? Could it be that our understanding of health promotion as a discipline, rather than as a social and political practice, influences the way it is socially produced?

Health Promotion in Latin-America: A Shared Vision – Manifest, a Social Movement, a Political Challenge, a Field of Practice, or Just a Dream?

During the past few decades, Latin America has been under the influence of a paradigm of economic and social development driven by neo-liberal policies. The strength of these policies lies in the economic power of developed countries and in their interaction and leveraging with international organisms that somehow define the policies of the Latin American governments, using the foreign debt and the financial dependency of those countries and the great uncertainty regarding their insertion into the world market.

The tendency is to reduce the state in such a way that its participation in the economy and in society would be as little as possible. No doubt this paradigm leads to the prevailing valuing of efficiency measurements centered on reducing expenses and privatization of public services.

To speak about inequality and to fill ourselves with tables and indicators on social urban-rural inequality among those so called "social stratum", genders, et cetera, could be considered rhetoric, if the knowledge of said inequalities is not accompanied by the studies of the inequalities of power that generates them. The distribution of inequities and the way they affect both outcomes and implementation of the intervention are good reasons to advocate for evaluations that respond to population and territories' needs. Inequities are related not only to the risk of having a condition but also with the effectiveness of the intervention. The question to be answered is, whether the socio-economic status is associated with the implementation of the intervention protocol, and if they are evenly distributed among the population receiving the intervention, these probabilities affect the effectiveness of the intervention.

The search for evidence of effectiveness of health promotion interventions developed in non-favourable structural situations has a considerable risk. This is the case for the evaluation of interventions that have not been implemented or the time to see results has not been sufficient. The results of these evaluations could serve as an input to justify abandoning the intervention or hindering the search for conditions and capabilities in order to apply the principles and values that promote it; to change the system of values by favouring the practices of those who display power; to keep a status quo under the pretence that the institutions are inoperable; to reorient the state's and governmental institutions' mission who represent it towards what can be accomplished and not towards what must be accomplished. The abovementioned aspects have been taken into consideration in the health sector reforms.

The previous paragraph raises the question, "What type of evidence do we require in health promotion? Who determines it? For what purpose and how will it be used? Who determines what is successful and what is not? Success indicators are a topic that should be taken into account. In this regard, Samaja (2004), sustains that what is normal and abnormal is not derived from a passive normal or abnormal registration of the facts themselves, according to a physical, chemical or biological perspective, but from an active proposal of interpretation or practical intervention derived from the subject's symbolic models, congruent with the actual social order to which it belongs, in such a way that knowledge is valued more by its interpretational virtues than by its operational values.

The topic of evidence goes into dimensions that pick up the contextual, the ideological, the territorial, the political, the social, and the temporal-conjuncture, converting itself into a function of variables that are dynamic and modified in time. The acknowledgement of this fact brings up the need for establishing differences between the impacts and outcomes that sum up the effectiveness, on a regional, national and local level.

Is there Evidence of Effectiveness of Health Promotion in the Latin American Region?

The answer to this question goes though the analysis of the following aspects:

The Sectoral: A common constraint found in many countries is the sectoral approach in practice, despite the integrated approach that has been seen as the solution in order to "bridge government boundaries and bureaucracies divisions". This constraint of the sectoral approach has been mentioned several times but there are no responses, and on the contrary, the health system reforms advocate not only for a sectoral, but a curative approach.

If the evaluation of the promotion of health concentrates only on the results that have to do with changes in health status, the probabilities of showing evidence of its effectiveness are slim, and not seen in the short term. In fact, as we mentioned earlier, great advances in the region have been discovered that have taken time to build, starting from the positioning of the topic on the region's political agenda, and ending in successful experiences which, although slight, give account of important advances. There is a need to understand the complex interdependencies that exist among institutions within and outside the health sector and to build strategies that account for its cultural and political nature.

The Territorial: Effectiveness measures how well an intervention works in real settings and systems. Community effectiveness is often substantially lower than efficiency because of a staircase effect, which is the result of lower compliance, access, coverage, adherence and awareness about their risk and responses available to face them (Tugwell, Savigny, Hawker & Robinson, 2006). Knowing this information it is important to tackle the factors reducing the effectiveness.

The local level has a limited governability to modify what comes vertically from higher structures, therefore, power and negotiating capability in each territory is different and influenced by diverse factors. Are we aware of the power and feasibility of local government to make sustainable changes, beyond successful pilot studies?

This analysis should include other issues such as the influence and interference of international cooperation agencies; their funding policies; private sector; government responsibility and governability, among others. We should not continue "blaming the victim" and looking for reasons or causalities only inside the health sector or inside a territory – local governments and communities.

If we compare the accomplishments in the region with the accomplishments in the countries and towns, we are going to encounter differences or manifestations of the briefly described aspects mentioned earlier that contradict each other. The local accomplishments have a lot to do with the governability and ability to intervene and negotiate. Milio (2001) assures that negotiation requires taking into account the interests of governments and other stakeholders, and being willing and able to trade away some valued interests to gain others in the foreseeable future.

On the other hand, regional indicators have shown effectiveness if we look at health promotion as a political process, not only as a health result, but also as social movements that are not tied to the sectorial, such as the rising of theories founded and supported by political commitments for social change. Max Neef, on the other hand, maintains that "the region could do a lot to reduce the consequences of the neo-liberal model if it acted as a block."

The Political: The political and ethical side of evaluation of effectiveness has been raised by Ray & Mayan (2001) bringing up the question – who determines what counts as evidence, the right indicators and appropriate standards in evaluation research of health programs? The other concern is related to how different stakeholders with profound differences and perspectives can reach an agreement about criteria to establish effectiveness of an intervention that benefits each of them differently.

The need to tailor policies to the institutional contexts in which they are implemented is recognized (Inter-American Development Bank, 2006). The structural conditions influencing the implementation and results of health promotion interventions in most of the Latin-American countries have not changed, and more important, we have not oriented our work to address them, despite the fact that the need to confront social structures that promote social inequalities has been widely recognized.

Only in recent years have public health workers become aware of the importance of working more closely with policymakers and the public to implement their findings in political arenas. The growing interest in linking knowledge, policy and action has been reflected in the literature, but not in actions taken to accomplish this purpose (Stivers, 1991; Brint, 1990). Competing priorities is another issue that merits attention, needless to say in countries that are facing wars or other political and social situations, as well as the differential influences of international policies and phenomenon, such as globalization and urbanization.

Many factors have influenced the above situation: evaluators are not aware that the evaluation is conducted in a political environment, which demand negotiation skills; information is provided that does not meet the criteria of relevance and sufficiency; the questions asked do no respond to the needs of those who will use the results; poor strategies to disseminate the results, among others.

It is well known that decisions are supported not only by information about effectiveness, but also by information about when and how the intervention works and what makes the changes possible. Decisions are also supported by information about the characteristics of the life cycle of the intervention, the interrelations among actors, the strengths and limitations, the changes, and factors that are responsible for outcomes, and very importantly, stakeholders' gains making a given decision; among others. In other words, decisions are based upon "context-bounded knowledge" that serves to judge the reproducibility or extension of the intervention.

The rationale of evaluators could differ from decision makers, so the main questions here are whether we need scientific research (evaluative research) to obtain evidence of effectiveness in health promotion, or do we need evidence to act? For this purpose, we must characterize the political processes by identifying the key actors; the powers and roles with which they are endowed; preferences, incentives, and capabilities; time horizons; and the nature of the dealings and/or the transactions they perform. Development depends not so much on choosing the right policies from a technical standpoint, but on negotiating, approving, and implementing them in a way leading to their political survival and their effective application.

The Technical-Scientific: It has been recognized (Dowie, 2001) that evaluation for scientific purposes is fundamentally different from evaluation for decision making, being differentiated from deciding whether something is true. Evidence of effectiveness is judged in different ways ranging from scientific to empirical studies. Waters, Doyle, Jackson, Howes, Brunton & Oakley (2006) and others, such as Lomas (2006), say that scientific evidence can be categorized into context free (absolute truth) and context sensitive (context in the guidance of decision making process); on the other hand, Oxman argues that "all evidence is context sensitive" since all observations are made in a specific context.

The critical point to retain here is – what are the contextual factors that influence evidence of effectiveness? Are they the same everywhere? In fact "sensitive evidence" is influenced by political and social factors, while personal and institutional factors influence more the "scientific evidence"; the definition of evidence covers qualitative and quantitative data.

Although there is a wide acknowledgement that evidence of effectiveness is linked to facts of context, in practice, the criteria to judge and value effectiveness is standardized. The strategic problem is the utilization of information to convince target groups that their policy position is economically feasible, politically acceptable, and socially doable as well as administratively and technologically possible (Milio, 1992).

Evidence is often restricted to quantitative facts derived from large samples and randomized experimental designs, but does not capture the inherent complexity of health promotion (McQueen, 2000). Madjar & Walton (2001) argue that a broad notion of evidence also includes qualitative evidence in the form of lived experiences, case histories and stories. This kind of evidence is important because it enhances the understanding of human behavior; it promotes holistic thinking (Abma, 2005). On the other hand, ignoring the role of group or macro-level variables may lead to an incomplete understanding of the determinants of health (Diez-Roux, 1998).

According to WHO ("Bridging the Know-Do", 2005), evidence is context-sensitive, and policies and decisions should be informed by good evidence that is contextualized. This implies that "evidence is plural and that the implementability of good global evidence must be triangulated with local knowledge." This issue raises other types of concerns, such as should we standardize and produce generalizable evidence of effectiveness in health promotion? Should the definition of evidence be flexible to be adjusted according to the type of inquiries, to the context where decisions will be made? Or rather, is the given evidence definition unsuitable for the judgment of effectiveness of complex social interventions and to the demands of information for decision-makers?.

To what Extent is Effectiveness Evaluation in Health Promotion Different in Developing Countries?

The answer to this question depends on how different the countries are. Effectiveness evaluation in health promotion should consider, among other things, the fact that health promotion initiatives respond to dynamic processes that are context bounded, which are political, participative, multi-factorial and multi-dimensional in nature; the existence of concomitant and diverse interventions oriented to reach specific but complementary objectives; its focus on groups and communities rather than individuals; its short and long term effects and often intangible benefits; its articulation to development and inter-sectoral plans more than health plans alone, in order to address health determinants that require actions beyond the health sector and an inter-sectoral planning approach instead of sectoral.

The above characteristics are reflected in the evaluation of health promotion initiatives: the need to articulate political, social and biologic sciences in the analysis and interpretation of results; the limitation to define in measurable terms the main driven health promotion principles and values; the potential need and also difficulty to generalize and predict results; the trade off between credibility, opportunity, relevance, replicability of evaluation results; the diverse and sometimes opposite interests of stakeholders – including evaluators, users and theorists; and ways to conduct evaluation under circumstances of resource constraints.

There is a need to analyze the practicability of the research approaches for searching evidences of effectiveness and to address the success of policies, processes and programs to apply principles and values such as equity, empowerment, and the right to health, following processes that are developed under adverse and contradictory conditions, but with the pressure to show convincing results that can only be seen after a long period of time following sustainable processes.

The above mentioned aspects lead us into deliberation on whether the meanings of evidence of effectiveness are the same for all territories. If differences among countries exist, do they depend on their level of development and degree of economic and technological dependence? Should we base the evidence on health outcomes or should we look for evidence of the continuity and sustainability of the political process? If so, is this information of interest to decision-makers?

There is not one answer to all of the above concerns, and this paper does not pretend to produce it, but rather it aims to introduce new inputs to the evaluation debate, as well as new questions and a range of potential sources of answers, to bring together new and old arguments and proposals around health promotion effectiveness evaluation suited to different socio-political decision-making contexts. Another goal of this paper was to create awareness of the differences witnessed in Latin America in terms of the practical conception of health promotion as well as its evaluation.

References

Abma, TA. (2005). Responsive evaluation: Its meaning and special contribution to health promotion. *Evaluation and Program Planning* Vol. 28; 279–289.

Almeida-Filho, N. (2000) LA CIENCIA TÍMIDA Ensayos de Deconstrucción de la Epidemiología. Buenos Aires: Lugar Editorial.

Almeida-Filho N., Kawachi I., Pellegrini Filho A., Dachs N. (2003). Research on Health Inequalities in Latin America and the Caribbean: Bibliometric analysis (1971–2000) and descriptive content analysis (1971–1995), *American Journal of Public Health* peer reviewed by Latin American Social Medicine. December 2003, Vol. 93, No. 12, 2037–2043.

Bridging the "Know–Do" Gap Meeting on Knowledge Translation in Global Health. 10–12 October 2005 World Health Organization Geneva, Switzerland.

Brint, S. (1990). Rethinking the policy influence of experts: From general characterizations to analysis of variation. *Sociological Forum* 5(3): 361–385.

Carvalho A., Bodstein R., Hartz Z., Matida A.(2004). Concepts and Approaches in the Evaluation of Health Promotion. *Ciencia & Saude Colectiva*. Vol. 9(3): 521–529.

Diez-Roux, AV. (1998). Bringing Context Back Into Epidemiology: Variables And Fallacies In Multilevel Analysis. *American Journal of Public Health*, Vol. 88(2): 216–222.

Dowie, J. (2001) Analysing Health Outcomes. *Journal of Medical Ethics* Vol. 27(4): 245–250.

Fidler, P. (2001). The Globalization of Public Health: The First 100 Years of International Health Diplomacy. *Bulletin of the World Health Organization*. Vol. 79(9). World Health Organization.

Guba, E.G. & Lincoln, Y. (1989). *Fourth Generation Evaluation*. Newbury Park, CA: Sage Publications.

Lomas Cited By WHO (2006). Bridging the "know –Do" Gap. Meeting on Knowledge Translation in Global Health. World Health Organization WHO/EIP/KMS/2006.2

Madjar, I. & Walton, J. (2001). The Nature of Qualitative Evidence. In J. Morse, J. Swanson & A. Kuzel (Eds.), (pp. 28–45). Thousand Oaks: Sage.

Max-Neef, M. (2002). La Realidad Oculta tras los Tratados de Libre Comercio: lo que los ciudadanos y políticos ignoran. El utopista pragmático 101. En: http://www.primeralinea.cl/utopista/site/edic/20021230134956/pags/20021230135636.html

McQueen, D.V. (2000). V Conferencia Mundial de Promoción de la Salud. Informe Técnico 1. Bases Científicas para la Promoción de la Salud. Ciudad de México, 5 al 9 de junio de 2000.

Mehta, D. (2005). Health Promotion in an Urbanizing World: Healthy Slums UN-HABITAT-. 6th Global Conference on Health Promotion, Bangkok 7–11 August, 2005.

Milio, N. (2001). Glossary: Healthy Public Policy. *Journal of Epidemiology and Community Health* Vol.55: 622–623.

Milio, N. (1992). New Tools For Community Involvement In Health. *Health Promotion International*, Vol. 7(3): 209–217.

The Politics of Policies Economic and Social Progress in Latin America, 2006 Report Inter-American Development Bank.

Ray, L. D. & Mayan, M. (2001). Who decides what counts as evidence?. In J. M. Morse, J. M. Swanson & A. J. Kuzel (Eds.), *The nature of evidence in qualitative research* (pp. 50–73). Thousand Oaks: Sage.

Rychetnik L., Hawe P., Waters E., Barratt A., Frommer M. (2004). A Glossary for Evidence Based Public Health. *Journal of Epidemiology and Community Health*. Vol. 58: 538–545.

Samaja J. (2004). EPISTEMOLOGStake, R. E. & Abma, T. A. (2005). Responsive evaluation. In S. Mathison (Ed.), *Encyclopaedia of evaluation* (pp. 376–379). Thousand Oaks: Sage.

Stake, R. E. (Abma, T. A.) (2005). Responsive evaluation. In S. Mathison (Ed.), *Encyclopaedia of evaluation* (pp. 376–379). Thousand Oaks: Sage.

Stake, R. E. (1975). To evaluate an arts program. In R. E. Stake (Ed.), *Evaluating the arts in education: A responsive approach*, (pp. 13–31). Merrill: Colombus Ohio.

Stivers, C. (1991) The politics of public health: The dilemma of a public profession. In Litman, T and S Robins, eds, *Health politics and policy*, (pp. 356–369). Albany, NY: Delmar Pub.

Tetelboin, C. (2005). Conferencia "Medicina Social Pasado, Presente y Futuro". Memoria del Primer Seminario Internacional: Medicina Social y Política Sanitaria en Chile. Escuela de Medicina. Universidad de Valparaiso 9 y 10 de Julio de 2004. Valparaiso 2005.

Tugwell, P., De Savigny, D., Hawker, G. & Robinson, V. (2006). Applying Clinical Epidemiological Methods to Health Equity: The Equity Effectiveness Loop. *British Medical Journal*. Vol. 332: 358–361.

Waitzkin, H., Iriart, C., Estrada, A. & Lamadrid, S. (2001). Social Medicine Then and Now: Lessons from Latin America, *American Journal of Public Health*. Vol. 91, No 10, 1592–1601.

Waters E., Doyle J., Jackson N., Howes F., Brunton G. & Oakley A. (2006). Evaluating the effectiveness of public health interventions: the role and activities of the Cochrane Collaboration. *Journal of Epidemiology and Community Health*. Vol. 60: 285–289.

World Health Organization (1998). Health Promotion Glossary. Geneva, Switzerland.

21
Evaluating Equity
in Health Promotion

Louise Potvin, Pascale Mantoura and Valéry Ridde

The establishment in March 2005 by the World Health Organization (WHO) of an International Commission on the Social Determinants of Health with the goal "of supporting countries in placing heath equity as a shared goal" (WHO, 2006) constituted a global recognition of the existence of health inequalities and of the necessity for governments to take action to address the social determinants of such health inequalities. Indeed, during the past decade several countries have started to make the reduction of health inequalities an explicit goal of their health and public health policies. Four national health policy orientation documents from four leading Western countries formally identify both improving the health and quality of life of the citizens and reducing health inequalities as overarching public health goals. Those documents are the "Integrated Pan Canadian Healthy Living Strategy" (Secretariat for the Healthy Living Network, 2005), the Swedish Health on Equal Terms Public Health Policy (Hogstedt, Lundgren, Moberg, Pettersson & Ågren, 2004), "Tackling Heath Inequalities: A Program for Action" in the UK (Department of Health, 2003), and "Healthy People 2010" in the US (U.S. Department of Health and Human Services, 2000)[*]. These key documents stand at the forefront of the global preoccupation with health inequalities as a major population health challenge, recognizing that policies and programs that improve overall population health may also lead to increasing health disparities (Health Disparities Task Group of the Federal/Provincial/Territorial Advisory Committee on Population Health and Health Security, 2005).

Less well known, however, is the pioneering work of the early health promotion thinkers who sought recognition of health inequalities as a critical public health issue. Not long after the publication of the Black Report (Townsend & Davidson, 1982), which British Conservative Government of Margaret Thatcher shelved and disregarded (Macintyre, 1997), the task force that was put together by the WHO-EURO office clearly identified health inequalities as a core issue for

---

[*] Translating the rhetoric of health inequalities into action is often difficult. A close examination of the list of objectives in Healthy People 2010 and the recommendations for action in the Pan Canadian Healthy Living Strategy reveals more immediate preoccupations with improving overall health.

health promotion (WHO-EURO, 1984). Because discussions of the Charter often reduce this crucial document to a list of strategies for action, the commitments and values that are also part of the Charter are usually overlooked. It may be helpful to remind readers that in its final formulation the Charter stipulates that participants in the conference committed themselves "to respond to the health gap within and between societies and to tackle the inequities in health produced by the rules and practices of these societies" (WHO, 1986). From the outset, health inequality has been an integral part of health promotion rhetoric.

Consequently, it is somewhat surprising that twenty years later, the field of health promotion mostly uses criteria of effectiveness and efficacy when attempting to assign values to its achievements. Major health promotion evaluation synthesis endeavours have gathered and synthesized evidence primarily on health promotion effectiveness to improve overall health, seldom on its efficacy and efficiency to do so, and never to our knowledge on its capacity to reduce health inequalities and inequity (IUHPE, 1999; Zaza, Briss & Harris, 2005). A case in point is the report for which this chapter is being written. The IUHPE Global Program on Health Promotion Effectiveness pursues the "aims to raise standards of health promoting policy-making and practice worldwide by: reviewing evidence of effectiveness in terms of political, economic, social and health impact; translating evidence to policy makers, teachers, practitioners, researchers; stimulating debate of the nature of evidence of effectiveness." (IUHPE, http://www.iuhpe.org) Nowhere is it mentioned in the official program documentation that evidence on the effectiveness of health promotion to reduce health inequalities will also be gathered and analysed. In all fairness, we should mention that in the third edition (2001) of Tones and Tilford's initial "Health Education: Effectiveness and Efficiency"(1990), the authors have added in the title, "equity" as a value for health promotion. However, in his review of this book, Mittelmark (2002) rightly lamented that one of the book's major disappointments is its failure to give equity issues the same in-depth treatment that it accords the values of effectiveness and efficiency. In this regard, the field of health promotion evaluation does not differ from that of program evaluation in which equity is never discussed as a criterion for program evaluation.

As a critique of all of those efforts devoted to building a case for the effectiveness and efficiency of health promotion, this chapter proposes that the field re-examine the value base used for judging its impact. We argue that the question of which goal health promotion is (or should be) effectively contributing to must be addressed openly and explicitly. Increased health inequalities may be an unintended result of health promotion policies and programs that are effective in increasing population health. Unless there is a deliberate intention to address health inequalities and to build up evaluations that purposefully use equity as a value criterion, the field of health promotion may go astray regarding its underlying commitments to equity in health. With the aim of steering the field of health promotion evaluation toward broader reliance on equity as a value criterion, this paper discusses and illustrates how issues of equity can be built into evaluation studies. As a first step, we present distinctions between notions of effectiveness, inequality and equity proposing that the latter is essentially a value judgment about the fairness of observed inequalities. We then review indicators of inequalities that can be used in equity evaluations of health promotion.

Equity and Distributive Justice

Effectiveness[*] is usually defined as a program's ability to produce effects that correspond to the objectives that planners set beforehand (Mathison, 2004). Some authors make a distinction between efficacy and effectiveness. The former refers to the establishment of program effects when conditions are controlled in order to maximize the results' internal validity. Effectiveness refers to efficacy as tested in the real world in order to emphasize the external validity of the conclusions (Glasgow, Lichtenstein & Marcus, 2003). Efficiency, in the realm of program evaluation is understood as the relationship between the effects produced and the resources used to this end. While the definitions of effectiveness and efficiency are fairly straightforward, the exercise of defining equity is less obvious given the polysemic nature of this concept.

Equity is a concept related to that of social justice (Braveman & Gruskin, 2003; Wagstaff & Van Doorsaler, 1993). When the principles of social justice are not applied in a society, inequalities and fractures along the axes of social stratification are created. Disparities in health status across social groups are among the key consequences of these justice deficits. In order for these differences or inequalities to be understood as an injustice that must be remedied, the notion of equity must be invoked and a value judgement made.

However, such a judgment is often ambiguous. A number of inequalities in health status are perceived as "natural" and caused by fate. In such cases, the judgement is "objective" and is based on the observation of facts. Alternatively, deeming certain inequalities to be inequitable implies a "subjective" value judgment in which the principles of distributive justice are used to confirm that the health inequalities observed stem from a complex process of social inequalities. The situation is further complicated because the outcome of the judgment exercise can differ according to the notion of distributive justice adopted. Indeed, there are several distribution theories and models to attain the ideal of social justice and equity and to judge what is fair in a society (Krasnik, 1996; Mooney, 1987; Olsen, 1997). Table 21.1 indicates the most frequently cited distributive justice models in relation to health systems and their definitions.

Effectiveness in Health Promotion and Distributive Justice

Neglecting equity issues in health policies is a consequence of the predominance of libertarian theories (Gilson, 1998). However, public health in general and research on efficacy in health promotion in particular are often rooted in the

---

[*] In this chapter, we will not examine the differences between different types of effectiveness (i.e. population-based, use, trial, theoretical and so on), or between technical efficiency (cost efficiency) and allocative efficiency (cost-benefit).

TABLE 21.1. Most Frequently Cited Distributive Justice Models

Distribution models	Definition
Ownership/libertarian theory	The freedom to own property and use it according to one's choices.
Egalitarian model	All individuals are equal and must be treated in the same manner.
Needs-based model	Care is part of the basic needs that must be satisfied.
Classical utilitarian model	We must ensure a maximum of goods for a maximum number of people, regardless of how those goods are distributed.
Maximin theory	We must ensure an acceptable threshold for those who possess only the minimum.

classical utilitarian model. Thinkers faithful to this model are not interested in the distribution of utilities but in overall utility (Gilson, Kalyalya, Kuchler, Lake, Oranga & Ouendo, 2000). These utilitarian values underpin arguments for the use of the cost-effectiveness ratio criteria to select interventions. Indeed, this ratio seeks to maximize the overall benefits stemming from an intervention regardless of their distribution (Ubel, DeKay, Baron & Asch, 1996). While this model has been criticized (Farmer & Castro, 2004), public health project managers continue to pursue utilitarian values (de Savigny, Kasale, Mbuya & Reid, 2004) following the famous 1993 World Bank report "Investing in health."

This utilitarian vision also appears to underpin several recent or older interventions (IUHPE, 1999; Thurston, Wilson, Felix, MacKean & Wright, 1998) pursuing effectiveness in health promotion. The proceedings of the symposium devoted to this topic in Paris in late 2003 do not mention the problem of equity (IUHPE, 2004), nor does recent Canadian or African research mention equity or health inequalities (Amuyunzu-Nyamongo, 2005; Hills & Carroll, 2004). Concerning these two regional examples, the analytical frameworks that promoters use to assess effectiveness clearly stipulate that the objective of health promotion interventions is the enhancement of health, overlooking the principle of a reduction in health inequalities advocated by the Ottawa Charter. More precisely, it must be noted that the Canadian conceptual framework has changed. In its initial form equity appeared as a contextual condition and one of the numerous criteria for potential effectiveness mechanisms, while in the model's latest iteration, the reduction in health inequalities is appended to the utilitarian objective of health improvement (Hills & Carroll, 2004). This example simply reveals the gulf that has yet to be bridged in order for equity to be given better consideration in attempts to demonstrate health promotion program effectiveness.

Difficulties Regarding Fair Redistribution

Addressing health inequalities and attempting to eliminate them is neither a spontaneous nor a universal process. It varies across societies. One must first acknowledge the plurality of these principles and theories of justice (Culyer, 2001;

Dubet, 2006). Then come difficulties associated with the subjective nature of the notion of equity (Ubel, DeKay, Baron & Asch, 1996). Some authors believe that relying on fair (re)distribution is an ideological objective. Others, like Rawls (1971), are of the opinion that society's resources must be used to enhance the lot of the worst-off. It is inequalities, inevitable in all societies according to the author, but unacceptable, that the principles of justice wish to tackle to achieve greater equity. For Rawls (1971), inequalities thus engender the need to improve the chances of those who have the fewest chances. However, Mooney (1999) criticizes this position since it only takes into account the specific needs of the most disadvantaged individuals and positive discrimination is only directed toward them. Economists regard equity and particularly vertical equity which consists in applying a different treatment to different people, as imposing the obligation to find a fair solution, not only for the worst-off but for everyone. This vision of justice has practical consequences since acting against poverty and its effects on the worst-off does not solve the problem of health inequalities stemming from belonging to specific social groups. This political focus on poverty instead of health inequalities is not new, as the French case reveals and to a lesser extent, the Quebec case (Ridde, 2004). To adopt a charity and assistance policy does not call into question the foundations of an unjust society which can only be addressed through social justice policies.

Given the diversity of theories of distributive justice, to take into account equity in intervention implementation supposes discussions and prior agreement on the manner in which resources or goods must be distributed to satisfy the specific theory of justice that prevails in the situation. Who decides to channel an intervention toward certain subgroups in the population? Who decides that some practitioners and not others participate in the implementation process? The notion of equity is a reflection of the values of the society in which the interventions are undertaken (Mooney, 2002). Both the political context and the plurality of values influence definitions of equity (Peter, 2001; Popay, Williams, Thomas & Gatrell, 1998). Therefore, local populations must participate in defining criteria of equity in health (Peter, 2001). Here are five examples of different perspectives on distributive justice: (a) the Anglo-American neo-liberalist tradition of equal opportunities (Labonte, 2004, p.119); (b) the desire among Swedish politicians to avoid sacrificing equity to efficiency (Lindholm, Rosen & Emmelin, 1998); (c) the rejection in Australia of a policy aimed at maximizing health results if people in poor health must curtail their access to care (Nord, Richardson, Street, Kuhse & Singer, 1995); (d) the Rawlsian vision of social justice among public health practitioners in Quebec who believe public health should devote much of its resources to specific subgroups of the population (worst-off, groups from Aboriginal Descent, drug addicted) who are considered disadvantaged because of socially created injustices (Massé & Saint-Arnaud, 2003), and (e) the rhetorical precedence of egalitarianism among the Mossi of Burkina Faso (Fiske, 1990; Ridde 2006), who believe like their neighbors the Haoussa in Niger, that inequality is constitutive of the social order (Raynault, 1990, p.139).

Equity is thus a value that appears to be as difficult and tricky to define as effectiveness and is an empty concept that must be fleshed out, along with that of performance or quality. An extreme position would be to qualify as effective for health promotion only those interventions that address the problem of equity and achieve a certain reduction in health inequalities. To this end, health promotion evaluation would have to incorporate criteria of equity and rely on indicators of inequalities. Experiences have shown that health promotion evaluation can measure inequalities and be conducted with criteria of values of equity (Gepkens & Gunning-Schepers, 1996; Mackenbach & Stronks, 2002). In an attempt to systematize the evaluation of equity in health promotion we will examine in the sections that follow how evaluation can provide insights regarding whether and how health promotion contributes to reducing health inequalities. In so doing, we will also review some of the most salient technical issues that have to be dealt with in order to quantify inequality in a distribution and to assign an equity value to those inequalities.

How can Health Promotion Decrease Health Inequalities and Where Should Evaluation Focus in Order to Demonstrate this Capacity?

There is no question that the health sector, including public health, has been, and continues to be, very effective in increasing the overall health in Western societies[*] (Detels & Breslow, 2002). Despite an already high level, life expectancy is still increasing in Western Europe and in the Americas. However, this overall success masks important variations across various groups. If, on average, everyone seems to have enjoyed health gains, these gains have been distributed differently between segments of the population. Often interventions leading to improvements in average health may have had no effect on inequalities. Furthermore those inequalities could have been widened by policies and programs that had a greater impact on the better-off (Acheson, 1998; Braveman, 2000; Braveman, Krieger & Lynch, 2000; Gwatkin, Bhuiya & Victora, 2004; Gwatkin, 2000; Gwatkin, 2005; Starfield, 2006; Wagstaff, 2002).

Smoking is a case in point. In Canada, where the overall prevalence of smoking has been cut by more than half over the past forty years, data show that this habit is now four times more prevalent among people who have not finished secondary school compared with those with a university degree (Choinière, Lafontaine & Edwards, 2001). In Canada and the U.S., while people in higher socioeconomic strata are still reducing their tobacco consumption, smoking cessation is stagnating among lower classes (Barbeau, Krieger & Soobader, 2004;

---

[*] Having to make this distinction about the geographical dimension of public health's progress constitutes in itself a statement of failure on the global health equity issue, that we cannot address here for lack of space.

The National Strategy, 2005). Differences observed in the results of health interventions suggest that the latter might contribute to widening the gap in morbidity and mortality between the rich and the poor (G.A. Kaplan, 2001; G.A. Kaplan, Everson & Lynch, 2000).

A health promotion evaluation rhetoric centered exclusively on values of effectiveness and efficiency for judging interventions without specifying also values of equity can, therefore, inadvertently mask increases in health inequities. We suggest that there are potentially four sources of inequalities and inequities associated with health promotion interventions. Those sources are related to: (a) the planning process; (b) the implementation process; (c) the effect of intervention; and (d) the impact of those effects on the health of the population. Each of these potential sources could be the focus of evaluations that use equity as a criterion.

Evaluating Inequalities and Inequities Associated with the Planning Process

Examining inequalities potentially resulting from the intervention planning process amounts to conducting a strategic evaluation that examines whether an intervention was decided and designed with a view to reducing disparities between various groups. Unless interventions are explicitly and intentionally designed to address heath inequities, they are very unlikely to reduce health inequalities. At best, such interventions contribute to the reproduction of health inequity.

Evaluating inequities related to the planning process requires that the normative basis and values that prevailed throughout planning are examined. This issue is, indeed, directly linked to the public health dilemma of planning interventions targeting the overall population or specific groups. Although both strategies have pros and cons, it is important to remember that Rose's (1992) goal in advocating for a population approach was not to reduce health inequities but to pursue a utilitarian goal of increasing overall population heath. As evaluators concerned with equity, our task is to provide information as to whether or not the planning of an intervention fosters the reproduction or alteration of health inequities and inequalities.

As for the construction of the problematic situation, equity-sensitive strategic evaluations would attempt to determine to what extent and how data related to the determinants of heath were considered. In most countries, however, there is no complete population data set linking individual health or mortality/morbidity indicators with the social determinants of health. Health planners must either use survey data when available or aggregate census data. Under an equity perspective, the evaluation of health promotion planning strategy would, therefore, start by questioning whether an initial assessment of areas of inequality regarding a specific health objective was performed. Such an assessment would involve, at the outset, a measurement of health or health determinants. In pursuing the evaluation, it could be asked what constituents of health or health related factors were considered. For health, it is suggested that the full range of aspects of health status itself be considered, not only morbidity and mortality but functional status or disability, suffering, and quality of life (Braveman, 2006; Macinko & Starfield, 2002; Measuring Inequalities in Health Working Group, 2003). For health determinants, this entails considering the many conditions that produce different consequences in different groups of people (Braveman, 2006; Braveman, Egerter, Cubbin & Marchi, 2004).

Moreover, evaluation could examine whether complexities in the measurement of inequalities have been taken into account. Such complexities concern firstly the fact that health status inequality appears to be sensitive to the type of health measure used. Various measures of morbidity or health exist each leading to varying conclusions about inequality (Clarke, Gerdtham, Johannesson, Bingefors & Smith, 2002; Turrell & Mathers, 2001). In addition, inequalities related to different social groups vary whether health measures concern the occurrence or progression of illness (Starfield, 2006). Phelan et al. (2004) demonstrated that the more preventable the causes of death, the more strongly socioeconomic status is associated with mortality, because prevention is more accessible to those in socially advantaged groups. Also, people at lower levels of income have both more illness and more co-morbidity. Differences in health between social groups can hence at times be greater for indicators of severity than for those of appearance of new cases.

Once proper indicators are identified, measuring them across different social groups or generally across individuals in the population (Murray & Gakidou, 1999) essentially reflects the distinction between "inequity" and "inequality", respectively (Kawachi, Subramanian & Almeida-Filho, 2002). The former reflects the assumption that the relevant differences are those between better- and worse-off social groups, selected in light of which groups are known to be more and less advantaged in society (Braveman, 2006), while the latter reflects that the important differences are those between the individuals and the population average.

If the population is stratified into subgroups, evaluation should also take into account interactions between various determinants of health (Reagan & Salsberry, 2005). It should consider whether the population has been stratified into relevant subgroups as well as which particular health outcome was targeted for change (Starfield, 2006). It is proposed that socioeconomic, racial/ethnic, gender, and geographic groups should always be considered as potentially relevant (Braveman, Egerter, Cubbin & Marchi, 2004). The recent approach to study inequalities in health and health care devised by Braveman et al., (2004) proposed that it is necessary to examine indicators of health separately for each social group, comparing all other social groups with the most-advantaged group (Braveman et al., 2004). Such measures that reveal inequalities between social groups should facilitate the elaboration of interventions which would better target certain subgroups according to the particular health or health determinant improvement objectives.

From the standpoint of the elaboration of interventions, evaluators should identify the type of intervention be it specific or generic, individual or structural that was proposed and the justification for its selection as regards equity considerations. On the one hand, given that morbidity clusters in vulnerable subgroups, planning for overall improvements in equity in health is likely to require the elaboration of integrated interventions rather than interventions geared to specific manifestations of ill health (such as disease) (Starfield, 2006). On the other hand, it is recognized that structural changes at the population level provide greater improvement and equity than interventions targeted at individual behaviour. The latter interventions are less effective for individuals with limited social resources (Starfield, 2006).

Evaluation of planning could also examine whether life stages were considered. The literature reveals that good health in earlier life stages represents an opportunity for good health in later stages in life (Braveman, 2005; Kawachi, Subramanian & Almeida-Filho, 2002; Power, Matthews & Manor, 1998). It also demonstrates that the roots of many types of inequities in health appear in early life (Davey-Smith & Lynch, 2004; Galobardes, Lynch & Davey Smith, 2004). Evaluation could, therefore, examine if priority is given to effective interventions at younger ages (Starfield, 2006) or to other priority areas justified by an equity perspective.

Evaluating Health Inequalities and Inequities Associated with the Implementation Process

Evaluators interested in inequities associated with intervention implementation should examine whether the intervention is reaching vulnerable populations to the same extent that it reaches other segments. To answer this question, we need to monitor the social characteristics of participants, which is rarely done. Indeed, very few published evaluation studies have systematically documented differential intervention coverage across various groups. To the extent that the heath care sector reflects the capacity for public heath to reach vulnerable populations, there is mounting evidence that traditionally vulnerable populations such as people of low SES and people of Aboriginal descent are under-represented among those who take advantage of preventive health services available through medical care, such as screening and immunization (Lees, Wortley & Coughlin, 2005). This is so even in jurisdictions where these services are covered by universal Medicare programs (Hagoel, Ore, Neter, Shifroni & Rennert, 1999; Wain, Morrell, Taylor, Mamoon & Bodkin, 2001). With specific reference to health promotion, there are indications that participation in health promotion intervention trials is lower among people from deprived areas (Chinn, White, Howel, Harland & Drinkwater, 2006). Monitoring of program implementation is generally regarded as a secondary and less noble function of evaluation. Furthermore, most discussions on process evaluation focus on the sequence of events that need to take place for the program to produce the intended effect (Scheirer, 1994). Documenting intervention implementation of population programs among specific vulnerable groups poses various sorts of problems. The most obvious methodological problem is to operationally define and assess whether program participants or intervention beneficiaries belong to vulnerable groups. Less obvious but as important is to be able to obtain estimations of group denominators to provide rates of program penetration into those various groups.

Evaluating Inequalities and Inequities Associated with Intervention Effects

A third source of inequalities and inequities that can be taken into account in health promotion evaluation relates to intervention effects. It requires that evaluators examine whether the intervention effects are the same for all groups in the population. Technically this means testing interaction effects between the intervention, the intended effects and one or more social determinants. Although such a requirement may appear to be easily met, there are some technical difficulties especially in cases where the evaluation studies were not specifically designed to test the hypothesis of differential effects. One such difficulty is the issue of sample size; there are often not enough people in some of the interaction cells to provide sufficient power to test for interaction effects. First, there are fewer people from vulnerable groups than from the mainstream population so, even if all groups were equally proportionately represented in the program, there would be a numerical imbalance favouring non-vulnerable groups. This imbalance is further aggravated by the above-mentioned coverage deficit of people from vulnerable groups. Another difficulty arises with the requirement for a longitudinal evaluation design, meaning that the same subject units (individuals or aggregated units such as classrooms or neighborhoods) are tested at baseline and at post test. Indeed, testing for interaction involves that individual unit effects are regressed on other individual characteristics. Longitudinal designs are infrequent in health promotion interventions and community interventions usually involve too few community units to allow for community-level analyses.

To our knowledge, only a few evaluation studies have reported interaction effects showing that people from vulnerable populations gain more from population interventions. One such intervention is water fluoridation. Data show that in jurisdictions where water fluoridation is introduced, children from low SES families experience a greater reduction of dental decay compared with children from higher SES families (Riley, Lennon & Ellwood, 1999). Indeed, this interaction effect is explained by the fact that higher SES children experience lower rates of dental cavities in situations where water is not fluoridated. However, as most interventions initially reach those of higher socioeconomic status and only later affect the poorer segments of society, there are early increases in morbidity and mortality disparities that must be considered in evaluating interventions (Victora, Vaughan, Barros, Silva & Tomasi, 2000).

In assessing what works for the reduction of health inequalities, tension arises between absolute and relative measures and their implications for policy and program evaluation (Gilson, Kalyalya, Kuchler, Lake, Oranga et al., 2000; Macinko & Starfield, 2002; Starfield, 2006; Yip & Berman, 2001). Improvement in equity in health, as measured by decreased absolute differences, may appear as increases in relative differences (Measuring Inequalities in Health Working Group, 2003; Wagstaff, 2002). Thus, the extent to which goals are met depends on how they are stated, that is, as percentages or absolute reductions (Starfield, 2006). The relative difference between any two groups is calculated by dividing the rate of a given indicator in one group by the rate in the other group (rate ratio). The rate difference is obtained by calculating an absolute difference in rates. Expressing inequality in relative terms therefore implies a relation to a benchmark (Alleyne, Castillo-Salgado, Schneider, Loyola & Vidaurre, 2002). Both relative and absolute measures are meaningful and provide complementary information (Asada, 2005; Braveman, 2003, 2006; Mackenbach & Kunst, 1997; Wagstaff, Van Doorslaer & Paci, 1991). For some, relative measures constitute the most appropriate method for measuring inequality (Measuring Inequalities in Health Working Group, 2003). For others, it is essential to combine both relative and absolute measures because the meaning of a large relative gap between two groups varies depending on how the absolute difference compare with some minimum adequate level (Braveman, 2003, 2006). Relative measures are most often used as they are more stable and easier to understand. Absolute measures are more useful for decision-makers because they permit a better appraisal of the magnitude of the public health problem (Schneider et al., 2004).

Another measurement classification method is the simple and complex dichotomy. Simple measurements refer to the previously explained rate ratios or rate differences, which involve comparing only two groups, preferably those at the extremes. In order to reflect comparisons among more than two groups, or to address changes in group size over time, or to reflect both absolute and relative differences across social groups, more complex methods may be used (Braveman, 2006; Macinko & Starfield, 2002; Schneider et al., 2004). Examples of such methods are the population attributable risk (PAR), the slope index of inequality (SII), the relative index of inequality (RII), the concentration curve and index and the index of dissimilarity. Mackenbach and Kunst (in Schneider, 2004) and Braveman (2003) recommend that decision-makers use simple methods, but that investigators confirm the results using more complex ones.

Evaluating Inequalities and Inequities Associated with Intervention Impacts

Finally differential impact constitutes the fourth potential source of inequities and inequalities associated with health intervention. It is usually assumed that a given effect has the same health impact regardless of the characteristics of individuals. For example, in physical activity promoting interventions, this would amount to assuming that there is no interaction between health, the degree to which an individual is physically active and characteristics that affect this person's vulnerability. There are two reasons to question such an assumption. The first is the multiplicative nature of the interactions between most risk factors coupled with the fact that by definition people in vulnerable populations cumulate a higher number of risk factors. In other words, the more numerous the risk factors one is exposed to, the less predictable is the impact on one's health following the alleviation of one risk factor. The second reason is related to the growing evidence of the effects of contextual characteristics on health. Most of the vulnerable groups live in impoverished neighborhoods, the characteristics of which may interact with known risk factors. The impact on health of smoking cessation for someone living in a heavily polluted environment might be marginally lower than that for someone not exposed to pollution. In order to rule out differential impact as a source of inequity resulting from a population intervention, evaluators must design longitudinal studies in which data regarding the entire sequence of events leading from intervention exposure to effect on risk factors to health impact are collected.

Regarding indicators, measurement of impact of socioeconomic inequalities on health "takes into account the actual socioeconomic situation and measures changes in health conditions that are to be expected as a result of potential interventions" (Alleyne, Castillo-Salgado, Schneider, Loyola & Vidaurre, 2002, p. 391). Measures of impact are therefore "particularly relevant for decision-making and for public health aimed at achieving equity." (Alleyne, Castillo-Salgado, Schneider, Loyola & Vidaurre, 2002, p. 391).

The population attributable risk (PAR) is one of the most widely used indicators of overall impact, which can be both relative and absolute. In simple terms, the PAR is defined as "the (level of) reduction in ill health in a population that could be achieved if all social groups experienced the level observed in the most advantaged group." (Braveman, 2003, p. 189). This indicator is easy to calculate and interpret (Alleyne, Castillo-Salgado, Schneider, Loyola & Vidaurre, 2002). Braveman (2003) suggests that although the PAR is categorized as a complex indicator, it remains an intuitive and useful one to present information on equity to policy-makers.

The index of dissimilarity (ID) has also been proposed to measure the magnitude of disparities across diverse groups (Pearcy & Keppel, 2002) and is another example of an impact measure (Schneider et al., 2004). "The ID for a given health indicator sums differences between rates in each subgroup and the overall population rate, expressing the total as a percentage of the overall population rate." (Braveman, 2006, p179). This method has been criticized because it implies comparing to the population average. This is problematic when important proportions of the population are disadvantaged (Braveman, 2006).

Conclusion

The Ottawa Charter for Health Promotion (WHO, 1986) proposed an agenda for action that is much more ambitious than simply improving population health. It forcefully advocated that public health interventions and programs pursue the goal of reducing those health inequalities that are unfair and unjustifiable from a distributive justice perspective. Although the Charter does not identify the principles and models of justice that should be promoted in the name of health, it clearly rejects the utilitarian goal of insuring maximum health for a maximum number of persons if this means that large groups of people are neglected and do not benefit from public health initiatives. Furthermore, the Charter challenges public health practitioners to take action on those social determinants of health that result from social inequities and are at the root of social health inequalities.

Unless evaluation projects clearly and explicitly search for indicators of health promotion effects and impacts on the reduction of health inequalities, they will contribute little to the central agenda of health promotion. Under certain conditions such projects may even contribute to promote interventions that increase health inequalities. Effectiveness is an empty shell and indeed a monograph on health promotion effectiveness begs for someone to ask the critical question: effectiveness for what?

As we have seen, equity is not an easy value to assess and use as a criterion for evaluation. It involves subjective judgements, collective discussions of values and the use of very complex indicators and statistical techniques. True, it is much easier to assess intervention effectiveness in terms of overall improvement in population health indicators than in terms of changes in the distribution of health determinants, health services or health outcomes. In addition, because the inequalities at the root of health inequities result from the ways in which our societies are organized and from the mostly libertarian ideologies that guide governance, it comes as no surprise that little effort is made to overcome the enormous difficulties that would plague evaluating the equity of health promotion interventions.

Authors' Note. A part of the writing of this article was made possible through funding from the Canadian Institutes for Health Research (CIHR): Doctoral Fellowship (MFE-58109) obtained by Pascale Mantoura, and the Global Health Research Initiative Post-Doctoral Fellowship (FGH-81565) obtained by Valéry Ridde. Louise Potvin holds the Canadian Health Services Research Foundation Chair in Community Approaches and Health Inequality (CHSRF/CIHR CP1-0526-05).

References

Acheson, D. (1998). *Independent Inquiry into Inequalities in Health Report*. London: The Stationery Office.

Alleyne, G. A., Castillo-Salgado, C., Schneider, M. C., Loyola, E. & Vidaurre, M. (2002). Overview of social inequalities in health in the Region of the Americas, using various methodological approaches. *Revista Panamericana de Salud Pública/Pan American Journal of Public Health, 12*(6), 388–387.

Amuyunzu-Nyamongo, M. (2005). *Health Promotion and Education: African Programme on Effectiveness (APE). Working Paper*: IUHPE.

Asada, Y. (2005). A framework for measuring health inequity. *J Epidemiol Community Health, 59*(8), 700–705.

Barbeau, E. M., Krieger, N. & Soobader, M. J. (2004). Working class matters: socioeconomic disadvantage, race/ethnicity, gender, and smoking in NHIS 2000. *American Journal of Public Health, 94*(2), 269–278.

Braveman, P. (2000). Round table discussion. Combining forces against inequity and poverty rather than splitting hairs. *Bulletin of the World Health Organization, 78*(1), 78–79.

Braveman, P. (2003). Monitoring Equity in Health and Healthcare: A Conceptual Framework. *Journal of Health Population Nutrition, 21*(3), 181–192.

Braveman, P. (2005). The question is not: "is race or class more important?" *Journal of Epidemiology & Community Health, 59*(12), 1029.

Braveman, P. (2006). Health disparities and health equity: concepts and measurement. *Annu Rev Public Health, 27*, 167–194.

Braveman, P., Egerter, S. A., Cubbin, C. & Marchi, K. S. (2004). An Approach to Studying Social Disparities in Health and Health Care. *Am J Public Health, 94*(12), 2139–2148.

Braveman, P. & Gruskin, S. (2003). Defining equity in health. *Journal of Epidemiology and Community Health, 57*, 254–258.

Braveman, P., Krieger, N. & Lynch, J. (2000). Health inequalities and social inequalities in health. Feedback. *Bulletin of the World Health Organization, 2000, 78*(2), 232–233.

Chinn, D. J., White, M., Howel, D., Harland, J. O. & Drinkwater, C. K. (2006). Factors associated with non-participation in a physical activity promotion trial. *Public Health, 120*, 309–319.

Choinière, R., Lafontaine, P. & Edwards, A. C. (2001). Distribution of cardiovascular disease risk factors by socioeconomic status among Canadian adults. *Can Med Assoc J., 162* (suppl.9), S13–S24.

Clarke, P. M., Gerdtham, U.-G., Johannesson, M., Bingefors, K. & Smith, L. (2002). On the measurement of relative and absolute income-related health inequality. *Social Science & Medicine, 55*(11), 1923–1928.

Culyer, A. J. (2001). Equity – some theory and its policy implications. *J Med Ethics, 27*(4), 275–283.

Davey-Smith, G. & Lynch, J. (2004). Commentary: Social capital, social epidemiology and disease aetiology. *Int. J. Epidemiol., 33*(4), 691–700.

de Savigny, D., Kasale, H., Mbuya, C. & Reid, G. (2004). *In Focus: Fixing Health Systems.* Ottawa: IDRC.

Department of Health. (2003). *Tackling health inequalities: a program for action.* London UK: Department of Health.

Detels, R. & Breslow, L. (2002). Current scope and concerns in public health. In R. Detels, J. McEwen, R. Beaglehole & H. Tanaka (Eds.), *Oxford textbook of public health. The scope of Public Health* (Fourth ed., Vol. 1, pp. 3–20). Oxford, UK: Oxford University Press.

Farmer, P. & Castro, A. (2004). Pearls of the Antilles? Public Health in Haïti and Cuba. In A. Castro & M. Singer (Eds.), *Unhealthy health policy: a critical anthropological examination* (pp. 3–28). Walnut Creek, Calif.; Toronto: AltaMira Press.

Fiske, A. P. (1990). Relativity within Moose culture: Four incommensurable models for social relationships. *Ethos 18*, 180–204.

Galobardes, B., Lynch, J. W. & Davey Smith, G. (2004). Childhood Socioeconomic Circumstances and Cause-specific Mortality in Adulthood: Systematic Review and Interpretation. *Epidemiol Rev, 26*(1), 7–21.

Gepkens, A. & Gunning-Schepers, L. J. (1996). Interventions to reduce socioeconomic health differences: a review of the international literature. *European Journal of Public Health, 6*, 218–226.

Gilson, L. (1998). In defence and pursuit of equity. *Social Science and Medicine, 47*(12), 1891–1896.

Gilson, L., Kalyalya, D., Kuchler, F., Lake, S., Oranga, H. & Ouendo, M. (2000). The equity impacts of community financing activities in three African countries. *The International Journal of Health Planning and Management, 15*(4), 291–317.

Glasgow, R. E., Lichtenstein, E. & Marcus, A. C. (2003). Why don't we see more translation of health promotion research to practice? Rethinking the efficacy to effectiveness transition. *Am J Public Health, 93*, 1261–1267.

Gwatkin, D., Bhuiya, A. & Victora, C. G. (2004). Making health systems more equitable. *The Lancet, 364*(9441), 1273–1280.

Gwatkin, D. R. (2000). Health inequalities and the health of the poor: what do we know? What can we do? *Bulletin of the World Health Organization, 78*(1), 3–18.

Gwatkin, D. R. (2005). How much would poor people gain from faster progress towards the Millennium Development Goals for health? *The Lancet, 365*(9461), 813–817.

Hagoel, L., Ore, L., Neter, E., Shifroni, G. & Rennert, G. (1999). The gradient in mammography screening behavior: a lifestyle marker. *Social Science and Medicine, 48*, 1281–1290.

Health Disparities Task Group of the Federal/Provincial/Territorial Advisory Committee on Population Health and Health Security. (2005). *Reducing health disparities – Roles of the health sector: Discussion paper.* (No. ISBN 0-662-69313-2).

Hills, M. & Carroll, S. (2004). Health promotion evaluation, realist synthesis and participation. *Ciência & Saúde Coletiva, 9*(3), 530–543.

Hogstedt, C., Lundgren, B., Moberg, H., Pettersson, B. & Ågren, G. (2004). *Scandinavian Journal of Public Health, 32*(suppl. 64), 3–64.

IUHPE. Global Programme on Health Promotion Effectiveness (GPHPE). PROMOTING EFFECTIVE HEALTH PROMOTION [Electronic Version]. Retrieved 8 September 2006 from http://www.iuhpe.org

IUHPE (Ed.). (1999). *The Evidence of Health Promotion Effectiveness: Shaping Public Health in a new Europe. Part Two.* Brussels – Luxembourg: ECSC-EC-EAEC. 1st edition. Paris: Jouve Composition & Impression.

IUHPE (Ed.). (2004). *Efficacité de la promotion de la santé. Actes du colloque organisé par l'Inpes avec la collaboration de l'UIPES. Promotion & Education.* Hors série 1.

Kaplan, G. A. (2001). Economic policy is health policy: Findings from the study of income, socioeconomic status and health. In B. Auerbach & J. Krimgold (Eds.), *Income, socioeconomic status, and health: Exploring the relationships* (pp. 137–149). Washington DC: National Policy Association.

Kaplan, G. A., Everson, S. A. & Lynch, J. W. (2000). The contribution of social and behavioral research to an understanding of the distribution of disease: A multilevel approach. In B. Smedley & S. Syme (Eds.), *Promoting health. Intervention strategies from social and behavioral research* (pp. 37–80). Washington DC: Institute of Medicine

Kawachi, I., Subramanian, S. V. & Almeida-Filho, N. (2002). A glossary for health inequalities. *J Epidemiol Community Health, 56*(9), 647–652.

Krasnik, A. (1996). The concept of equity in health services research. *Scandinavian Journal of Social Medicine, 24*(1), 2–7.

Labonte, R. (2004). Social inclusion/exclusion: dancing the dialectic. *Health Promotion International, 19*(1), 115–121.

Lees, P., Wortley, S. & Coughlin, K. (2005). Comparison of racial/ethnic disparities in adult immunization and cancer screening. *American Journal of Preventive Medicine, 29*, 404–411.

Lindholm, L., Rosen, M. & Emmelin, M. (1998). How many lives is equity worth? A proposal for equity adjusted years of life saved. *J Epidemiol Community Health, 52*(12), 808–811.

Macinko, J. & Starfield, B. (2002). Annotated Bibliography on Equity in Health, 1980–2001. *International Journal for Equity in Health 1*(1), 1.

Macintyre, S. (1997). The Black Report and beyond: what are the issues? *Social Science & Medicine, 44*, 723–745.

Mackenbach, J. P. & Kunst, A. E. (1997). Measuring the magnitude of socio-economic inequalities in health: An overview of available measures illustrated with two examples from Europe. *Social Science & Medicine, 44*(6), 757–771.

Mackenbach, J. P. & Stronks, K. (2002). A strategy for tackling health inequalities in the Netherlands. *BMJ, 325*(7371), 1029–1032.

Massé, R. & Saint-Arnaud, J. (2003). *Éthique et santé publique: enjeux, valeurs et normativité*. [Québec]: Presses de l'Université Laval.

Mathison, S. (2004). *Encyclopedia of Evaluation*. Newbury Park, CA: Sage Publication.

Measuring Inequalities in Health Working Group. (2003). *Inequalities in Health – Report of the Measuring Inequalities in Health Working Group*

Mittelmark, M. (2002). Health promotion: Effectiveness, efficiency and equity, 3rd edition. *Health Promotion International, 17*, 376–377.

Mooney, G. (1987). Qu'est-ce que l'équité en matière de santé. *Rapport trimestriel statistique sanitaire mondial*, 296–303.

Mooney, G. (1999). *Vertical equity in health care resource allocation* (Vol. 3/99). Sydney: Department of public health and community medicine, University of Sydney.

Mooney, G. (2002). Reply to Barbara Starfied UK Health Equity Network, http://www.ukhen.org.uk/ Sent: Sun 10/13/2002 9:42 AM.

Murray, C. & Gakidou, E. J. F. (1999). Health inequalities and social group differences: what should we measure? *Bull World Health Organ 77*(7), 537–543.

Nord, E., Richardson, J., Street, A., Kuhse, H. & Singer, P. (1995). Maximizing health benefits vs egalitarianism: an Australian survey of health issues. *Social Science and Medicine, 41*(10), 1429–1437.

Olsen, J. A. (1997). Theories of justice and their implications for priority setting in health care. *Journal of Health Economics, 16*, 625–639.

Pearcy, J. N. & Keppel, K. G. (2002). A summary measure of health disparity. *Public Health Rep, 117*, 273–280.

Peter, F. (2001). Health equity and social justice. *J Appl Philos, 18*(2), 159–170.

Phelan, J.C., Link, B.G., Diez-Roux, A., Kawachi, I. & Levin, B. (2004). Fundamental Causes of Social Inequalities in Mortality: A Test of the Theory. *Journal of Health and Social Behavior 45*: 265–285.

Popay, J., Williams, G., Thomas, C. & Gatrell, A. (1998). Theorising inequalities in health: the place of lay knowledge. In M. Bartley, D. Blane & G. D. Smith (Eds.), *The sociology of health inequalities* (pp. 59–83). Oxford: Blackwell Publishers.

Power, C., Matthews, S. & Manor, O. (1998). Inequalities in self-rated health: explanations from different stages of life. *The Lancet, 351*(9108), 1009–1013.

Rawls, J. (1971). *Justice as Fairness*. Cambridge: Harvard University Press.

Raynault, C. (1990). Inégalités économiques et solidarités sociales. Exemples haoussa au Niger. In D. Fassin & Y. Jaffré (Eds.), *Sociétés, développement et santé* (pp. 136–154). Paris: ELLIPSES.

Reagan, P. B. & Salsberry, P. J. (2005). Race and ethnic differences in determinants of preterm birth in the USA: broadening the social context. *Social Science & Medicine, 60*(10), 2217–2228.

Ridde, V. (2004). Une analyse comparative entre le Canada, le Québec et la France: l'importance des rapports sociaux et politiques eu égard aux déterminants et aux inégalités de la santé. *Recherches Sociographiques, XLV*(2), 343–364; accessible à http://www.erudit.org/revue/rs/2004/v2045/n2002/index.html.

Ridde, V. (2006). *Efficacité ou équité? Les politiques de santé à l'épreuve des inégalités au Burkina Faso*. Paris: L'Harmattan.

Riley, J. C., Lennon, M. A. & Ellwood, R. P. (1999). The effect of water fluoridation and social inequalities on dental caries in 5-year-old children. *International Journal of Epidemiology, 28*, 300–305.

Rose, G. (1992). *The Strategy of Preventive Medicine*. Oxford: Oxford University Press.

Scheirer, M. A. (1994). Designing and using process evaluation. In J. S. Wholey, H. P. Hatry & K. E. Newcomer (Eds.), *Handbook of practical program evaluation* (pp. 40–68). San Francisco: Jossey-Bass.

Schneider, M. C., Castillo-Salgado, C., Bacallao, J., Loyola, E., Mujica, O. J., Vidaurre, M., et al. (2004). Methods for measuring health inequalities (Part 1). *Epidemiological Bulletin PAHO, 25*(4), 7–10.

Secretariat for the Healthy Living Network. (2005). The Integrated Pan-Canadian Healthy Living Strategy. Retrieved September 8, 2006, from www.phac-aspc.gc.ca/hl-vs-strat/pdf/hls_e.pdf.

Starfield, B. (2006). State of the Art in Research on Equity in Health. *Journal of Health Politics Policy and Law, 31*(1), 11–32.

The National Strategy. (2005). *Moving Forward: The 2005 Progress Report on Tobacco Control*. Retrieved. from.

Thurston, W. E., Wilson, D. R., Felix, R., MacKean, G. & Wright, M.-F. (1998). *A review of the effectiveness of health promotion strategies in Alberta*.

Tones, K. & Tilford, S. (2001). *Health Promotion: Effectiveness, Efficiency and Equity* (3 ed.). Cheltenham: Nelson Thornes.

Tones, K., Tilford, S. & Robinson, Y. K. (1990). *Health Education: Effectiveness and Efficiency*. London: Chapman & Hall.

Townsend, P. & Davidson, N. (1982). *Inequalities in heath: The Black Report*. Harmondsworth, UK: Penguin.

Turrell, G. & Mathers, C. (2001). Socioeconomic inequalities in all-cause and specific-cause mortality in Australia: 1985–1987 and 1995–1997. *Int. J. Epidemiol., 30*(2), 231–239.

U.S. Department of Health and Human Services. (2000). *Healthy People 2010: Understanding and Improving Health* (2d ed.). Washington, DC: US Government Printing Office.

Ubel, P. A., DeKay, M. L., Baron, J. & Asch, D. A. (1996). Cost-effectiveness analysis in a setting of budget constraints–is it equitable? *N Engl J Med, 334*(18), 1174–1177.

Victora, C. G., Vaughan, J. P., Barros, F. C., Silva, A. C. & Tomasi, E. (2000). Explaining trends in inequities: evidence from Brazilian child health studies. *The Lancet, 356*(9235), 1093–1098.

Wagstaff, A. (2002). *Inequalities in health in developing countries – swimming against the tide?*: The World Bank-Policy Research Working Paper Series 2795.

Wagstaff, A. & Van Doorsaler, E. (1993). Equity in the finance and delivery of health care: concepts and definitions. In A. Wagstaff, E. Van Doorsaler & F. Rutten (Eds.), *Equity in the finance and delivery of health care, an international perspective* (pp. 7–19). Oxford, New York, Tokyo: Oxford University Press.

Wagstaff, A., Van Doorslaer, E. & Paci, P. (1991). On the measurement of horizontal inequity in the delivery of health care. *Journal of Health Economics, 10*(2), 169–205.

Wain, G., Morrell, S., Taylor, R., Mamoon, H. & Bodkin, N. (2001). Variation in cervical cancer screening by region, socio-economic, migrant and indigenous status in women in New South Wales. *Australian & New Zealand Journal of Obstetrics & Gynaecology, 41*, 320–325.

WHO-EURO. (1984, 9–13 July). *Health Promotion: Concepts and Principles. A selection of papers presented at the Working Group on Concept and Principles*, Copenhagen.

WHO. (1986). The Ottawa Charter for Health Promotion. Retrieved September 8, 2006, from www.euro.who.int/AboutWHO/Policy/20010827_2.

WHO. (2006). Commission on Social Determinants of Health. Retrieved September 8, 2006, from http://www.who.int/social_determinants/resources/csdh_brochure.pdf

Yip, W. & Berman, P. (2001). Targeted health insurance in a low income country and its impact on access and equity in access: Egypt's school health insurance. *Health Economics, 10*(3), 207–220.

Zaza, S., Briss, P. A. & Harris, K. W. (2005). *The Guide to community preventive services. What works to promote health?*. New York: Oxford university Press.

22
Evaluation of Empowerment and Effectiveness
Universal Concepts?

VALÉRY RIDDE, TREENA DELORMIER AND GHISLAINE GOUDREAU

L'important est de savoir si certaines phrases, certains énoncés vous induisent à penser, vous emménent, même éventuellement, dans une rêverie . . .

(Guattari, Spire, Field & Hirsch, 2002)

The question of the effectiveness of health promotion (HP) interventions has captured the attention and energy of a number researchers, superseding the continual debates on delineating the field of HP vis-à-vis that of public and community health. The central problem is the following: how can we claim that a HP intervention is effective? The informed reader will understand that this includes subject matter which cannot economize on paradigm-oriented reflections, given four separate yet intertwined ontological, epistemological, teleological, and methodological dimensions (Gendron, 2001). The interplay of all these beliefs and values, previously stated by Kuhn, leads to a situation where our vision of the world and our relationship with it conditions both the methodological arsenal useful for considering the effectiveness of an intervention, and our vision of the concept of effectiveness itself.

Some think that HP is not founded upon any disciplinary epistemology, and therefore it is illusionary to develop *"evidence rules"* (McQueen & Anderson, 2001). Others seek to adapt HP vocabulary to that of bio-medicine (Green & Glasgow, 2006) preferring terms like external validity for example, a richly meaningful term to positivists, to terms such as the nature of transferability of conclusions, one used more frequently by constructivists. These ponderings upon scientific criteria, which are specific to the HP discipline, are echoed in the discipline of program evaluation. The epistemological suggestions given by the defenders of "Real World Evaluation" (Bamberger, Rugh & Mabry, 2006) take up Guba's and Lincoln's notorious propositions of a method for evaluating the effectiveness of actions, mirroring those of their colleagues in the health field (Carvalho, Bodstein, Hartz & Matida, 2004; Lock, Nguyen & Zarowsky, 2005). This suggests for example, studying the *contribution* of certain factors, and not the *determinants* on the effects of interventions. The issues surrounding the evaluation of HP effectiveness are numerous. Considering the current state of our reflection on the subject, this chapter is centred on two essential concepts according to the authors, but which have not been sufficiently addressed in the literature on HP effectiveness.

The first section is dedicated to the proposition linking the methodological and teleological elements of HP, specifically the concept of empowerment, which remains central to HP practice. The debates on this concept are as old as the tools available for the evaluation of HP effectiveness which are still rare. But, if empowerment is a process, it is also an intended outcome of HP the extent to which requires verification in order to determine the effectiveness of HP. How can one then evaluate empowerment as an outcome of an HP program*, recognizing that it is a right of passage which is obligatory in order to demonstrate effectiveness. This section focuses on the quest *"for appropriate indicators for health promotion success"* (McQueen & Anderson, 2001). The second section features an epistemological and ontological discussion concerning the concept of effectiveness itself. Above and beyond the paradigmatic issues, which imply an understanding of effectiveness, and the manner by which one can account for it scientifically is the core question of the universality of the effectiveness concept.

Before delving into the crux of the subject, it is prudent to state that this chapter does not have any other aim aside from soliciting debate and reflection around HP effectiveness. It consists purely of an attempt to broach the subject in an exploratory fashion. We hope that this effort is understood as a way to share our initial thoughts in order to enrich the existing dialogue and which could eventually be used to advance the state of knowledge through a dialogue between different academic disciplines, cultures, societies and languages.[†]

How to Evaluate Empowerment as a Health Promotion Outcome?

We will not reiterate here the multitude of existing discussions regarding the definition of HP, since the literature on this topic is abundant. For the purpose of this chapter, we will therefore adopt a definition proposed by the experts, for it is useful in initiating our discussion:

health promotion is fundamentally about ensuring that individuals and communities are able to assume power to which they are entitled [. . .and] the primary criterion for determining whether a particular initiative should be considered to be health promoting, ought to be the extent to which it involves the process of enabling or empowering individuals or communities (Rootman et al., 2001).

---

[*] The same question is posed by the defenders of "empowerment evaluation" (Ridde, 2006).
[†] We have, although in vain, made an effort to involve academics from other contexts in the development and drafting of this chapter, in order to ensure a broad representation of the various concepts from a perspective in the Arab-Muslim context and that of West Africa. We hope that this will be possible in a future exercise of this nature.

If empowerment, a flagship value of HP for over 25 years and recognized as such in the Ottawa Charter, is at the heart of this definition, then it is interesting that we can also find its dual nature hidden herewith. In fact, empowerment is on the one hand a process, and on the other, it is an expected outcome of such a process. It is precisely this particular process which differentiates HP from public health, which relies heavily on a technocratic process as Ridde (2007) argue, and from community health, which employs a participatory approach. In terms of generating change, we conceive empowerment as a proximate effect of an HP process, the distal effect being that of the reduction of social inequalities in health (Ridde, 2007). The challenge of evaluating empowerment as a proximal outcome is that this concept remains *"in the early stages of development [. . .] requiring the development of new research procedures and technologies"* (Rootman et al., 2001). Very little ground has been covered in this area since this fact was documented nearly 15 years ago (Boyce, 1993) and that others still demand the *"refinement of measurement tools"* (Wallerstein, 2006). It therefore remains an essential sphere since as long as we are unable to verify that a HP intervention has achieved this outcome, we will not be able to make any statement about its effectiveness. The demonstration of the effectiveness of empowerment as a *process* has already been attempted, now we must dwell upon the *outcomes*. Obviously in different contexts and cultures, the understanding and interpretation of such a concept is delicate, as is also the case for its operationalization for evaluation purposes. Indeed, the evaluation of a concept requires its transformation into different components/dimensions/variables (according to the school of thought), and the consideration of construct validity. Is the concept of empowerment, as for that of effectiveness, a universal one? One must even further explore and reflect upon this question given that the majority of scientific literature comes from an epistemic community writing in the English language, and hence the only existing source of the final analysis on the effectiveness of the process of empowerment (Wallerstein, 2006). Notwithstanding, some recent attempts have been made to translate this concept or suggest useful dimensions for its evaluation, generally carried out on three planes: individual, organizational, and community. For each one of these levels, many authors have developed, with varying degrees of detail and differing epistemological positions, the origins of a list of indicators to study in substantiating the reach of empowerment. Wallerstein (2002) proposes that the outcomes at the community level are of three types: participation, control and critical conscience. Still looking at the community level, Rifkin (2003) suggests six dimensions: capacity building, human rights, organizational sustainability, institutional accountability, contribution, and a positive environment. Peterson and Zimmerman (2004) attempted the same type of analysis, but with regard to organizational empowerment, picking up the different expected outcomes (and processes) noted by many other authors.

The objective of this chapter is not to present a review of the literature, but rather to illustrate that it is imperative that empirical work in this area is developed, namely in other languages and cultures where use of such indicators has already been made. Studies show that theoretical constructs of empowerment as an outcome are as rare as the cultural and social diversity of their attempts. But, diverse attempts are not absent because, for example, Nepalese villagers have already tried to account for the dimensions of community empowerment with community competencies and with changes at the social structural level (Purdey, Adhikari, Robinson & Cox, 1994). Since this chapter is written according to a perspective of change, it is therefore useful to relate two recent developments that differ from the epistemological point of view of empowerment evaluation as an outcome. Neither are well known yet because they were both conducted in the French language.

The first pertains to individual empowerment, which has been more widely studied than organizational and community empowerment (Peterson & Zimmerman, 2004). In order to evaluate the outcomes of a program targeting the promotion of well-being for children under three years of age and their parents, Le Bossé and his colleagues (Le Bossé, Dufort & Vandette, 2004) developed a specific tool. A measurement scale for psycho-sociological markers for empowerment of parents – empowerment being translated into French as *"pouvoir d'agir"*, i.e. "power to act" – was created following many theoretical and empirical evaluation steps over a five year period. The creators of this instrument, which is still in the experimental stage, believe that it could be used in contexts different from the one for which it was created as long as the items for each of the dimensions are adapted accordingly to the relevant context of the study. The tool is composed of three dimensions and twenty-two items measuring the propensity to act, the critical conscience, and finally the perception of self-efficacy. The psychometric performance of this exploratory instrument seems to be interesting, with the three factors explaining 65% of the variance.

The second attempt is of a different paradigmatic nature and relates individual, organizational and community empowerment. For Ninacs (2002), individual empowerment corresponds to a succession of steps working together, like four threads of the same rope, according to four dimensions: participation, technical competencies, self-esteem, and critical conscience. The transition through these steps, along with their interaction, permits their mutual strengthening, and allows an individual to go from one step without much power[*] to a state where s/he is able to act as a function of his/her own choice. The four threads (dimensions) corresponding to organizational and community empowerment are sensibly the same as those of individual empowerment (Figure 22.1).

Each one of these four dimensions has been specified with regard to numerous (more or less) precise indicators. For example, the seminal work of Arnstein (1969) was of great benefit in order to develop the manner by which the extent of individual participation is evaluated. Communication at the community level per-

---

[*] Ninacs said that the process for people is from a disempowered position to a powered one. But it's not clear for us if it possible that someone can be completely disempowered for everything in one's life. This is why we preferred to say that an individual starts from one step without much power and not disempowered.

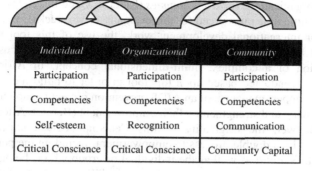

Individual	Organizational	Community
Participation	Participation	Participation
Competencies	Competencies	Competencies
Self-esteem	Recognition	Communication
Critical Conscience	Critical Conscience	Community Capital

FIGURE 22.1. Dimensions of empowerment
Source: Adapted from (Ninacs, 2002)

tains to i) the effective circulation of general information, ii) access to information required for successfully completing specific projects, and iii) transparency in decision-making processes. We will not present a list of all the indicators here, due to space limitations, but most importantly because a number of theoretical efforts from this view point remain to be rendered. This theoretical proposal including the four dimensions has recently inspired many evaluators in applying it.[*] For example, borrowing the empowerment evaluation (EE) approach, we have used it to analyze, *a posteriori*, an evaluative process undertaken for a street workers program in Quebec (Ridde, Baillargeon, Ouellet & Roy, 2003). In fact, one of the main criticisms of this approach is the difficulty of being able to *"conceptualize outcomes of EE in this way and to demonstrate the links to EE processes"* (Cousins, 2005). Also in Quebec, the indicators suggested by Ninacs (2002) were adapted in order to better grasp the context of a collective kitchens community program (Racine & Leroux, 2006). The authors found it significant to assure that empowerment is not a generalized state and that it consists of being able to qualify it to then evaluate it. Evaluating empowerment of one's own life, as a global concept, is indeed a very delicate exercise, assuredly an impossible one. Likewise, the evaluators of empowerment in this project specified that it is contingent on the program itself, that is to say empowerment on food security. In this way researchers were able to obtain, in a concrete and observable way, the four components of empowerment and to propose corresponding indicators. The practical competencies at the individual level manifest themselves through i) strategies for food security utilized outside the kitchens, ii) capacities to cook, iii) communication skills and team work (tolerance), and iv) the ensemble of the capacities developed by the participants. In contexts very different from the one it which it was created, this tool has already been used in two other cases. In Haiti, it proved useful for evaluating the expected outcomes of a program implemented

---

[*] These experiences are in part re-grouped in a special issue of the Canadian Journal of Program Evaluation (2006, Vol 21, n°3).

by a Swiss organization, *Terre des hommes* (Ridde & Queuille, 2006). Taking into account the little time outsourced for this evaluation (two weeks), as is frequently the case for international development work, the use of this tool was greatly appreciated by participants allowing them to have a simple and useful visual representation of a complex, multi-dimensional concept. In Africa, training courses were conducted based upon this tool in order to build the capacities of community support managers of an AIDS prevention project to support sex workers in improving and strengthening their empowerment (Bernier, Arteau & Papin, 2005). Moreover, the originality of this Canadian-African experience was characterized by a double process to empowerment, including the person who is providing the support as well as the individual or group who is being supported. The four components of empowerment were mobilized in parallel in a support process based upon four axes of practice: personal and structural context, involvement of those who are impacted, the coinciding of "here and now", and finally the stimulation of critical conscience.

In this first section, we wanted to succinctly convey the relatively few new attempts at evaluating empowerment outcomes and show that much more territory remains to be explored, namely in the construct validation of these proposals and the accuracy of empowerment indicators. While these experiences are encouraging, the advancement of knowledge in this respect seems urgent and an integral part of any reflection on HP effectiveness.

The Meaning of the Effectiveness Concept

As we stated in the introduction, current initiatives to reflect on HP effectiveness all start from the same postulate: that effectiveness would be the achievement of objectives that were established at the beginning of the intervention.[*] Is it possible to think of effectiveness differently? Without any other pretension than that of stimulating debate, the aim of this section is to show that it is possible to envisage that the emic perspectives (i.e. insider perspectives) of effectiveness vary from one society to another. We will not venture into the realm of cultural relativism which at times has done harm to public health (Fassin, 2001). We simply wish to stimulate this reflection from two philosophical standpoints and with two examples which illustrate that the understanding of effectiveness can be specific to a society.

In general, it is appropriate to credit the mechanical vision of effectiveness (the activities/output must meet their objectives/outcomes), and its lot of performance indicators, to the defenders of *New Public Management*, most certainly rationalists. But maybe things are not as simple as that, they actually appear more

---

[*] In chapter 21 (Potvin, Mantoura & Ridde), we also think that the other postulate which predominates in these initiatives on effectiveness consists of a utilitarian vision of effectiveness, frequently putting the notion of equity to the side.

complex since "*as soon as an individual undertakes an action, whatever it might be, it then begins to escape his intentions*" (Morin, 2005). We are looking to the idea that the programs themselves are trivial, which in the words of Edgard Morin (2005), signifies that "*if you know the inputs, you know the outputs; you can predict the behavior as soon as you know that which goes into the machine.*" Input and output are words in the everyday vocabulary of evaluators and planners who master the widespread use of logical frameworks and other management models which center on intervention results.

But could the effectiveness of an intervention, rest upon an analysis of its capacity to adapt itself, taking into account the context and the environment regardless of initial intended objectives? Piaget said yesterday and Le Moigne reiterates today, action and knowledge go hand in hand, they are inseparable (Saillant, 2004). The recourse to philosophy can certainly help us here, and the conference lecture on effectiveness delivered by Jullien (2005) is definitely of assistance. Without going into the details of Jullien's arguments, his presentation demonstrated that the notion of effectiveness itself is culturally and socially con-structed. Looking to China in order to "*put some distance between the thinking from which we come*", the author distinguishes two ways of conceiving effective-ness (Figure 22.2).

On one side, the classical European school of thought, of Greek heritage, conceives effectiveness as being the capacity to standardize, to create an ideal model, a plan setting out a goal that one will try to achieve through a heroic act according to a means-to-an-end relationship. An ideal model is thereby projected onto reality.[*] For readers accustomed to program evaluation approaches and concepts, they will

In order to be effective, one must . . .	
Classic European School of Thought	Classic Chinese School of Thought
. . .*Modelling* • Building a model, an ideal • Draft a plan, establish a goal • Means-End • Heroism of the act	. . .*Surfing* • Rely upon the supporting factors • Take advantage of the circumstances • Acknowledging the potential of a situation • Transform

FIGURE 22.2. Two different understandings of effectiveness

Source: Adapted from (Jullien, 2005)

---

[*] Jullien (2005) moderates his dichotomy by saying that we keep this typical ideal model to render our reasoning more understandable, by taking up Aristotle's propositions on the notion of caution (*phronésis*) as a way to mediate between the plan and its implementa-tion, or the notion of *métis* present in ancient Greek and translated as the capacity to take advantage of the circumstances. For a recent critic of the dichotomy, see Billeter, 2006.

immediately and instinctively make a link to the suggestions of those who adhere to *theory-driven evaluation* (Chen, 2005), logic models and results-based management. The ideology of performance (Heilbrunn, 2005) underlies this worldview and its related planning processes. From another perspective, the classical Chinese school of thought maintains that the effectiveness of action is determined by the capacity of its managers to adapt, to benefit from and take advantage of circumstances which present themselves by relying upon the supporting factors. Non-knowledge, or the absence of knowledge, is at the core of this vision, which poses serious difficulties to Cartesian thinkers. As stated by another traditional Chinese specialist, "*to listen without knowledge is not a failure, but rather a learning method [which permits] perceiving the possibilities*" (Eyssalet, 2006). Here, "*the strategist is thus invited to use the situation as the starting point, not necessarily a situation such as I would for-mulise it beforehand, but rather a more fitting situation in which I am engaged and deep within which I try to seek or locate the potential and how best to harness it*" states Jullien (2005). All managers have read Sunzi's famous classic text "The art of war" in which the first chapter addresses evaluation (or rather *evaluability assess-ment*). Jullien has done a rereading and interpretation of this work to show that vic-tory, or otherwise stated, effectiveness, is understood as the result of the potential offered by a situation, and not as the application of a plan corresponding to a pre-designed model to achieve an objective at all costs. "*You miss the outcome because you forced it*" whereas you should "*let it (the process) flow and take its course, yet without neglecting it either*" (Jullien, 2005). Thereby, we are reminded by the differ-entiation between the determinants of health and the "contributors" to it, that it is about transforming (in an indirect way) rather that acting compulsorily (in a direct way). Edgard Morin, surely having been influenced by Chinese thinking, states that "*the development of a strategy entails the undeviating vigilance of the person at the core of the activity, takes into account the potential hazards, modifies the strategy in progress and underway, and possibly, if need be, torpedoes the activity which might have taken a dangerous path. Strategy is like navigating with a rudder on uncertain seas*" (Morin, 2004). Those who are familiar with evaluation trends will have most certainly made the connection between the realist approach (which is not against the-ories) and namely the Pawsonian equation where $M + C = O$, that is to say that the evaluation of effectiveness must be capable of locating which mechanism (M) works is which context (C) to produce what particular outcome (O) (Pawson, 2006). If this realist approach to evaluation is still theoretical and unclear, a distinct number of attempts are currently underway in the HP field to apply and sidestep the deadlock of evidentiary data and classical European thought. We will not go into the details of the related theoretical propositions and practical considerations here as far as the evaluation of HP effectiveness is concerned, as they are already widely debated in a number of other publications (Hills, Carroll & O'Neill, 2004; Potvin, Gendron & Bilodeau, 2006).

This reflection around two philosophical traditions now brings us to two examples of the way in which HP effectiveness can be very specific to one distinct society: an Indigenous perspective within Canada. First, it must be said that the current health status of indigenous people, and the health disparities they suffer, are understood as rooted in the colonial relationships experienced with Canada (Adelson, 2005). Therefore, the promotion of health in indigenous communities is intricately tied to the revitalization of indigenous peoples' communities through self-governance efforts. Indigenous understandings of health are holistic, rooted in relationships to family, community, all living things, the earth, and all of creation. Traditional, indigenous understandings of health go beyond physical health of the individual, and consider mental, emotional and spiritual health. This holistic model can be referred to as the "Circle of Life" and extends beyond the individual to include relationships to the community. The model teaches that everything and everyone has something to contribute to the circle, which can be understood as the community. In the "Circle of Life" everything is connected and equally important where one's well-being is related to the community and connected to elements of the earth. Building on the strengths of the circle makes it strong and healthy for the next seven generations. Seven generations is a concept that signifies the long term impacts that should be considered when making decisions. Holistic and positive concepts of health are shared with those of health promotion. As well, the values of social justice, community control of the determinants of health through empowerment and participation echo those of indigenous communities. From an indigenous perspective, HP is simply a newer term to describe the traditional way of life that indigenous communities are striving to revive today.

Effectiveness in health promotion would therefore be reflected in approaches which support self-governance efforts to revitalize and build strong communities. Effectiveness can be sought in endeavors that are based upon indigenous understandings of health which build on the strengths of the community and support the broader goals of self-governance. Two examples of effective HP interventions are provided. The first, from northern Ontario, is an urban indigenous women's hand drumming circle which has been demonstrated as effective in promoting health (Goudreau, 2006). Through participating in this cultural practice, these women are reviving their culture and building on existing strengths in their community. In this study, women hand drummers found physical, mental, emotional, and spiritual benefits of drumming as well as cultural and social support within the hand-drumming circle. They expressed finding healing, their voice, empowerment, renewal, strength, and *Mino-Biimadiziwin* (an Ojibwe word that translates into "good life"). Another example is the Kahnawake Schools Diabetes Prevention Project, where the Kanien'kehaka (Mohawk) community of Kahnawake mobilized efforts to prevent diabetes with the long term goal of healthy future seven generations. The result was a community-directed and owned research and intervention collaboration that has promoted healthy lifestyles, built capacity and created meaningful knowledge that continues to serve current health promotion efforts to address high rates of diabetes in the community (Bisset, Cargo, Delormier, Macaulay & Potvin, 2004; Delormier, Cargo, Kirby & McComber, 2003). Therefore, what one must keep in mind from this indigenous perspective is that effectiveness, in this particular social context, cannot be limited or contained to a simple confirmation of some indicators of loose environmental outcomes. Effectiveness must be studied and seen in a holistic sense, taking into account a myriad of elements, of which empowerment and self-governance are central concepts. This of course poses some serious methodological problems and concerns given the discussion included in the first section of this chapter. In order to link this indigenous perspective to the philosophical reflections of this section, the concept of ecosophy (social ecology) from the philosopher Guattari (1989) can be useful to qualify this vision of effectiveness. In fact, "ecosophy" postulates that it is impossible to transform environments without changing mentalities and rebuilding the social fabric at the same time. We do not have the space available here to go further in-depth, but we would simply add that "ecosophy" pitches a "rhizome" which spreads its roots and grows under the surface, more than an arranged logical, hierarchy as a tree, pushing up and out. And to attest to this link between HP and post-modern philosophy, this same bulb came to the rescue of the last book on HP in Canada, for which it was used as the image to depict HP (Dupéré et al., 2007; Kickbusch, 2007); therefore, clearly an analogy and image whose link to HP should be carefully watched and followed in the future.

The comparative approach presented here, starting from two different schools of thought and elaborating an indigenous perspective, presents a true methodological challenge. In fact, the transition through a Weberian creation of such general ideal-types is a delicate matter and presents the risk of creating *"barriers which can become impossible to overcome and constitute truly solid logical walls which on the one hand help to protect us, and on the other can confine us"* (Jacquard, 2006). That being said, this section's primary aim was to reconsider the implications of a universal nature of the effectiveness concept, similar to the case of equity (see Potvin, Mantoura and Ridde chapter in this book), as a debate that could be further pursued.

What if Effectiveness became Responsiveness?

Realists perceive social change as transformational and the social system as an "open system" which is a product of literally endless components and forces (Pawson, 2006). So, if we accept to adhere to a realist position for the evaluation of effectiveness and to a mode of thinking where permanent and on-going adaptation of a program to its environment has precedence over meeting an objective, then to be effective is to be responsive.[*] Responsiveness is considered as one of the objectives of health systems by WHO and as one of the evaluation criteria of HP programs (Potvin, Haddad & Frohlich, 2001). This vision with regard to programs which should adapt, contradicts that which describes the life of a project characterised by an unavoidable cycle from the needs assessment to steps for planning and implementation. The understanding of such a step-by-step process surely finds its roots in the 1950's study of public policy by American *stagists* (deLeon, 1999). Evaluation often

---

[*] Experts in organizational theory, following Parsons, try to show that the performance of organizations (and through the expansion of programs) can be judged on the scale of the balance between four interconnected dimensions: i) achieving goals (effectiveness), ii) production, iii) maintaining values and iv) adaptation (Champagne & Guiset, 2005).

becomes the ultimate step. Others sometimes add sustainability or even capitalization to close the circle. However some believe, on the contrary, that the process of HP practice is neither linear nor cyclical. Rather, one could conceive of these practices as a series of four sub-processes which are both concurrent and interdependent: *planning, implementation, evaluation, and sustainability.* Although the definitions of the first three terms are well-known, those of sustainability are less understood. In French, we have two words to describe the sustainability process (*pérennisation*) or level (*pérennité*). The first one is concerned with the process which permits for the continuation of activities and outcomes related to programs. And contrary to what one would normally think, actions and interventions which are conducive to high sustainability levels must begin simultaneously with the implementation of the program, and not at the end (Pluye, Potvin, Denis, Pelletier & Mannoni, 2005). The second one (sustainability level) is the result of this process – manifesting itself in the organizational routines – which can be evaluated as a function of various degrees, the highest being that of standardization (the integration of these routines as programmatic outcomes of public policy). We will not go any further into this proposal, undoubtedly new to the field, but of which the conceptual details and empirical illustrations from Quebec and Haiti are presented elsewhere (Pluye, Potvin & Denis, 2004; Ridde, Pluye & Queuille, 2006). Let us then retain that these four sub-processes are concomitant for when we implement a program (implementation), we are constantly asking ourselves about what is happening (evaluation), we are consistently monitoring what was scheduled to happen (planning) with an on-going preoccupation with the way to proceed in support all the aforementioned processes, (the sustainability process) often understood as the program's weakest link.

Conclusion

The elements for reflection suggested in this chapter offer three research avenues, or at the least, three interesting subjects for further investigation by those working in HP effectiveness. The first research path, and the most urgent in our opinion, addresses the evaluation of the intended proximal outcome of HP interventions, otherwise stated, empowerment. We have demonstrated that certain theoretical and empirical initiatives are under way, but there remains a great deal of distance to be covered. We hope that this chapter will serve as a window to better see and acknowledge the work which has been done in Quebec in order for these assumptions to be tested in multiple contexts, the only useful approach for their eventual validation.

The second research path is related to the concept of effectiveness itself. It requires a true epistemological and interdisciplinary dialogue between HP academics, scientific theorists and practitioners working in the field. The reflections related to HP effectiveness cannot, in our estimation, overlook an interdisciplinary, and most importantly, an intercultural dialogue. The understanding of effectiveness as a concept (is this a transdisciplinary term?) should supersede any epistemological or geographic boundaries.

The final suggestion most certainly demands research related to the conceptualization of HP interventions. The topics that we have covered in the previous pages seem to converge in the same direction and summon the necessary re-definition of HP interventions and their evaluation according to a realist paradigmatic perspective. We should organize ourselves so that the interventions target the reduction of social inequalities in health, as the distal outcome, through the intermediary of an empowerment process which rests upon the five pillars of HP. Above and beyond the "objective" verification of the scope of reducing social inequalities in health, the production of other proximal outcomes should be considered by the implementation of HP interventions. The effectiveness of these HP interventions should be studied with respect to their capacity to adapt to the surrounding environment, to take advantage of the altering circumstances and benefit from the events in sight to reduce social inequalities in health. It involves being aware that these interventions are implemented according to an intertwined process comprised of four elements, all of which are equally important, and should follow an empowerment approach, which is also composed of four other inter-related elements. With reference to Buddhist philosophy, we would even dare to qualify the HP process as the *noble eightfold path* which leads to the reduction of social inequalities in health. Indeed, in Buddhism, the noble eightfold path refers to the way which carries one to the suspension of suffering, to Nirvana, these eight elements not be followed sequentially but *simultaneously* by the disciple. This dual image of four elements of HP can at last be illustrated by Figure 22.3 which incorporates three temporal levels, which should be read from the top to the bottom, either for the process, the proximal outcome, or the distal outcome.

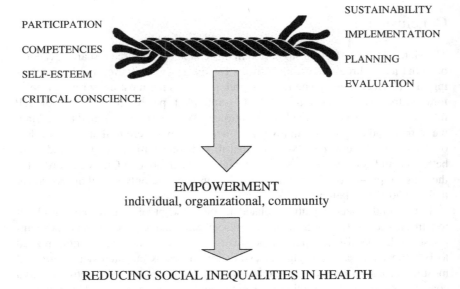

FIGURE 22.3. An attempt to illustrate the process, the proximal and the distal outcomes of health promotion interventions

Authors' Note. We would like to sincerely thank Catherine Jones for her support and most of all for her translation of the Francophone portions of this chapter. The suggestions and comments of the two readers of the outline for this chapter were also very useful. Part of the writing of this chapter was made possible through funding from the Canadian Institutes for Health Research (CIHR): Global Health Research Initiative Post-Doctoral Fellowship (FGH-81565) obtained by Valéry Ridde. Ghislaine Goudreau is the 2007 recipient of the Western Association of Graduate Schools (WAGS) Distinguished Master's Thesis Award for her research. The Aboriginal Women's Hand Drumming (AWHD) Circle of Life framework, which is a modification of the traditional medicine wheel, is an outcome from the thesis work. This framework will aid in studying other traditional Aboriginal activities and will support Aboriginal researchers to continue to gather evidence of their merit.

References

Adelson, N. (2005). The embodiment of inequity: Health disparities in aboriginal Canada. *Canadian Journal of Public Health, 96*(S45), Suppl 2:S45–61.

Arnstein, S. R. (1969). A Ladder of Citizen Participation. *Journal of American Institute Planners, 35*(4), 216–224.

Bamberger, M., Rugh, J. & Mabry, L. (2006). *RealWorld Evaluation. Working Under Budget, Time, Data, and Political Constraints.* Sage Publications. Thousand Oaks, CA.

Bernier, M., Arteau, M. & Papin, C. (2005). *Palabres sur le pouvoir d'agir. Outil d'accompagnement sur l'empowerment.* Québec: CCISD Inc.

Billeter, J-F. (2006). Contre François Jullien. Paris: Allia.

Bisset, S., Cargo, M., Delormier, T., Macaulay, A. C. & Potvin, L. (2004). Legitimizing diabetes as a community health issue: A case analysis of an aboriginal community in Canada. *Health Promotion International, 19*(3), 317–326.

Boyce, W. (1993). Evaluating participation in community programs: an empowerment paradigm. *Canadian Journal of Program Evaluation, 8*(1), 89–102.

Carvalho, A. I., Bodstein, R. C., Hartz, Z. & Matida, A. H. (2004). Concepts and approaches in the evaluation of health promotion. *Ciência & Saude Coletiva, 9*(3), 521–529.

Champagne, F. & Guiset, A.-L. (2005). The Assessment of Hospital performance: Collected Background Papers, R05–04. Montréal GRIS-Université de Montréal.

Chen, H.-T. (2005). *Practical program evaluation: assessing and improving planning, implementation, and effectiveness.* Thousand Oaks, Calif.: Sage.

Cousins, J. B. (2005). Will the real empowerment evaluation please stand up? A critical friend perspective. In D. M. Fetterman & A. Wandersman (Eds.), *Empowerment evaluation principles in practice* (pp. 183–208). Thousand Oaks: Sage.

deLeon, P. (1999). The stages approach to policy process: what has it done? Where is it going? In P. A. Sabatier (Ed.), *Theories of the policy process. Theoretical lenses on public policy* (pp. 19–32). Boulder, Colo.: Westview Press.

Delormier, T., Cargo, M., Kirby, R. & McComber, A. (2003). Activity implementation as a reflection of living in balance: The Kahnawake Schools Diabetes Prevention Project. *Pimatziwin: a journal of aboriginal and indigenous community health, 1*(1), 45–63.

Dupéré, S., Ridde, V., Carroll, S., O'Neill, M., Rootman, I. & Pederson, A. (2007). Conclusion: the rhizome and the tree. In M. O'Neill, A. Pederson, I. Rootman & D. S. (Eds.), *Health Promotion in Canada: Critical perspectives* (2nd ed.). Toronto: Canadian Scholars Press Inc.

Eyssalet, J. M. (2006). Communication personnelle, Montréal, août 2006.

Fassin, D. (2001). Le culturalisme pratique de la santé publique. Critique d'un sens commun. In J. P. Dozon & D. Fassin (Eds.), *Critique de la santé publique. Une approche anthropologique* (pp. 181–208). Paris: Balland.

Gendron, S. (2001). *La pratique participative en santé publique: l'émergence d'un paradigme.* Unpublished PhD Santé publique option promotion de la santé, Montréal.

Goudreau, G. (2006). *Exploring the connection between aboriginal women's hand drumming and health promotion (mino-bimaadiziwin).* Edmonton: University of Alberta.

Green, L. W. & Glasgow, R. E. (2006). Evaluating the relevance, generalization, and applicability of research: issues in external validation and translation methodology. *Eval Health Prof, 29*(1), 126–153.

Guattari, F. (1989). *Les trois écologies.* Paris: Éditions Galilée.

Guattari, F., Spire, A., Field, M., & Hirsch, E. (2002). La philosophie est essentielle à l'existence humaine. La Tour d'Aigues: L'Aube.

Heilbrunn, B. (2005). *La performance, une nouvelle idéologie?: critique et enjeux*: La decouverte. Paris.

Hills, M. D., Carroll, S. & O'Neill, M. (2004). Vers un modéle d'évaluation de l'efficacité des interventions communautaires en promotion de la santé: compte-rendu de quelques développements nord-américains récents. *Promotion & Education, Spec no 1,* 17–21, 49.

Jacquard, A. (2006). Le regard d'Albert Jacquard. Emission de France Culture le 19 Avril 2006.

Jullien, F. (2005). *Conférence sur l'efficacité.* Paris: PUF-Centre Marcel Granet. Institut de la pensée contemporaine.

Kickbusch, I. (2007). Health promotion: the rhizome. In M. O'Neill, A. Pederson, I. Rootman & D. S. (Eds.), *Health Promotion in Canada: Critical perspectives* (2nd ed.). Toronto: Canadian Scholars Press Inc., in press.

Le Bossé, Y., Dufort, F. & Vandette, L. (2004). L'évaluation de l'empowerment des personnes: développement d'une mesure d'indices psychosociologiques du pouvoir d'agir (MIPPA). *Revue canadienne de santé mentale communautaire, 23*(1), 91–114.

Lock, M., Nguyen, V.-K. & Zarowsky, C. (2005). Global and Local Perspectives on Population Health. In J. Heymann, C. Hertzman, M. L. Barer & R. G. Evans (Eds.), *Healthier Societies. From Analysis to Action* (pp. 58–82). New York: Oxford University Press.

McQueen, D. V. & Anderson, L. M. (2001). What counts as evidence: issues and debates. In I. Rootman, M. Goodstadt, B. Hyndman, D. V. McQueen, L. Potvin, J. Springett & E. Ziglio (Eds.), *Evaluation in health promotion: principles and perspectives* (pp. 63–81): WHO Regional Publications. European Series, No. 92.

Morin, E. (2004). La méthode 6. Ethique. Paris: Seuil.

Morin, E. (2005). *Introduction à la pensée complexe* (Nouv. ed.). Paris: Seuil.

Ninacs, W. A. (2002). *Types et processus d'empowerment dans les initiatives de développement économique communautaire au Québec.PhD Thesis, Ecole de service social.* Québec: Université Laval.

Pawson, R. (2006). *Evidence-based Policy. A Realist Perspective.* London: Sage Publications.

Peterson, N. A. & Zimmerman, M. A. (2004). Beyond the individual: toward a nomological network of organizational empowerment. *Am J Community Psychol, 34*(1–2), 129–145.

Pluye, P., Potvin, L. & Denis, J. L. (2004). Making public health programs last: conceptualizing sustainability. *Evaluation and Program Planning, 27*(2), 121–133.

Pluye, P., Potvin, L., Denis, J. L., Pelletier, J. & Mannoni, C. (2005). Program sustainability begins with the first events. *Evaluation and Program Planning, 28*(2), 123–137.

Potvin, L., Gendron, S. & Bilodeau, A. (2006). Três posturas ontológicas concernentes à natureza dos programas de saúde: implicações para a avaliação. In M. Bosi & F. J. Mercado (Eds.), *Avaliação Qualitativa de programas de saude. Enfoques emergentes* (pp. 65–86). Petropolis, Brazil: Vozes Editorial.

Potvin, L., Haddad, S. & Frohlich, C. (2001). Beyond process and outcome evaluation: A comprehensive approach for evaluating health promotion programmes. In I. Rootman, M. Goodstadt, B. Hyndman, D. V. McQueen, L. Potvin, J. Springett & E. Ziglio (Eds.), *Evaluation in health promotion: principles and perspectives* (pp. 45–62): WHO Regional Publications. European Series, No. 92.

Purdey, A. F., Adhikari, G. B., Robinson, S. A. & Cox, P. W. (1994). Participatory health development in rural Nepal: clarifying the process of community empowerment. *Health Educ Q, 21*(3), 329–343.

Racine, S. & Leroux, R. (2006). L'animation de groupe: une pratique à redécouvrir afin de développer le pouvoir d'agir des individus! *Revue canadienne d'évaluation de programme, 21*(3), 137–162.

Ridde, V. (2006). Suggestions d'amélioration d'un cadre conceptual de l'évaluation participative. *Revue canadienne d'évaluation de programme, 21*(2), 1–23.

Ridde V. (2007). Reducing Social Inequalities in Health: Public Health, Community Health or Health Promotion? *Promotion & Education.* XIV (2): in press.

Ridde, V., Baillargeon, J., Ouellet, P. & Roy, S. (2003). L'évaluation participative de type empowerment: une stratégie pour le travail de rue. *Service Social, vol 50*(1), 263–279.

Ridde, V., Pluye, P. & Queuille, L. (2006). Evaluer la pérennité des programmes de santé publique: un outil et son application en Haïti. *Revue d'Epidémiologie et de Santé Publique, 54*(5), 421–431.

Ridde, V. & Queuille, L. (2006). Evaluer l'empowerment: tentative d'application d'un cadre d'analyse en Haïti. *Canadian Journal of Program Evaluation, 21*(3), 173–180.

Rifkin, S. B. (2003). A framework linking community empowerment and health equity: it is a matter of CHOICE. *Journal of Health Population Nutrition, 21*(3), 168–180.

Rootman, I., Goodstadt, M., Hyndman, B., McQueen, D. V., Potvin, L., Springett, J., et al. (Eds.). (2001). *Evaluation in health promotion: principles and perspectives*: WHO Regional Publications. European Series, No. 92.

Saillant, F. (2004). Constructivisme, identités flexibles et communautés vulnérables. In F. Saillant, M. Clément & C. Gaucher (Eds.), *Identités, vulnérabilités, communautés* (pp. 19–42). Québec: Editions Nota bene.

Wallerstein, N. (2002). Empowerment to reduce health disparities. *Scandinavian Journal of Public Health, 30*, 72–77.

Wallerstein, N. (2006). *What is the evidence on effectiveness of empowerment to improve health?* Copenhagen: WHO, Regional Office for Europe, Health Evidence Network.

23
Enhancing the Effectiveness and Quality of Health Promotion
Perspectives of the International Union for Health Promotion and Education

MAURICE B. MITTELMARK, CATHERINE M. JONES, MARIE-CLAUDE LAMARRE, MARTHA W. PERRY, MARIANNE VAN DER WEL AND MARILYN WISE

Introduction

This chapter on the future of health promotion has the perspective of the *International Union for Health Promotion and Education* (IUHPE). Since its founding during the international development movement that followed the close of World War II, the IUHPE has worked at several levels to advance health promotion quality, effectiveness and equity. Here, the recent record of IUHPE activities is summarized briefly,[*] to set the context for the rest of the chapter. Our main aim is to prompt discussion of the question, "what needs to happen if health promotion is to contribute to its full potential to improve health?" Our overarching premise is that health promotion has yet to contribute to "equity in health" to its full potential. Our approach is therefore self-critical, notwithstanding the IUHPE's many documented achievements.

IUHPE Initiatives for Quality, Effectiveness and Equity

Abundant research makes a convincing case for the effectiveness of health promotion. However, we in health promotion have not communicated well enough to completely allay decision-makers' doubts about the wisdom of investing in health promotion. Therefore, the IUHPE has as one of its central tasks the development of clearer and more compelling ways to summarize and to disseminate evidence about health promotion's effectiveness. In pursuit of this, the IUHPE draws on the multiple skills and competencies of its global network, to manage the initiatives that are described next.

Over the past decade, the IUHPE has developed its flagship journal, *Promotion & Education* into a peer reviewed scholarly publication with contributions in English, French, Spanish, and most recently, Portuguese. We have gone into a partnership with Oxford University Press involving *Health Promotion International*, and *Health*

---

[*] Since the Ottawa Charter for Health Promotion in 1986.

Education Research, which are today official research journals of the IUHPE. In these journals and at our regional and global conferences, dialogue is encouraged about what counts as evidence of health promotion effectiveness. Inappropriate standards are challenged, and alternative standards are developed. In Europe, for example, six conferences explicitly on the theme of health promotion quality and effectiveness have been held since the first one in Rotterdam in 1989.[*] The volume in which this chapter appears illustrates the way in which our early efforts in Europe have been used to spearhead a global programme for health promotion effectiveness that has had many manifestations in the various regions of the world where the IUHPE operates.

Fundamental Challenges

One of the most fundamental challenges that the IUHPE faces today is that the health promotion knowledge base is very unevenly developed across the globe. In the southern hemisphere, health promotion is often practiced quite differently from practices in the northern hemisphere, and with great innovation, to fit diverse regional and local contexts. However, the knowledge base from this experience is hardly accessible outside the circles of health promoters that are immediately involved. The classical ways of generating, assembling and disseminating scientific knowledge – ending with publication in a few English language journals with stiff styles – excludes many who have important experience to share. Responding, the IUHPE's journal *Promotion & Education* has launched collaboration with other key journals in the field, to ease the path to publication for researchers whose native language is not English. Much more innovation is needed, however. The Internet provides the possibility to break away from archaic print journal traditions that enforce rigid language, word and style limits. It is not desirable, nor is it possible, to write well in – say, scientific Spanish – in a way that mimics scientific English. With the concepts of page and word limits banished, and with ever-improving instant translation programmes coming online, Spanish-speaking health promoters, and those working in all the languages of the globe, can now communicate in the style that fits the contours of their cultures and the languages in which they best communicate. The liberating potential of emerging communications technology is a theme taken up again later in this chapter.

The challenge just described has led the IUHPE to prioritize the liberation of knowledge generated in the Global South, and the path from our original Euro-centric origins to having a truly global perspective has been arduous, but rewarding. Our initial step was indeed taken in Europe, dating to the Rotterdam conference in 1989, to which reference has already been made. A significant advance was also of European origin – a project funded by the European Commission (1998–2000) that brought together communications experts, policy and decision-makers, and health

---

[*] The other were held in Athens, Greece in 1992; Turin, Italy in 1996; Helsinki, Finland & Tallinn, Estonia, in 1999; London, United-Kingdom in 2002; Stockholm, Sweden in 2005.

promotion researchers and practitioners, to find a common language with which to advocate for investment in effective health promotion technologies. This ground-breaking European initiative resulted in a set of publications (IUHPE, 2000) that illustrate the IUHPE "blueprint" for documenting evidence and for communicating with a diverse range of target audiences in ways that they understand.

Today's IUHPE global effectiveness initiative used the European experience as a launching pad, but in each region of the world, the work has taken on flavors appropriate to the diverse contexts of the regions. However, the programme as a whole does share three hallmarks:

- The GPHPE illuminates evidence of effectiveness – we emphasize what is known, rather than what is not known;
- Inappropriate standards for judging the quality of evidence have been set aside – rigid attitudes placing the randomized controlled trial at the centre have no place in our framework;
- Wide-scale dissemination efforts breach geographic, linguistic, cultural and professional boundaries.

Health Promotion's Proven Technologies

The effectiveness of some health promotion practices is so well documented, that these practices can be recommended with confidence. In this chapter, such practices are referred to as technologies. In its simplest sense, technology is the application of knowledge to solve problems, and using the term to describe proven-effective health promotion methods has advantages. Many who are outside of health promotion are puzzled by health promotion's "insider" terminology, and that makes it harder to communicate with decision-makers than it needs to be – but everyone is comforted knowing that cutting-edge technology is being applied to their problems!

So, what is meant by the term health promotion "technology"? One example is that of health impact assessment (HIA), by which policies and programmes, at all levels from national to local, can be systematically and rigorously evaluated for their positive, neutral and negative impacts on health. HIA can be used to document the need for healthy policy, both public and private. Another example is that of community-based public health action, to strengthen communities' ability to take effective action at the local level, including methods to map and mobilize local resources, activate citizens, governments and the commercial sectors, manage positive change, and transform homes, schools, hospitals and work places into health-promoting environments.

Perhaps the best developed amongst health promotion's technologies is settings-based action, in places such as schools, workplaces and hospitals. When this technology is applied with high quality, it works. Yet the vast majority of settings have not had the advantage of systematic application of this technology, and a challenge for health promotion is its more equitable use in communities where it is needed most.

Settings are ubiquitous in our lives, as they are the physical and social environments within which we carry out our daily activities, and settings themselves can influence our health directly and indirectly. Individual settings (such as a single school or workplace or church or sporting club) are microcosms of society – structures within which tasks are carried out, places within which individuals and groups negotiate social relationships and carry out the actions mandated by society to achieve specific goals. The technology of health promotion in settings includes participative processes that help organizations decide on and implement their policies, use research-derived evidence to inform policy development, and undertake routine measurement of progress and outcomes.

The Problem of Exclusion

Health promotion in settings has been developed in scattered, relatively small-scale local projects and programs. Exemplars can be found today all around the world, but the vast majority of communities are untouched. The goal now is to spread the technology to all schools and all workplaces, but no matter the degree of success in reaching this goal, many people will be excluded from health promotion because there are no schools and workplaces for them. Children who have no school to attend, and adults who have no workplace, can hardly benefit from even the most successful settings-based health promotion programme. Human development initiatives that create schools and create jobs are fundamental. The best approach is one in which these new creations are established from the start as health promoting environments, using the lessons learned from converting existing settings into health promoting places.

Changing systems and settings on the scale and in the ways required to achieve equity requires effective action at all political levels. Success in influencing the goals, policies, practices of the education, health and employment sectors requires the engagement of practitioners and researchers who understand – and are willing to engage in – the politics of building and implementing public policy for health in *all* policy arenas. This last point is vital: health promotion cannot succeed in its aim to achieve equity in health based on the efforts of professional health promoters alone. We need to train professionals in education, welfare, economics, public administration, to name but a few fields, so that health promotion becomes part-and-parcel of their professional lore. This would not require particularly dramatic changes in curricula, and the feasibility of such change is evident: today, every business management school in the world includes courses on corporate social responsibility, a result of decades of pressure to produce business leaders who take social responsibility seriously. Advocacy to require some training in health promotion in all the professions is required, but no organized efforts are yet underway, signaling an unmet need that should be prioritized. Since all professions have requirements of one sort or another for continuing education, the development of model curricula for short courses suitable for continuing education could be a reasonable way to launch efforts.

The IUHPE in the New Communications Age

Health-related international non-governmental organizations (INGOs) play a vital role in the interplay of government, commerce and civil society. Governments seek to manage the distribution of society's (always too meager) resources in ways that serve citizens, but also maximize their own longevity. Commerce seeks to maximize profit and competitive advantage, sometimes with social responsibility in mind, but oftentimes not. In this powerful brew, NGO's are the critical voices of the people, holding governments and commerce accountable to work in ways that promote social justice. The playing field is not even; governments and commerce command resources (people, tools, finances) that are beyond the dream of even the most richly endowed INGO. Therefore, INGO's must use the resources they do have in the most effective and efficient manner possible. The one resource that INGOs *do* have, that does not pale in comparison to government and commerce, is dedicated people. The ability of those people to communicate well with one another and with others helps to even the playing field considerably.

Hardly any evidence of INGO potential to sway the power brokers in government and commerce is more compelling than The Ottawa Convention banning anti-personnel landmines (signed in 1997). After just two years of INGO-led lobbying and civil action, governments from 122 countries signed the Convention, formally titled the *Convention on the Prohibition of the Use, Stockpiling, Production and Transfer of Anti-Personnel Mines and on their Destruction.*[1] Such Spectacular "wins" such as this demonstrate the power of civil society, as personified by NGO's, and are mostly a demonstration of the power of *communication*. All this is highly relevant to the IUHPE. Central to the mission to promote equity in health is our capacity as a global, independent and professional organization to share experience, exchange information, stimulate dialogue and be advocates for social justice. Because our membership spans the world, we are able to advocate for health in all corners of the planet. Our ability to do this well is improving all the time, due to developments in information and communications technologies (ICT).

ICT helps the IUHPE overcome the cultural, language, distance and economic barriers that any global organization must reckon with (Perry and Mittelmark, 2006). For example, we are beginning to explore the utility of automatic machine translation to allow multi-lingual communication and knowledge acquisition from resources in other languages than our own. The best programmes translate material well enough to communicate the gist of the original, giving the term "gisting" to describe the process, and the term "gist" for the product of a machine translation. For all practical purposes, the gist may be good enough, even if amusing due to grammatical contortions. Gisting and other new developments seem to

---

[1] An archive of material related to the Convention is to be found at
http://www.mines.gc.ca/VII/menu-en.asp, last accessed 28 September 2006.

be only the beginning of the communications revolution. Already under development are seamless, "ubiquitous networks" (Murakami, 2003) that connect people to people, people to objects and objects to objects. An example of the complexity that is already feasible is the way that people, computers, autos, roads, and satellites are connected by navigation systems.

Rising cost is a key factor restraining the IUHPE's complete involvement in the communication revolution. Well-endowed governments and successful commercial enterprises have the resources to invest in top-of-the-line technology, while under-resourced institutions must often depend on hand-me-downs, if lucky. This is contributing to a growing gap between the digital haves and the have-nots, the signs of which are evident within the IUHPE itself. Some of us enjoy access to virtually the full range of ICT, while others are not connected at all. There is the natural tendency for those who are connected to work in ways that exclude those who are not connected, a seriously disturbing development in a "union"!

Responding to the growing divide, there is today a global effort led by the United Nations to connect the unconnected communities by 2015. A challenge for the IUHPE is to eliminate our own digital divide as fast as possible. There are signs that this may not be as hard a task as one might think. In every part of the world, the pre-digital generations are fading and all young professionals are children of the digital age in one way or another. Today, it can be easier to communicate with a colleague via the internet and satellite than via the telephone. The newest technology is jumping over the gaps, because in a wireless world, the lack of wires is no hindrance. These developments provide the means to accumulate evidence of health promotion's effectiveness no matter where in the world the evidence is generated.

IUHPE's Accountability for its Own Effectiveness

As a knowledge-based, professional organization, the IUHPE needs to be actively engaged in knowledge production. With a flourishing network of health promotion researchers, practitioners and policy-makers at its fingertips, the IUHPE has the resources and expertise available to carry out research on a wide range of fronts. Over the past decade, there has been an increasing awareness of the organisation's strategic position on the academic health promotion map, since many IUHPE members are academicians whose main links to one another is via the IUHPE. The IUHPE work programme is constructed in part on this academic foundation, and the IUHPE ability to participate in science is growing. In concert with this, knowledge development as well as knowledge dissemination should become integral to all the operations of the IUHPE.

This requires a shift, now underway, towards an IUHPE whose management philosophy embraces the ideal of the "learning organization", alongside long-existing commitments to professional networking and service provision. Whilst learning and doing are complementary – the very ideal of action research – they do require different sets of skills, techniques and resources for their support, development and implementation. Of course, the IUHPE cannot and should not aspire to become an academic organization, nor "compete" with its own academic members in the research arena. However, two knowledge development niches fit neatly with IUHPE priorities. These are: (a) IUHPE research using the resources of members, and (b) optimizing and ensuring IUHPE's effectiveness. Each of these is touched on briefly, below.

IUHPE Research Using the Resources of Members

In 2005, the first IUHPE Research Associates were appointed to connect graduate student research to IUHPE priorities. In 2006, the first three issues of the IUHPE Research Report series were issued, containing the results of IUHPE Research Associates efforts. These efforts are supported entirely by IUHPE members with academic credentials and academic institutional backing. The Research Associates and the Research Reports provide mechanisms by which the IUHPE can coordinate a global team of researchers by recruiting them from the IUHPE network itself, commissioning research on topics that are priorities for the IUHPE. As Walker, Ouellette and Ridde (2006) point out, graduate student researchers " . . .have the potential to make a unique and valuable contribution to global health". The early experience shows that when graduate students have the opportunity to do thesis and dissertation research on topics of high priority to the IUHPE, their motivation and seriousness of purpose grows to new heights. Research of this type serves not only the IUHPE's growth as a knowledge-producing agency; it serves also to bring the work of IUHPE student members to the global readership. To date, three such research projects have been completed, the reports of which are available at (www.iuhpe.org).

Optimizing and Ensuring IUHPE's Effectiveness

There is a need for evaluation research to examine the degree to which the IUHPE is accomplishing its mission to promote global health, and to contribute to the achievement of equity in health between and within countries of the world. The organization continues to search for ways to operationalize these goals, and incorporate assessments of progress into everything we do, striving to make concrete responses to the question, how effective are we at meeting our stated goals, for every specific task we take on? As a knowledge-based organization, the IUHPE must itself pose hard questions about our own effectiveness and impact, rather than relying solely on positive performance indicators and successful implementation of work. Three main activities comprise the growing IUHPE programme for optimizing effectiveness: (1) develop and implement evaluation components in all projects; (2) use evaluation data to identify possibilities to enhance performance and effectiveness; (3) conduct operational research on one of our main methods of working, which is the tailored use of dialogue methodology (DM). The IUHPE has utilized DM in a number of projects such as the European Effectiveness project (International Union for Health Promotion and Education, 2000), HP-Source.net

(Mittelmark, Fosse, Jones, et al., 2005), and most recently the Indo/EU dialogue on public-private partnerships for health (Gupta, 2006). Briefly, DM brings together experts from a variety of fields in order to have extended, managed dialogues about significant health promotion issues, such as how to maximize the effectiveness of public-private partnerships for health. IUHPE evaluation research is now underway, to study DM processes, with the aim of strengthening our capacity to use DM in a wide range of applications.

Advocacy for Health Promotion and for Equity in Health

The IUHPE has advocated for health education and health promotion for over 50 years. Through our journals, other publications, website, triennial world conferences, regional workshops and conferences, research program, and regional structures, we have worked to be a powerful advocate for health promotion training, practice and research.

However, advocacy for health promotion as a professional arena is not sufficient. Advocacy for equity in health is of crucial importance, because the world is changing in ways that threaten to worsen – not reduce – health inequity. As was the case during other eras of major economic development (e.g. the industrial revolution; Szreter, 2003), the post-cold war period of globalization has produced fast-moving, disruptive shifts in production, in labor supply and demand, in trade (volume and practices), and in economic regulation. Among major barriers to improvements in health are the growth of corporate power among industries whose products are demonstrably unhealthy (such as the tobacco, sugar and soft drink industries), and industries that resist changing products and production methods, to reduce negative impact on health and the environment. The equity gap is not closing, and in many places it is actually widening (Marmot, 2004).

Responding, the IUHPE has since 1998 been actively involved in advocacy for the inclusion of social clauses in trade agreements. The work is done by the IUHPE Working Group on Social Clauses and Advocacy, led by Ron Labonte. Declarations and commitments associated with the annual G7 (now G8) Summit meetings have direct and indirect impacts on health, and the three most recent Summits included discussions and commitments related to health and development in poor countries. The IUHPE advocacy in this arena includes the production of a series of briefs on social clauses in trade agreements, and participation in the Non-Governmental Initiative on International Governance and World Trade Organization Reform.

Another example of sustained IUHPE advocacy is our work in the tobacco control arena. We advocate for global tobacco control via various activities, including the production of a manual on tobacco control legislation, to assist governments the world over to enact effective tobacco control policy and to implement the Framework Convention on Tobacco Control in their own political and legal context. These and our other advocacy initiatives are fully described at www.iuhpe.org. As we gain experience and confidence in our ability to orchestrate our global resources to advocate for equity in health, the IUHPE will be able to expand its work in the advocacy arena. Through the planned evaluations of the entire IUHPE program of work, we will identify our strengths and weaknesses as advocates for health, and work to eliminate the weaknesses. The IUHPE's commitment to excellence in this area is signaled by the establishment of the post Vice President for Advocacy, and our work on social clauses in trade agreements and tobacco control provides convincing evidence that we have the capacity to mount sustained advocacy campaigns on a widening range of issues.

A particularly efficient way to expand IUHPE advocacy is to participate in the growing number of global health networks. Our work in the tobacco arena shows us the way, and we are joining with others to advance the cause of health at all levels from the individual to the societal. Examples include the provision of technical support to the WHO Commission on the Social Determinants of Health, and participation in networks on physical activity, nutrition, obesity and injury prevention. Through such collaboration, we continue to create synergy with long-time partners such as the WHO and the CDC in the United States, and create new ties with organizations such as the People's Health Movement, and the Global Forum for Health Research. At the core of all IUHPE advocacy efforts is our aim to contribute to equity in health within and among nations. As mentioned elsewhere in this chapter, we hold ourselves accountable to contribute to this aim, and a high priority in the coming period will be to document how and to what degree we are succeeding.

Learning from Others

Despite the significant influence on health promotion of a few extraordinarily visionary social and political scientists – the name Ilona Kickbush will come immediately to the minds of many readers – health promotion is populated mostly by health professionals. Our professional training takes place mostly in health faculties, our conferences and journals are health-oriented, and our key partners are health organizations such as the World Health Organization. While our health "cocoon" is stimulating enough in some regards, health promotion may gain much energy and invigoration by reaching out to the broader world of human development and to academic communities with which we have much in common, but little contact.

As used here, the term "human development" refers to all efforts to create equitable social and physical conditions that enable people to experience satisfying and meaningful lives, in harmony with a thriving natural environment. Health promotion certainly fits the description, but so too do women's and children's advancement movements, fair work and labor practices movements, peace and security movements, environmental protection movements, and so on. The World Health Organization fits the description, but so too does UNICEF, UNESCO, UNIFEM, and so on. In this sense, health promotion has a warm and potentially welcoming ideological "home" in the human development arena that it seems not to know exists!

There is a need also for new alliances with academic arenas "on and beyond the periphery of health promotion." Health promotion's key contributory disciplines include medical and public health sciences, health psychology, sociology and education. Generally missing from the health promotion mix are gender studies, feminist scholarship, pedagogy of the oppressed, ethics, community psychology, economic development, informatics, international development, cultural epidemiology and political ecology. The opportunities for enrichment at every level – philosophical, theoretical, and empirical – are too appealing to be missed, yet we do not have the mechanisms for real cross-fertilization. Serious barriers stand in the way, including disciplinary stiffness and professional constellations that do not touch. With separate research standards, conferences and journals, academic arenas that have much to offer one another are at a loss about how to take advantage of the potential that seems just out of reach.

This is where enlightened leadership must step in. Conference organizers need to invite speakers who may know very little about health promotion but have priceless ideas to offer. Journal editors need to solicit papers from the best-of-the-best in fields beyond health promotion, to inject new thinking onto their pages. Training institutions need to create cross-training opportunities, providing academic credit to those who dare cross over for visits into strange territory.

Keeping Faith with IUHPE's Stakeholders

Like all international professional organizations with democratic traditions and a mix of activities including knowledge development and dissemination, education and advocacy, the IUHPE has a myriad of stakeholders. Being accountable to many different parties presents the IUHPE with a formidable challenge: how to do the right thing when the demands for accountability are so many and so diverse. Positively, the IUHPE has conducted a self-study of its accountability mechanisms that shows what aspects of stakeholder accountability seem well addressed, but also illuminates areas for improvement. This is highly relevant to the aim of this chapter, to stimulate critical discussion about the quality and effectiveness of our efforts to contribute to the achievement of equity in health.

What did the IUHPE self-study teach us? The areas of accountability that were probed were those of the One World Trust GAP framework (Blagescu, de Las Casas and Lloyd, 2005):

- Transparency – openness about organizational activities and operations. A flow of information is not sufficient; the organization must open up for dialogue with stakeholders.
- Participation – the process whereby stakeholders are enabled to play an active part in the organization. Participation should relate to policies and activities, and must lead to change. A passive variant of participation is in other words only sub-optimal
- Evaluation – processes whereby the organization, in collaboration with relevant stakeholders, monitors and reviews progress and results against goals and objectives, feeds learning from this back into the organization, and reports on the

results. Evaluation should not be confined to end-results, but should also examine if activities are done in a socially responsible manner.
- Response/complaint mechanisms – means whereby stakeholders may address complaints. Stakeholders should be able to address complaints against practice and policies.

Positively, the analysis revealed a number of accountability mechanisms worthy of note; an on-line journal open to all without editorial interdiction; the possibility at General Assemblies for members to speak to any issue; a code of practice about partnership, collaboration and sponsorship; special efforts to engage young members; a sliding membership fee scale based on ability to pay.

Opportunities to improve accountability were also identified, especially the need to evaluate and document IUHPE activities, processes and effectiveness in achieving its mission and related sub-goals. Some progress has been made – see for example Corbin and Mittelmark's chapter on partnership processes in the GPHPE – and the intention is that the IUHPE shall be a learning organization, not only disseminating knowledge generated by others, but also generating knowledge from its own programmatic activities.

Summary

The quest for effective health promotion should not be limited to interventions, projects and programmes. The organizations for health promotion, governmental and non-governmental alike, should strive for effectiveness and efficiency in everything they do. The resources devoted to health promotion are extraordinarily meager, considering the ambition to contribute to equity in health at local, national and global levels, so making resources count to the maximum is not just a matter of practicality, but also a matter of ethics. The IUHPE response has to be two-fold: to do more of everything we do well, and to improve that which can be improved. This chapter has addressed both these aims:

- The Global Programme for Health Promotion Effectiveness provides a blueprint for how the IUHPE can effectively participate in, and lead, global networks for health. Now we need to expand our collaborations to embrace the wider world of human development, and enrich health promotion with new impulses from academic fields that have much to contribute.
- Health promotion research is well organized and productive in most of the Northern hemisphere, but important wells of health promotion knowledge in the Southern hemisphere are not widely-enough disseminated. The IUHPE needs to help liberate knowledge producers everywhere from unnecessary strictures, and find innovative ways to illuminate knowledge for all to see.
- We have developed and proven the effectiveness of a range of technologies such as settings-based health promotion. However, the vast majority of communities are untouched, and the IUHPE needs to be a leader in finding ways to better disseminate effective health promotion practice.

- The IUHPE is a vigorous and effective advocate for health promotion training, practice and research. Now we need to expand our advocacy for equity in health, building on our effective work on social clauses in trade agreements and on tobacco control.
- The IUHPE is an effective deliverer of services that support health promotion training, practice and research. Now we need to advance our capacity to be a learning organization, hold ourselves accountable for the goals we set, and evaluate and improve what we do, so that as an organization we can deliver services with better quality and greater efficiency.

These answers to the question *"what needs to happen if health promotion is to contribute to its full potential to improve health?"* do not comprise a position taken by the IUHPE's Board of Trustees. Rather, they emerge from the authors' collective, critical consideration of opportunities for improvement, taking as the starting point the IUHPE's considerable strengths and achievements. Perhaps more important for their existence than for their content, the observations and comments of this chapter illustrate that thinking about quality and effectiveness can be brought to bear not only on what health promotion does, but also on organized health promotion itself.

References

Blagescu, M., Las Casas, L. de & Lloyd, R. (2005): *Pathways to Accountability. The GAP Framework*. London: One World Trust.

Gupta, A. (2006). Public-Private Partnerships in Health. *Health for the Millions*, 32 (6&7), 7–13.

International Union for Health Promotion and Education. (2000). *The Evidence of Health Promotion Effectiveness: Shaping Public Health in a New Europe*. 2nd edition. Paris: Jouve Composition & Impression.

Marmot, M. (2004). *Status syndrome: how your social standing directly affects your health and life expectancy*. London: Bloomsbury Publishing.

Mittelmark, M.B., Fosse, E., Jones, C., Davies, M. & Davies, J.K. (2005). Mapping European capacity to engage in health promotion: HP-Source.net. *Promotion & Education, Supp 1*, 3–39.

Murakami, T. (2003). Establishing the ubiquitous network environment in Japan" *NRI Papers*, No. 66, July. Viewed February 26th, 2006 <www.nri.co.jp/english/opinion/papers/2005/pdf/np200597.pdf>

Perry, M. & Mittelmark, M. B. (2006). The use of emerging technology to build health promotion capacity in regions with diversity in language and culture. *Promotion & Education XIII* (3), 197–202.

Szreter, S. (2002). The McKeown Thesis: Rethinking McKeown: the relationship between public health and social change. *American Journal of Public Health* 92(5): 722 – 725.

Walker, S., Ouellette, V. & Ridde, V. (2006). How can PhD research contribute to the global health research agenda. *Canadian Journal of Public Health, 97* (2), 145–148.

Global Programme on Health Promotion Effectiveness

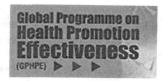

Coordinated by the International Union for Health Promotion and Education

The Global Programme for Health Promotion Effectiveness (GPHPE) is a multi-partner initiative, coordinated by the International Union for Health Promotion and Education (IUHPE) in collaboration with the World Health Organization, and supported by a number of partners from across the world. The work carried out under the GPHPE is guided by a Global Steering Group (GSG) made up of representatives from each region and from major partner organisations.

> *The rationale of the Global Programme on Health Promotion Effectiveness is to focus on the principles, models and methods that relate to the evaluation of effective health promotion practice, taking regional and cultural variations into consideration.*

The GPHPE aims to raise the standards of health promoting policy-making and practice world-wide by reviewing, building and translating evidence of effectiveness while stimulating debate on the nature of evidence of health promotion effectiveness.

Fundamentally, the GPHPE is concerned with how to:

- stimulate the evaluation of effectiveness,
- champion the development of appropriate tools and methods to do so, and
- support the implementation of this body of knowledge for use in practice and for advocacy.

Why is Evidence of Health Promotion Effectiveness Needed?

We need evidence:

- to identify the best possible ways to promote health;
- to make decisions for policy development and funding allocation;
- to demonstrate to decision-makers that health promotion works and is an effective strategy in public health;

413

- to support practitioners in project development and evaluation;
- to show the wider community the benefits of health promotion actions;
- to advocate for health promotion development.

Distinguishing features of the GPHPE include that it:

➢ operates as a world-wide programme;
➢ advocates the importance of effectiveness to researchers, practitioners and decision-makers;
➢ cultivates regionally specificity, encouraging input from the developing world with a larger focus on non-Western views of effectiveness;
➢ promotes the development of unique evaluation approaches to accomodate emerging areas of interest; and
➢ employs the diversity emanating from the regional projects to foster opportuninties for regions to exchange and learn from each other.

Volume I of the GPHPE Monograph series *Global Perspectives on Health Promotion Effectivness* aims to :

- Provide a broad overview of issues of evidence, evaluation and effectiveness in health promotion.
- Compare and contrast regional variations.
- Codify commonality where warranted and emphasize differences where indicated.
- Underline some key areas considered critical to health promotion throughout the world.
- Serve as a background and companion document to the various regional project products.

Some Indicators of Achievement by the GPHPE

1. Representativeness
  o the extent to which health promotion initiatives from a diversity of countries, cultures, languages and peoples is represented in the monograph series and throughout the overall programme;
  o the extent to which health promotion interventions and projects are distinctively recognised.

2. Quality of reflection
  o the ability of the monographs to propose analyses developed to distinguish the specific features of effective health promotion;
  o the ability of an adequate number of critical examples from practice and other contexts to be sought out and presented, as well as the reviews of effectiveness which will take place.

3. **Relevance of knowledge for use**
   o the extent to which the knowledge obtained from the programme is documented in the monograph series and then translated into use by practitioners in the field;
   o the extent to which the knowledge obtained influences research priorities, as well as impact on advocacy for policy and decision making;
   o the general improvement in the knowledge-base for better education, training and capacity buildcing of health promotion professionals.

Programme Leaders and Contact Persons

Global Programme management team:

▶ **David McQueen** (Global Programme Leader)
IUHPE Vice-President for Scientific and Technical Development
E: dvmcqueen@cdc.gov

▶ **Catherine Jones** (Global Programme Coordinator)
IUHPE Programme Director
E: cjones@iuhpe.org

▶ **Global Programme Secretariat:**
IUHPE
42 Boulevard de la Libération
93203 Saint-Denis Cedex, France
T: +33 (0)1 48 13 71 20
F: +33 (0)1 48 09.17 67
W: www.iuhpe.org

GPHPE Regional Effectiveness Project Coordination:
▶ **Africa**
Leader & Coordinator: Mary Amuyunzu-Nyamongo
E: mnyamongo@aihd.org

▶ **Europe**
Co-Leaders: Viv Speller and Ursel Broesskamp-Stone
E: viv.speller@healthdevelopment.co.uk / ursel.broesskamp@promotionsante.ch

▶ **Latin America**
Leader & Coordinator: Ligia de Salazar
E: lsalazar@emcali.net.co

▶ **North America**
Co-leaders: Steve Fawcett and Marcia Hills
E: sfawcett@ku.edu/mhills@uvic.ca
Coordinator: Marilyn Metzler
E: mom7@cdc.gov

▶ **Northern Part of the Western Pacific**
Leader & Coordinator: Albert Lee
E: alee@cuhk.edu.hk

▶ **South East Asia**
Leader & Coordinator: Alok Mukhopadhay
E: vhai@vsnl.com

▶ **South West Pacific**
Leader & Coordinator: Jan Ritchie
E: j.ritchie@unsw.edu.au

GPHPE supporters

- Health Promotion Switzerland
- Ministry of Health and Social Services, Quebec
- National Institute for Health and Clinical Excellence, England (NICE)
- The Netherlands Institute for Health Promotion and Disease Prevention (NIGZ)
- Public Health Agency of Canada
- Spanish Ministry of Health and Consumption
- United Kingdom Department of Health
- US Centers for Disease Control and Prevention (an agency of the Department of Health and Human Services)
- World Health Organization (WHO Geneva)

GPHPE collaborators

- African Institute of Health and Development
- African Medical and Research Foundation
- Brazilian Association of Post-graduate studies in Collective Health (ABRASCO)
- Canadian Consortium for Health Promotion Research (CCHPR)
- Center for the Development and Evaluation of Public Health Policy and Technology (CEDETES), Colombia
- Center for Health Promotion and Health Education, The Chinese University of Hong Kong
- French Health Directorate
- French Institute for Prevention and Health Promotion (Inpes)
- NHS Health Scotland
- Oswaldo Cruz Foundation - National School of Public Health, Brazil
- Pan-American Health Organization (PAHO)
- University of Bergen, Norway
- Victorian Health Promotion Foundation (VicHealth)
- Voluntary Health Association of India (VHAI)
- WHO Collaborating Centre for Community Health and Development, University of Kansas
- World Health Organisation African Region (WHO/AFRO)

GPHPE interested parties

- Cochrane Collaboration Health Promotion and Public Health Field The Community Guide
- Getting Evidence into Practice European Evidence Consortium
- IUHPE/EuroHealthNet Joint Special Interest Group on Health Promotion Evidence, Effectiveness and Transferability

Scientific and Technical consultants to the GPHPE

- Hiram Arroyo
- Anne Bunde Birouste
- Simon Carroll
- Spencer Hagard
- Saroj Jha
- Maurice Mittelmark
- Michel O'Neill
- Louise Potvin
- Marilyn Rice
- Valéry Ridde
- Hans Saan
- Kwok-cho Tang
- Elizabeth Waters
- Mabel Yap
- Pat Youri

Index